EXPOSED: From the Files Of...

Health Confidential

DR. AL SEARS, MD

America's #1 Anti-Aging Pioneer

ISBN 13: 978-0-9968102-0-3

Published by:
Al Sears, MD
11905 Southern Blvd., Royal Palm Beach, FL 33411
561-784-7852
www.AlSearsMD.com

Dr. Al Sears wrote this book to provide information in regard to the subject matter covered. It is offered with the understanding that the publisher and the author are not liable for any misconception or misuse of the information provided. Every effort has been made to make this book as complete and accurate as possible. The purpose of this book is to educate. The author and the publisher shall have neither liability nor responsibility to any person or entity with respect to any loss, damage, or injury caused or alleged to be caused directly or indirectly by the information contained in this book. The information presented herein is in no way intended as a substitute for medical counseling or medical attention.

Al Sears, MD

President/Medical Director, Wellness Research Foundation, Dr. Sears' Center for Health and Wellness, Primal Force, and Ah-Ha Press, Royal Palm Beach, Florida; and Wellness Research and Consulting, Kampala, Uganda.

After entering private practice, Dr. Sears was one of the first to be board certified in anti-aging medicine. As a pioneer in this new field of medicine, he is an avid researcher, published author, and enthusiastic lecturer.

Dr. Sears is also board certified as a clinical nutrition specialist (CNS) and is a member of the American College of Sports Medicine (ACSM), the American College for Advancement in Medicine (ACAM), the American Medical Association (AMA), the Southern Medical Association (SMA), the American Academy of Anti-Aging Medicine (A4M), and the Herb Research Foundation (HRF). Dr. Sears is also an ACE-certified fitness instructor.

As the founder and director of Wellness Research Foundation, a non-profit research organization, Dr. Sears travels the globe to bring back to his patients the latest breakthroughs in natural therapies. Trips to Peru, Brazil, India, Jamaica, Uganda, South Africa, Ecuador, and Bali have yielded important new discoveries in nutrition, traditional herbal treatments, anti-aging, and alternative medicine.

Dr. Sears currently writes and publishes the monthly newsletter *Confidential Cures* and daily email broadcast *Doctor's House Call,* and contributes to a host of other publications in the field. He has appeared on over 50 national radio programs, ABC News, CNN, and ESPN.

Dr. Sears has published 14 books and reports on health and wellness with a readership of millions spread over 163 countries. His bestselling titles include *The Doctor's Heart Cure, The 12 Secrets to Virility, Rediscover Your Native Fitness, Your Best Health Under the Sun, High-Speed Fat Loss in 7 Easy Steps, PACE: The 12-Minute Fitness Revolution,* and *Reset Your Biological Clock.*

Dr. Sears is currently working on three additional books. He has started writing his discovery of incredible healing herbs in the *Healing Herbs From Paradise.* Dr. Sears is also penning his uncensored revelation of a breakthrough cure the FDA doesn't want you to know about in *The Outlawed Cure for All Disease.* And he is writing about traditional healing systems that are about to be lost to the West in *Healing Roots of Africa.*

Introduction

You and I have a problem.

The pristine, natural world we were meant to live in is gone.

We now live on an alien and highly toxic planet. And no, this is not the plot of a sci-fi movie. *This is our new reality.*

Today, we are born into a poisonous world. Even while still in the womb, we are bombarded by toxins, contaminants, chemical compounds, heavy metals, and even "alien molecules" that have never existed on this planet before.

It's important that you understand this. Not so you can fret and worry about the state of the world and your health, *but so you can do something about it.*

The purpose of Health Confidential is to arm you with real solutions you can use RIGHT AWAY.

In the following pages of ***EXPOSED: From the Files of Health Confidential,*** I'll reveal the problems of modern food production, the rise of Big Pharma and modern medicine, and their profit-driven model that sacrifices your health and well-being.

The average Western diet is now packed with so many toxic additives, and overloaded with so many processed carbohydrates and refined sugars, our bodies are no longer able to function as they were intended to.

You and I did NOT ask for this toxic plague. But like Dr. Frankenstein's monster, these creations escaped from the lab and are running amok in our environment.

And in spite of near-miraculous advances in modern medicine and technology, we have not become healthier.

Technology and progress are positive accomplishments, and I would never advocate we go back to living in the forest or hunting for our food. But when you solve one problem, you create another.

We're no longer slaves to the predator-prey survival model of our ancestors, but we're faced with new survival challenges.

To thrive in this alien world, we need a deeper awareness of nutrition and how our bodies work. At the same time, we have to second-guess the medical establishment, and their cozy collusion with the U.S. government and Big Agra.

It pains me to say it, but you can't fully trust mainstream medicine. While medicine was once about curing ailments and making people better, it's now about the management of disease in the most profitable way possible.

Thanks to Big Pharma's constant barrage of aggressive and deceptive marketing, you're pressured to accept a laundry list of drugs with unknown toxicity, and submit to dangerous and often unnecessary surgeries.

In other words, your life is put at risk without your knowledge or consent.

Your doctor may be well-intentioned, but he or she is locked into a system that puts profit before your health.

And when multinational corporations pull in $23 billion a year for just a single class of drug, your health and well-being is no longer a concern. That's exactly what's happened with statin drugs. The most profitable drug ever made is propped up by the myth of lowering cholesterol to "save" your heart.

Curing heart disease is a noble pursuit. Except it can't be done with statins, and the medical establishment has known it for decades.

But when they're making a 40,000% profit on each prescription, the CEOs of the world's biggest pharmaceutical companies don't care if you die prematurely as a result.

Now, don't get me wrong. There's nothing wrong with making a profit in business. But when profit is valued more than human life, it's time to take matters into your own hands.

No, you don't need another book to scare you. You need real solutions to this modern crisis, and that's the big point of this book.

I want you to know that for every disease there is a natural, non-toxic, non-drug cure.

But natural cures can't be patented, and that means no mega-profit potential. But thanks to Big Pharma and Big Agra's propaganda machine, doctors are largely kept ignorant of natural treatments.

In the pages that follow, you'll discover:

- How to beat diabetes in three simple steps WITHOUT risky drugs;

- The 12-minute cure for heart disease and congestive heart failure;

- How to fight Alzheimer's with the cure Big Pharma buried;

- Why higher cholesterol will make you live better for LONGER;

- How to release the toxic overload spawned by Big Agra's insatiable greed;

- How to kick osteoporosis to the curb and build bones of steel;

- How modern "health food" is making you sick, and why steak and eggs are a much better idea;

- The original cancer medicine, and new strategies for keeping cancer out of your body for good;

- How to control and lower high blood pressure without beta blockers and ACE inhibitors;

- And much more.

To get the most out of this book, you don't need to read it from beginning to end. You can skip to the sections that are most relevant to you.

But it's full of good advice, and backed with peer-reviewed studies from some of the most prestigious universities and research centers in the world. You'll even discover ancient wisdom and remedies that have been tried and tested for thousands of years.

But remember, any health improvement strategy can only be successful if you actually do it.

You'll have to do the work yourself.

I've made sure each section has what I call "actionable advice." In other words, things you can actively fix on your own. And I've tried to make it as easy as possible.

I recommend you start off with a few things you can do easily, and then build on them. As you move forward, you'll take more control of your health.

Good health is more of a perpetual journey than a destination, but all journeys start with a single step.

To Your Good Health,

Al Sears, MD, CNS

Table of Contents

PART 2 / A PLATE FULL OF LIES

PART 3 / DITCH THE DIET ADVICE AND FEAST ON THE FATTY FOODS YOU LOVE

PART 4 / NATURAL CURES TRUMP THE PRESCRIPTION PAD

PART 5 / THE FORGOTTEN KEYS TO HEART HEALTH

PART 6 / ELIMINATE THE THREAT OF DEADLY TOXINS

PART 7 / ANCIENT WISDOM FOR MODERN HEALTH AND WELLNESS

PART 8 / WHERE TO AVOID TRADITIONAL MEDICINE

PART 9 / THROW AWAY YOUR JOGGING SHOES

PART 10 / CALCIUM DOING MORE HARM THAN GOOD?

PART 1

THE PHARMACY OF RISK

Chapter 1

How You Can Prevent Hair Loss

Most men and women watch their hair slowly thin with age. It is one of the most apparent signals of your age to people you meet. But you may be among the first generation of men that can actually do something about it.

We do not lose our hair because of wear and tear from the environment. New scientific discoveries have led to a very important revelation about why hair thins with age. Your hair falls out on commands from hormones. The secret to keeping a naturally thick, lustrous, full head of hair is to change that hormonal command.

We have known for some time that male hormones were involved. They provide a genetically programmed signal for hair thinning to begin, and they control how it progresses as you age. Convention made a big mistake, however, in blaming testosterone. As it turns out, high testosterone levels throughout life can *protect* you from hair loss.

The real culprit has turned out to be a different male hormone called dihydrotestosterone or DHT. This hormone also exists in women, where it also causes hair loss. In fact, most women I've treated with the pattern of receding hair lines and hair thinning over the crown have high DHT levels in their blood.

I have seen high blood levels of DHT induce hair loss in young athletes who abuse anabolic steroids. In some cases, there was not a genetic predisposition to baldness. When we employ strategies to lower DHT levels, their hair loss stops.

You can use these same strategies to lower your DHT. They have been recently proven to reduce hair loss, preserve your current head of hair, or even induce new hair growth.

You may have seen ads for the prescription drug Propecia. It has been a significant balding treatment breakthrough. Propecia has been associated with a number of side effects though. It's also very expensive, is not covered by most health insurances, and has not been approved for women. There are safer, less expensive natural alternatives that can do the same thing. In fact, they can work with exactly the same mechanism.

Propecia works by blocking the conversion of testosterone to DHT. This is the perfect point of attack. It has the effect of both decreasing DHT and increasing testosterone. Propecia inhibits the enzyme *5-alpha reductase,* necessary for this conversion. A number of plant-based nutrients also inhibit this enzyme.

The most powerful nutrient to block the conversion of testosterone to DHT is beta-sitosterol. Beta-sitosterol has been proven to inhibit 5-alpha reductase from converting testosterone into DHT.

A study published by the *Journal of Alternative and Complementary Medicine* examined beta-sitosterol's effectiveness in blocking the production of DHT. The study analyzed men between the ages of 23 and 64 with hair loss.

The participants received either beta-sitosterol or a placebo. The researchers found that 60% of the men receiving beta-sitosterol had an improvement in hair growth. They also lost less hair than the placebo group.[1]

You can also find beta-sitosterol in a few herbs at health food stores: saw palmetto, pygeum bark extract, and pumpkin seeds.

Another important nutrient is gamma-linolenic acid (GLA). It is an essential fatty acid found in natural plant oils. It is difficult to obtain healthy amounts through diet alone.

Gamma-linolenic acid is a proven 5-alpha-reductase inhibitor. The

Journal of Investigative Dermatology published one well-known study: researchers tested GLA's efficacy on hamsters.[2] GLA successfully inhibited the 5-alpha-reductase from converting testosterone into DHT.

Like most health issues, good nutrition serves as the foundation. Stress, abuse of drugs, poor health habits, and prescription drugs aggravate the problem and can accelerate the loss of hair.

6 Tips For Keeping Your Hair Youthful
Eat a healthy, high protein diet
Avoid too much stress
Do not use illegal drugs
Avoid prescription drugs
Limit hat wearing
Take a multivitamin

New technologies are rapidly emerging that will change the way older men look. From better hair grafts to hormonal manipulation to new prescription drugs, the options have changed from useless, vain and troublesome snake oils to a powerful armamentarium that can have a real effect.

Growing real hair takes time. There are no immediate solutions for a return of natural hair growth. But, if you have patience, you can expect to make a difference by sticking to a well-thought-out strategy.

---

[1] Prager N, et al. "A randomized, double-blind, placebo-controlled trial to determine the effectiveness of botanically derived inhibitors of 5-alpha-reductase in the treatment of androgenetic alopecia." *J Altern Complement Med* 2002 Apr; 8(2):143-152

[2] Liang T, et al. "Growth suppression of hamster flank organs by topical application of gamma-linolenic and other fatty acid inhibitors of 5 alpha-reductase." *J Inv Derm* 1997 Aug; 109(2):152-157

Chapter 2

Beat the Next Big Epidemic of Diabetes without Risky Drugs

I want to make one thing clear: *you don't have to rely on prescription drugs to prevent — even reverse — diabetes.* I'm going to reveal the first step to treat it safely, effectively, and naturally.

Despite what the medical establishment tells you, adult diabetes is NOT a genetic disease without a cure requiring treatment for life. I've helped hundreds of my own patients completely reverse their diabetes.

It's a problem of inadequate and unbalanced nutrition.

So rather than telling you to just learn to live with it, I'm going to give you two powerful minerals and one potent antioxidant to help you turn the tables on a disease that already afflicts 8.6 million Americans 60 or over.

By taking a few simple steps, you can:

- Return your blood sugar to healthy levels;
- Lower your blood pressure;
- Boost energy and lose weight;
- And so much more.

What Your Doctor May Never Tell You about Diabetes

Most people believe that diabetes is a problem of high blood sugar.

High blood sugar is a *symptom* of the diabetes. But it's not the root cause.

The major problem in adult diabetes is excess insulin. Insulin is the hormone that your body uses to move sugar from the blood into the cells where it's burned for energy. High-carb foods will spike your blood sugar. In response, your body will produce more insulin to move that sugar into your cells. But over time, the extra insulin makes your cells receptors less sensitive to insulin.

You then develop both elevated insulin and blood sugar levels, and your body compensates by producing more and more insulin. Your body becomes less sensitive to insulin. We call this condition ***insulin resistance***.

Too much insulin in the blood:[1]

- Converts excess glucose into fat stores causing you to gain weight.
- Triggers the creation of triglycerides, a risk factor for heart disease.
- Lowers HDL cholesterol levels increasing risk of heart disease and other diseases.
- Impairs the body's sodium balance, which raises blood pressure.
- Damages the kidneys.
- Damages the vascular system contributing to heart disease, retinopathy (eye damage), and neuropathy (nerve damage).

Big Pharma Puts You at Risk Again

The medical industry's response — to focus on lowering blood sugar — is appropriate for immediate care. But it ignores the cause — the insulin problem. Sometimes drugs make the cause worse by stimulating even more insulin production.

Hormones are powerful. When you have too much of any hormone, your body reacts by making your body less sensitive to it as a way of protecting itself. But over time, your body will lose the ability to respond altogether.

Big Pharma always is working on new, expensive drugs to treat your symptom of over production of insulin. Like when they created Avandia, or rosiglitazone, which at first seemed to address this problem. The manufacturer marketed its ability to help sensitize the body to insulin, and Big Pharma had a big hit. Avandia became another blockbuster, with total U.S. sales of $2.2 billion in 2006 as doctors and their patients rushed to embrace this latest treatment.

There's just one fly in the soup. A new study in the *New England Journal of Medicine* found that Avandia could kill you.[2]

Pooled results of several studies on nearly 28,000 people revealed a *43% higher risk of heart attack for those taking Avandia* compared to people taking other diabetes drugs or no diabetes medication.

So what can you do to treat diabetes without exposing yourself to the dangers of the drug industry?

Take Control with Three Simple and *Safe* Supplements

Here are my top three supplements for anyone with diabetes or at risk for diabetes:

Vanadium, a crucial trace mineral, mimics the action of insulin. This means it helps move glucose from the blood into the cells where it can be used as energy. It works by making cells more sensitive to insulin, which stimulates the movement of glucose into cells. It also inhibits the absorption of glucose from the gut, reducing damaging glucose and insulin spikes.[3] In one study, people with diabetes took a vanadium supplement for three weeks. After just three weeks the average participant's blood sugar levels dropped by 10%.

Chromium is another important mineral to help control and even reverse diabetes. In one study, participants took chromium picolinate and biotin for 30 days. All participants had diabetes. After 30 days, participants' cholesterol had dropped an average of 19 points, with LDL cholesterol (the kind that can contribute to heart disease) dropping by more than 10 points. Even more important, the average fasting blood sugar level fell by 26 mg/dL.[4]

Alpha-lipoic acid (ALA) plays a key role. ALA helps to control and prevent nerve and circulatory damage done by diabetes. In one study, people taking ALA showed improved blood pressure, reduced nerve damage, and better circulation.[5]

Alpha-Lipoic Acid

Use the easy chart below to guide you in making the best use of these three supplements.

Supplement	Dosage	When to take it
Vanadium	500 mcg. 3x daily (Do not take more than 10 mg. in a day.)	Take with meals
Chromium with biotin	500 mcg chromium 3x daily 2 mg. biotin daily	Take with meals
Alpha-Lipoic Acid	100 mg. twice daily	Take with meals

Chromium makes your cells more receptive to the action of insulin. ALA improves your body's use of glucose. Vanadium mimics insulin, lowering your body's overall need to produce insulin. Together, these three nutritional supplements give you a powerful support system to help permanently reverse diabetes and restore your good health.

Of course, curbing your carbohydrate intake and controlling the glycemic index of your carbs are important steps to reversing diabetes.

---

[1] "Novel Fiber Limits Sugar Absorption," *Life Extension Magazine*. September 2004.

[2] Nissen, Steven E., et al., â€œEffect of Rosiglitazone on the Risk of Myocardial Infarction, *New England Journal of Medicine*, 2007; 356(24): 2457-2471

[3] Presented at American Heart Association's Annual Conference on Arteriosclerosis, Thrombosis, and Vascular Biology, San Francisco, May 6-8 2004.

[4] Wallach, Joel D. and Lan, Ma. *Rare Earths: Forbidden Cures*. Bonita, CA: Double Happiness Publishing, 1994, pp 411-12.

[5] Tankova T., et al. "Alpha lipoic acid in the treatment of autonomic diabetic neuropathy," *Rom J Intern Med* 2004; 42(4): 457-64

Chapter 3

Here's Your Attention Prescription

Would you knowingly take potent amphetamines if you knew that they would help you focus your attention? Would you give them to a child?

That's exactly what the conventional common treatment has become for one of the most over diagnosed disorders in history — "Attention Deficit/Hyperactivity Disorder" (ADHD).

The medical establishment generously prescribes Ritalin, Adderall, and Dexedrine — drugs more powerful than cocaine. The fact is the drugs psychiatrists are handing out like candy for ADHD are entirely unnecessary and dangerous to you... and your children. Yet you don't hear about natural remedies that are just as effective as these dangerous and addictive drugs.

I'll offer some perspective on the "prevalence" of ADHD and give you treatment options that don't involve expensive, powerfully psychoactive drugs.

Is the ADHD "Epidemic" Real?

First, let's take a step back for a second. Before World War II, we just didn't diagnose ADHD at all. In 1985, about 500,000 people were diagnosed with ADHD. By 2000, that number had skyrocketed to *7 million.* To put this in perspective: about a *half million* people develop this disease every year, on top of those diagnosed the previous year.

Our National Institutes of Health (NIH) estimates that as many as

20% of children suffer from the syndrome. And by some estimates, approximately 30-70% of children who manifest symptoms of ADHD will continue to do so into adulthood.[1]

To many mental health practitioners ADHD is their "bread and butter." Yet as I write this, there is no objective test for the diagnosis of ADHD. Kind of makes you wonder, doesn't it? If we are in the midst of a new and sudden "epidemic" here, shouldn't someone be seeking out the cause?

A Windfall for the Legal Drug Cartel

Among the drugs that are prescribed for ADHD are Ritalin, Adderall, and Dexedrine — and these are at least as strong as methamphetamine and cocaine. And, if you compare brain scans of people on any of these drugs, you'll see that they light up the same areas of the brain — in *exactly the same way*.

Incredibly, the pharmaceutical giants, the medical mainstream, and even the U.S. government *have always known this*. In fact, the Drug Enforcement Administration (DEA) sets production quotas on these drugs as with any drug with potential to be abused recreationally.

And by the way, they do: The number of ER visits for these legal drugs is approaching the same number as visits for cocaine and heroin. Emergency rooms recorded 613,053 treatments involving cocaine and heroin in 2005, compared with 598,542 visits involving pharmaceutical abuse.[2]

The popularity of this treatment is turning more and more young people in this country — millions and millions — into "users." This has done nothing to put a brake on the prescription craze.

ADHD is a windfall for the pharmaceutical industry. Sales of methylphenidate (the chemical name for Ritalin) totaled $8 billion in 2012. Sales of stimulants to treat ADHD have more than doubled to $9 billion in 2012 from $4 billion in 2007, according to the health care information company IMS Health. Let's divorce ourselves from the "drug for everything model" and take a look at the real cause for the worsening behavioral symptoms responsible for the surging diagnosis… and find some safer solutions.

In a word, it's diet.

We're all "Fatheads"

The bad fats that make up a big part of the modern diet are sabotaging our body's capacity to build and maintain our brains. There's compelling evidence that many people have trouble focusing, paying attention, and thinking clearly… because of the kinds of fat they eat.

You've probably heard of "good" fats and "bad" fats. You have to get them in the right ratio. Many contemporary health problems are linked to a drastic reduction in the amount of omega-3s in the modern diet.

- Before the onset of modern animal husbandry techniques, beef contained more omega-3s than wild-caught salmon.

- Dietary sources of omega-3s have plummeted during the last 50 years.

- The average American currently consumes twenty times as much omega-6 as omega-3 fatty acids — 20:1 instead a healthy 2:1.

A number of recent studies have drawn a clear link between omega-3s and brainpower.

Two studies published in the *American Journal of Clinical Nutrition* found that a diet high in omega-3 fatty acids can actually prevent "cognitive decline," a fancy term for losing your ability to understand and think clearly.[3]

In the first, researchers examined diet and thinking ability in healthy men who were 79-89 years old. They reviewed the same group five years later. They found that men who ate fish regularly were mentally sharper than those who didn't. The benefit was the result of omega-3s, a nutrient found in abundance in fish.

In the other study on 2,200 older folks, those with high omega-3 blood levels had a better "way with words" those who didn't. They could recall words, names, and phrases without difficulty. And they were better able to keep track of what they and others were saying.[4]

So here's how to take the first step to get back your native source of omega-3s: Eat lean meats, preferably cold-water wild-caught fish or grass-fed, organic beef. Eggs and nuts are also good sources of omega-3s. Supplements in the form of cod liver oil are also a great source. A tablespoon a day is an excellent first line of defense against ADHD.

This also applies to the young. Boost levels of omega-3 in their diet, and you'll see results. In fact, I know a number of psychiatrists who prescribe pharmaceutical grade fish oil for patients suffering from mood disorders.

The Drug-Free Cure

Has your doctor or psychiatrist ever mentioned DMAE? I'd guess "no."

This is a natural, fundamental brain stimulant found in anchovies, sardines, and other fish. Studies show it increases levels of acetylcholine. Acetylcholine is a foundational compound of your brain's memory and learning capacity.[5]

DMAE provides a safe and non-addictive solution to a variety of cognitive and behavioral problems. DMAE can temper mood and ease behavioral and learning problems. In one study, hyperactive kids showed improvement in just 10 weeks.[6]

In another study, children with learning disabilities did better in concentration and skill tests.[7] And there were no side effects like an increase in heart rate and blood pressure as with drugs.[8]

Recent research has uncovered additional readily available, natural supplements that are highly effective in treating the symptoms of ADHD, including the amino acids 5-Hydroxytryptophan (5-HTP), Acetyl-L-Carnitine (ALC), glutamine, and tyrosine.

5-HTP is what's known as a serotonin "precursor." Serotonin is a chemical in the brain known as a "neurotransmitter" that regulates mood and alleviates anxiety and depression. I recommend doses of 50 to 100 mg. three times per day with meals.

Acetyl-L Carnitine, also known as ALC, increases the formation of acetylcholine. It also increases brain cell energy production and helps control impulsivity. The ideal dosage is 1,500 mg. twice per day between meals.

Tyrosine, another compound that supports mood by enhancing the production of neurotransmitters, has also been shown to be highly effective treating ADHD. The recommended dosage is up to 5,000 mg. per day for children and up to 10,000 mg. per day for adults.[9, 10, 11, 12, 13]

They're all available at your local vitamin shop.

[1] Strock, et al. "Attention Deficit Hyperactivity Disorder." *NIH Publication No. 3572*, National Institute of Mental Health (NIMH), 1996.

[2] Leinwand, D. "Misuse of pharmaceuticals linked to more ER visits," *USA Today*, 3/13/03.

[3] Strock, M., et al., "Attention Deficit Hyperactivity Disorder." *NIH Publication No. 3572*, National Institute of Mental Health (NIMH), 1996.

[4] Boukje M, et al. "Fish consumption, n–3 fatty acids, and subsequent 5-y cognitive decline in elderly men." *American Journal of Clinical Nutrition* (2007), 85(4):1142-1147.

[5] May A, et al. "Plasma n–3 fatty acids and the risk of cognitive decline in older adults." *American Journal of Clinical Nutrition* (2007), 85(4):1103-1111.

[6] Ward D."DMAE Cognitive-Enhancing, Life Extending Nutrient. *Vitamin Research News*, 18(2004),(8):1-4.

[7] Coleman N, et al. "Deanol in the treatment of hyperkinetic children." *Psychosomatics*, 17(1976):68-72.

[8] Geller S, et al., "Comparison of a tranquilizer and a psychic energizer." *Journal of the American Academy of Medicine*, 174(1960):89-92.

[9] Oettinger L, et al. "The use of Deanol in the treatment of disorders of behavior in children." *Journal of Pediatrics*, 53(1958):761-675.

[10] Lombardi R, et al., "ADHD: A modern malady." *Nutrition Science News.* July 2000.

[11] Adriani W, et al. "Acetyl-l-carnitine reduces impulsive behaviour in adolescent rats." *Psychopharmacology.* 2004 Nov;176(3-4): 296-304.

[12] Sahley B. "Natural control of ADD and ADHD." *Vitamin Research News.* 2000;14(10).

[13] McConnell H, et al. "Catecholamine metabolism in the attention deficit disorder." *Medical Hypotheses*, 17(4):305-311, 1985.

Chapter 4

Big Pharma Sets Its Sights on Spot and Fluffy

The big drug makers aren't satisfied with the global takeover of modern medicine…

Now they're gearing up their profit machine for a new conquest: *your pet.* Armed with the full support of the FDA, big drug makers are targeting your pets with the same drugs that are causing problems for us humans — and the same misleading propaganda.

I'll reveal the blueprint of their latest campaign and give you some easy-to-follow advice for keeping your four-legged friends happy, healthy, and drug free.

Just Say "No" to Doggie Drugs

This latest push by drug makers has been in the works for the last 20 years or so. The corporate heavyweights openly discuss the massive profits they can make by getting you to believe that your dog or cat needs chemical drugs to be "healthy."

Drug companies have spent millions of dollars aggressively rewriting vet schoolbooks and curricula. All for the sake of churning out vets who toe the party line. Just like they succeeded in training doctors to reach for prescription pad first, all across the United States vets are handing out pharmaceuticals for arthritis, diabetes, heart disease, cancer, and more. And earlier this year, the FDA approved Prozac for dogs!

Most of the problems your pet may run into are treatable — and avoidable — with good nutrition. But try telling that to a vet who's been taught to believe that drugs are the answer to everything.

And, some of the common products you buy for your pets may be doing them more harm than good. Most people trust their vets without question, and have no way of knowing they may recommend products that are dangerous.

If your pet is getting sick, it's likely it is being poisoned by commercial pet products. Some of the common culprits are:

- Pet food pumped full of chemicals and preservatives.
- Pet pharmaceuticals never intended for animals.
- Toxic flea and tick collars and medications.

Vets routinely prescribe powerful tranquilizers intended for humans. Drugs like Xanax and Valium are often given to dogs as a form of "behavior modification."

This is amazing to me. I did some digging on the Internet and in medical journals and I couldn't find any evidence that these drugs have even been tested on animals. In humans, these drugs are highly addictive and can have serious side effects, including death in the case of overdose.

When you give these powerful drugs to dogs, you have no way of knowing what kind of long-term physical effects they will have. Or how a particular dosage will affect a particular breed of animal.

Not to mention the fact that suppressing a dog's natural warmth and enthusiasm may create other personality disorders — the consequences of which are unknown.

Here's a brief list of some of the new doggie drugs hitting the market this year:[1]

Big Pharma's New Canine Meds		
Drug Name:	**Drug Maker:**	**Treatment for:**
Yarvitan	Johnson & Johnson	Weight Loss/Obesity
Slentrol	Pfizer	Weight Loss/Obesity
Cerenia	Pfizer	Vomiting
Reconcile (Prozac)	Eli Lilly	Depression
Vetmedin	Boehringer Ingelheim	Congestive Heart Failure

In many ways, this trend mirrors what's happening to people all over the world: People eat processed foods full of artificial ingredients and man-made fats, and then turn to drugs to help them lose weight.

Now we have dogs being fed processed dog food and then given drugs to help them cope with the side effects of an unnatural diet.

Even more alarming is a new push to have dogs vaccinated against diseases they have no history of ever having: Drug giant Merck is teaming up with Sanofi-Aventis for a new melanoma vaccine under their new company Merial.

In all my years of medicine, not once have I ever heard of a dog with skin cancer. Nor would a dog fed a healthy diet and given the room to exercise ever run the risk of skin cancer.

That's not to say that some animals don't get cancer. Sometimes they do. But cancer in animals is even easier to prevent than in humans. And avoiding processed foods and useless prescription drugs is the first step.

Give Your Pet What It Needs for Real Health and Happiness

I have a Springer Spaniel named Cosmo. He's 11 years old, but still has the same energy he did when he was a puppy. Taking care of him is easy. I simply create a natural, native environment for him.

That means a diet high in protein and omega-3 fats, and plenty of space to run around. I add raw eggs and cod liver oil to his food and often reward him with his favorite meal: raw grass-fed beef.

If your dog or cat has a problem with fleas or ticks — which is rare — I recommend an all-natural flea powder. The ingredients are peppermint oil, cinnamon oil, lemon grass oil, and thyme oil. These natural oils are harmless to dogs and cats, but they're deadly to biting pests. You can find similar products at the larger pet stores or on the Internet.

If your vet is insisting on prescription drugs for your pet, you may want to consider finding a holistic or naturopathic animal care expert. Unfortunately, Big Pharma controls many of the state licensing boards and some states are trying to de-license naturopathic vets. So you may have to do a little homework. They are out there in small numbers. You can find them with an Internet search.

---

[1] Petkewich R." Big Pharma Chases Dogs and Cats." *Chemical & Engineering News.* Jun 2007: 85(26)31-34.

Chapter 5

A Dangerous Game with Our Children

The other day I was picking up my nine-year-old son, D.S., from school and noticed some of the girls in his class were already wearing bras. My patients have been reporting the same thing to me more and more. Nowadays, some children are beginning to develop sexually *as early as seven.*[1] What's going on?

I have reason for concern over the hundreds of unnatural additives and pollutants in our food, water, air, and so many everyday household products. These "enviro-toxins" disrupt normal hormone levels in the body, causing weight gain, fatigue, infertility, and other serious health problems.

Now a growing body of evidence in the U.S. and Britain suggests that these chemicals are wreaking havoc in the lives of our kids. They're the main cause behind the alarming trend toward increasing "precocious puberty" — little girls prematurely growing breasts and pubic hair and going through all the other confusing changes that come with puberty.

And, research published in the *Archives of Pediatric and Adolescent Medicine* found that American boys are also hitting puberty earlier than in the past. A significant number of boys as young as eight showed signs of premature genital development.[2] A study in the U.K. found that about one in 14 eight-year-old British boys had developed pubic hair, compared to one in 150 boys in the last generation.[3]

In a major study of 17,000 American girls, 7% of Caucasians girls and a shocking 27% of African-American girls were either growing breasts or pubic hair by age seven. Even more upsetting, precocious puberty was seen in 3% of African-Americans and 1% of Caucasians by age three![4]

The Dangers of "Growing Up Too Fast"

What are the consequences of this bizarre phenomenon? Studies have shown that girls who go through puberty too soon also:

- Have sex earlier;
- Run greater risk of pregnancy;
- Suffer from behavioral problems;
- Have a lower IQ;
- Are more likely to drink, smoke;
- Are more likely to commit suicide.

They're also more likely to develop breast and ovarian cancer later in life, and to become infertile.[5]

In boys, precocious puberty can lead to more aggressive, violent behavior; learning disabilities; and greater risk of drug and alcohol abuse. As they mature, they're at increased risk for testicular cancer and low sperm counts.[6]

The Mainstream Response: Dangerous Drugs and Denial

An increasing number of experts agree with what I've been saying all along: the culprits are industrially produced hormones and chemical compounds. Most come from the food supply and household products, including plastics, cleaning solvents, vinyl flooring, even make up and hairspray.

Unfortunately, while the medical community has finally acknowledged this problem, their response is to put our children on yet another endocrine disrupting chemical. Lupron, their drug to treat precocious puberty blocks production of your own natural sex hormones and has 265 known side effects, including convulsions and cancer.

A separate physician's network has taken another wrongheaded approach to the problem, claiming that "precocious puberty" simply needs to be considered "normal." In other words, they're just defining down the right stage for the onset of puberty. This is just denial.[7]

Meanwhile, the U.S. government hasn't taken any steps to protect the public from these dangerous enviro-toxins, and the FDA allows cattle breeders to pump animals with hormones, steroids, and synthetic growth agents. All this stuff winds up in your body.

One researcher found hormone levels in industrially raised beef were *three hundred times greater than in normal or grass-fed beef.*[8] The same goes for the poultry industry, which uses synthetic proprietary feeds to make chickens grow mature and fat faster.

Household products can contain **phthalates** (pronounced THAL-ates) and **bisphenol-A**. These man-made chemicals have structures that look strikingly similar to estrogen. In Europe, industry has been banned from using phthalates, but they're still legal in the U.S.

Perfluorooctanoic acid (PFOA) is another common estrogen mimic. Industries use it to make Teflon for cookware and Gore-Tex for outerwear. The CDC recently tested for the presence of phthalates and PFOA in the general population. The results were sobering. Every person tested — without exception — had both chemicals in his or her bloodstream.[9]

Nine Simple Steps to Protect Yourself and Your Children *Right Now*

So what can you do to protect your child from this public health nightmare?

- Try to make your diet as organic as possible. Free-range organic chickens and grass-fed beef are free of most toxins. Small wild-caught fish are safe, although some larger fish contain heavy metals like mercury. Wild salmon, cod, halibut, mackerel, and sardines are your best bet.

- If you don't have access to organic meats, trim the fat off. Many of the worst chemicals are stored in the fat of the animal.

- Eat organic fruits and vegetables whenever possible. Be sure to wash those that aren't organic thoroughly, or peel off the skin.

- Try to avoid foods packaged in plastic, or remove the packaging as soon as you get home.

- Buy a high-quality water filter. Pesticides find their way into many municipal water systems.

- Don't let your children chew on plastic toys. Better yet, buy toys made of unfinished wood or other natural fibers.

- Avoid nonstick or plastic cookware. Stainless steel, cast iron, and glassware are all safe.

- Buy household products made from natural and organic ingredients. These are widely available in stores and online.

- Purify the air in your home with plants. Common household plants can filter dangerous chemicals from new carpets or curtains. For instance, Boston ferns can detoxify 1,000 micrograms of formaldehyde from the air in one hour.[10]

---

[1] Herman-Giddens, et al. "Secondary sexual characteristics and menses in young girls" *Pediatrics*, 1997, 99(4):505-512.

[2] Herman-Giddens, et al. "Secondary Sexual Characteristics in Boys," *Archives of Pediatric and Adolescent Medicine*, 155(2001):1022-1028.

[3] Golding, et al. "ALSPAC Study Team," *Paediatric Perinatal Epidemiology*, 2001, 15(1):74-87.

[4] Herman-Giddens, et al. "Secondary sexual characteristics and menses in young girls seen in office practice: a study from the Pediatric Research Office Settings Network." *Pediatrics*, 1997, 99(4):505-512.

[5] Willett W. "The search for the causes of breast and colon cancer." *Nature*, 338(1989):389-94

[6] Herman-Giddens, et al. "Secondary Sexual Characteristics in Boys: Estimates from the National Health and Nutrition Examination Survey III, 1988–1994," *Archives of Pediatric and Adolescent Medicine*, 155(2001):1022-1028.

[7] Rivkees S. "Monitoring Treatment of Children," Cares Foundation, 2014.

[8] Epstein. *The Breast Cancer Prevention Program*, New York: Macmillan, 1997, p. 193.

[9] Weise E. "Are Our Products Our Enemy?" *USA Today*. Aug 2, 2005.

[10] Seaman G. "The Top 10 Plants for Removing Indoor Toxins." Healthy Home, 2009.

Chapter 6

The Next Big Scandal Puts You in Danger

The *Wall Street Journal* called it "**Vytoringate.**"

In an effort to prove that their Vytorin is effective at reducing the arterial plaque that leads to heart disease, Merck/Schering-Plough conducted its own study on 750 patients. Much to Merck's disappoint-
ment, the study found that Vytorin was instead effective at doubling
the growth rate of arterial plaque![1]

So what did Merck do? They first hung on to the results, knowing full
well sales and prescriptions of the drug would plummet as soon as the
public found out.

And the organizations America trusts, the AHA and the ACC, both
made statements giving a supportive tone concerning Vytorin and the
ENHANCE trial. This has Congress looking into any financial ties
that exist between them and Merck.

As if that wasn't enough, it looks like the SEC is getting involved too.
Turns out top executives at Merck sold 900,000 shares of company
stock worth $28 million — before the ENHANCE trial went public.

Big Pharma Hid the Facts — Again

This is not the first time drug companies have hidden the facts they
didn't want you to know about.

Take GlaxoSmithKline, for instance, which in 2004 was found guilty
of hiding negative trial results of their antidepressant Paxil. Turns out

Paxil didn't do anything more for depression than a placebo did. Plus it increased the risk of suicide for those taking it. They held on to the information for up to four years before it became known.

A recent study published in the *New England Journal of Medicine* found nearly a third of the 74 industry-sponsored studies of antidepressants they examined were not published, most of which showed negative outcomes for the drug involved.[2]

Positive results were 12 times more likely to be published. And negative results were purposely written to show a favorable outcome. Put into perspective, of all the articles published, 94% show a positive outcome. But on further inspection by the FDA, only half were actually positive.

The *Journal of the American Medical Association* published a study as far back as 2004, stating that the reporting of trial outcomes are frequently biased and overstate the benefits.[3]

Whom Can You Trust?

Even doctors are misled by the drug companies into thinking the drugs they're prescribing are safe for their patients.

This is because once a drug receives FDA approval, it's pretty much a done deal. Drug companies are required to share any findings they get from studies to the FDA, but the FDA can't share the information with the public. It's because the study findings are considered "proprietary" information that belong to the drug companies.

To counteract this, Congress recently passed a new law, requiring drug companies to share all their findings. But there's one problem.

They've given them two years from the end date of the studies to make the information public. Critics are pointing out how even this new law wouldn't have stopped the Vytoringate scandal.

Nature's "Vytorin" — but Better

Nature has a substance that can do exactly what Vytorin was *supposed* to do. It's called folic acid and researchers have known about it for years.

See, Merck/Schering-Plough was looking to prove Vytorin effective by looking at how much it reduced the intima-media thickness of the carotid artery. The higher the thickness, the more likely a negative cardiovascular event such as heart attack, or stroke.

Recent studies show that folic acid supplementation significantly reduces the intima-media thickness of the carotid artery.[4]

Another study, published in the prestigious British medical journal the *Lancet,* found that folic acid reduces the risk of first stroke by as much as 18%.[5] Had Vytorin created results like these, Merck/Schering-Plough would be headed for a bigger payday.

But there's a bigger problem at work here. Mainstream medicine and the drug companies have got it all wrong. They're looking in the wrong places to find a solution to heart disease. They look to cholesterol as the panacea of curing heart disease. And they're missing the biggest indicators of heart disease, which are not high cholesterol, or even LDL cholesterol.

The two big indicators they're completely ignoring are homocysteine and C-reactive protein (CRP). But the links between them and heart disease are too strong to ignore.

One study found that levels of homocysteine were dramatically higher in men who died from heart attacks. They discovered that men with high levels were *four times* more likely to suffer a fatal heart attack than those with lower levels.[6]

And guess what? Folic acid can significantly reduce levels of homocysteine in the bloodstream.

The other indicator, CRP, isn't given enough attention.

The *New England Journal of Medicine* published a massive study on CRP. Almost 28,000 people participated in the trial. Researchers tried to predict cardiac events like heart attack and stroke by looking at LDL cholesterol and CRP levels in the blood. They found that CRP predicted cardiac events better than LDL cholesterol did.[7]

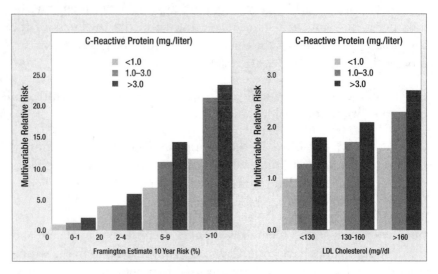

Here again, folic acid is proven to reduce levels of CRP. To get the benefits from folic acid, you should take 800 mcg. a day. You can find it at any health food or grocery store.

Nature Has Everything You Need to Keep Cholesterol under Control

When heart patients come to see me in my office, the first thing I do is wean them off any cholesterol drugs their doctors might've prescribed. It's because I know the inherent side effects that come with those drugs, including impotence, liver failure, and severe muscle pains, to name a few.

The most popular of these cholesterol-lowering drugs are statins. They work by blocking enzymes in the liver responsible for the formation of cholesterol. But again, nature already has its own substances that can lower LDL cholesterol, raise HDL cholesterol, and lessen hardening of the arteries.

And best of all, these substances are inexpensive, and free of side effects.

Four All-Natural, Powerful, and Safe Supplements to Lower Your Cholesterol

Ditch the cholesterol drugs, and use these four natural alternatives instead:

CoQ10 — You've heard of this one, I'm sure. Simply put, it's one of the best supplements you can take to protect your heart and raise "good" HDL cholesterol. Take 100 mg. per day if you're healthy. If you have heart problems, begin with 200 mg. and then get your doctor to check your blood levels.

Policosanol — This is an extract of plant waxes that naturally lowers high cholesterol. It's just as effective as FDA-approved drugs and is free of side effects. It's not toxic to your liver, even at extremely high doses. And it's safe if you have diabetes or liver disease.

One study found that after 24 weeks of supplementing with it, patients lowered LDL cholesterol by up to 28%, and reduced total cholesterol by 17%.[8] Other studies show it can raise your HDL cholesterol by up to 29%![9] Take 40 mg. daily to achieve optimal results.

Fenugreek — This herb has been used for centuries. The Ancient Greeks, Romans, and Egyptians used it for both culinary and medicinal purposes. Studies show this herb can significantly lower total and LDL cholesterol. Take 500 mg. a day to get the optimum cholesterol-lowering benefits of this herb.

Zinc — This is an underestimated, powerful antioxidant that can reduce plaque buildup in your blood vessels.

Researchers at the University of Singapore conducted an eight-week study in which they fed two groups of rabbits a high-cholesterol diet but gave only one group a natural zinc supplement.

The rabbits on a diet high in cholesterol along with a zinc supplement showed a substantially lower instance of hardening of the arteries and plaque buildup without a change in their blood cholesterol levels.[10]

The bad news is that you're probably not getting enough zinc from your diet alone. Sixty-five percent of Americans don't get even the minimum daily requirement. You can get zinc naturally, from eating red meat, oysters, clams, and fish. But ideally you should also take it as a supplement, to ensure you're getting enough. Take from 30 mg. to 60 mg. per day, for optimal heart health.

---

[1] "Merck/Schering-Plough Pharmaceuticals Provides Results of the ENHANCE trial." Business Wire press release, January 14, 2008.

[2] Turner H, Matthews A, Linardatos E, Tell R, Rosenthal R. "Selective Publication of Antidepressant Trials and Its Influence on Apparent Efficacy." *New England Journal of Medicine.* Volume 358:252-260, Jan.17, 2008. No.3.

[3] Chan A, Hróbjartsson A, Haahr M, Gøtzsche P,Altman G." Empirical Evidence for Selective Reporting of Outcomes in Randomized Trials," *JAMA.* 2004;(291):2457-2465.

[4] Vianna A, Mocelin A, Matsuo T, Morais-Filho D, Largura A, Delfino V, Soares A, Matni A."Uremic hyperhomocysteinemia: a randomized trial of folate treatment for the prevention of cardiovascular events," *Hemodial Int.* 2007 Apr;11(2):210-6.

[5] Wang X, Qin X, Demirtas H, Li J, Mao G, Huo Y, Sun N, Liu L, Xu. "Efficacy of folic acid supplementation in stroke prevention: a meta-analysis." *Lancet.* 2007 Jun 2;369(9576):1876-82

[6] Wald N, et al. "Homocysteine and ischemic heart disease: results of a prospective study with implications regarding prevention." *Arch Intern Med.* 1998; 158:862-7.

[7] Ridker P, et al. "Comparison of C-reactive protein and low-density lipoprotein cholesterol levels in the prediction of first cardiovascular events." *NEJM* 2002 Nov 14; 347(20): 1557-1565

[8] Castano G. et al. "Effects of policosanol 20 versus 40 mg/day in the treatment of patients with type II hypercholesterolemia: a 6-month double-blind study." *Int J Clin Pharmacol Res* 2001;21(1):43-57.

[9] Más R, Castaño G, Illnait J, Fernández L, Fernández J, Alemán C, Pontigas V, Lescay M. "Effects of policosanol in patients with type II hypercholesterolemia and additional coronary risk factors." *Clinical Pharmacology & Therapeutics* (1999) 65, 439–447.

[10] Jenner A, et al. "Zinc supplementation inhibits lipid peroxidation and the development of atherosclerosis in rabbits fed a high cholesterol diet." *Free Radical Biology and Medicine* 2007; 42: 559-566

Chapter 7

Drugs Can Rob You of More than Money

Popular prescription drugs can rob your body of many essential nutrients, doing you more harm than good.

The problems aren't limited to a handful of expensive, newly developed blockbusters like Lipitor. Scores of popularly prescribed drugs for all kinds of health problems have been proven to leach important vitamins, minerals, and key enzymes out of your body or prevent it from being able to absorb them. They can also effect metabolism and even make it impossible for your body to use certain nutrients.

For some reason, most doctors don't know this, or they simply forget to tell their patients. Until the word gets out, you're going to need to arm yourself with knowledge to protect your health. I'll explain just how bad the problem is and show you some easy, simple ways to sidestep it entirely.

These Common Culprits May Be in Your Medicine Cabinet

Some of the most commonly used drugs in America today can cause any one of the problems on this list.

Aspirin

You may be surprised to learn that aspirin makes it harder for your body to absorb vitamin C.[1] It can also decrease levels of iron and folic acid, leading to anemia, susceptibility to cold and flu, and a host of additional ailments.[2] And it's not even a prescription drug.

Oral Contraceptives

For my women readers, here's some news that should concern you: oral contraceptives have been shown to drain your body of vitamin B6. This can set a cascade of unwanted side effects in motion, including sleeplessness, mood swings, and depression.

That's because you need vitamin B6 to make serotonin, melatonin, and tryptophan.[3] These natural compounds powerfully affect your sense of contentment in life, your ability to rest, and your overall emotional stability. This is why so many women who come to my clinic complain of becoming someone they don't recognize while on "the pill" or "the patch."

What's more, oral contraceptives also rob you of B12, zinc, and blood magnesium levels, causing diarrhea, poor immune resistance, insomnia — even anorexia.[4]

Vitamin B12 in particular is vital to optimal health. I can't say enough how bad it is to be B12-deficient. It's crucial to brain function and the overall health of your nervous system. It's the engine behind your body's ability to make blood. Every cell in your body uses it to convert fuel into energy. It's also the key to DNA synthesis and regulation, and enables your body to produce life-supporting fatty acids.

I usually put my women patients suffering from these symptoms on supplements to offset nutrient imbalance: vitamin B (usually 50 mg. a day), zinc (60 mg.), and magnesium (200 mg.).

Acid Blockers

Attention men: if you're taking drugs to relieve heartburn or acid reflux, chances are you're shortchanging your body of zinc and iron.[5,6] You need zinc in abundance for its power to help your body recover from wounds and injury and fight off infectious diseases.

It's also one of the keys to prostate health, virility, and sexual performance. In fact, for men, the prostate gland is where most of the body's zinc is concentrated. This is one "rock" you can't do without.

Women ought to worry about acid blockers' effect on iron levels. We all need iron to enable our blood to deliver oxygen to every cell in our bodies. Most people get enough of it in their diet. Without enough of it, a host of problems set in, including anemia, fatigue, and greater vulnerability to illness. Women are particularly at risk because of blood loss during menstruation.

The ones to watch out for are "proton pump inhibitors" (PPI's) or "histamine-2 receptor antagonists" (H2 blockers). Prevacid (Lansoprazole) is one of the most popular PPIs, for example.

They've been linked to vitamin B12 deficiency, lower calcium absorption, and even lower beta carotene, a critical antioxidant.[7]

Even worse, they steal one of your body's most important nutrients — vitamin D. That means you'll suddenly be missing out on a long list of major health benefits, including:

- Elevated mood and boosting of your mental performance;
- Lower risk types of cancers including prostate, breast and ovarian;
- Reduced risk of melanoma, the deadly form of skin cancer;
- Prevention of bone diseases, including osteoporosis;
- Lower risk of depression and schizophrenia;
- Enhanced function of your pancreas
- Increased insulin sensitivity and diabetes prevention;
- Weight loss;
- Better sleep;
- Increased energy and stamina during the day;
- Significantly lower blood pressure;
- Lower blood sugar levels;
- Lower LDL or "bad" cholesterol levels;
- Increased white blood cells responsible for immunity.

Corticosteroids

Prednisone and hydrocortisone are some of the top drugs used to treat lupus, Crohn's disease, and other autoimmune or inflammatory conditions. Unfortunately, they also leach calcium from your body and increase its elimination, putting you at greater risk of bone fracture and osteoporosis.

Some studies have shown these drugs can also lower levels of key trace elements, including magnesium, selenium, zinc, copper, and potassium. You should be taking supplements to offset the loss of so many important nutrients.

Hormone Replacement Drugs

I've written about these before. The term "hormone replacement" is totally misleading: the drugs doctors are prescribing to millions every year to offset declining hormone levels aren't "replacing" anything. That's because drug makers derive them from animal hormones that are utterly foreign to your body.

They do this for profit, not patient health. They can't legally patent a naturally occurring substance, so they deliberately synthesize inorganic compounds your body was never meant to tolerate.

The health hazards range from relatively minor to severe. You may find yourself having trouble getting to sleep. That's because hormone replacement drugs prevent your body from making melatonin, the sleep hormone.

Studies show that these drugs deplete a long list of critical nutrients, including:

- Vitamin B2 (Riboflavin);
- Folic acid
- Vitamin B12 (Cobalamin);
- Vitamin C;
- Zinc;
- Magnesium.

Anti-Diabetic Drugs

Metformin, one of the most widely used medications to treat the symptoms of diabetes, robs your body of vitamin B12 and folic acid. It can attack heart health over time, partly because it also lowers CoQ10 levels. I've written at length about CoQ10. Every cell in your body needs it for metabolism, and it's especially crucial for the proper function of your vital organs, including the brain, heart, and liver. As you age, your body makes less and less of it.

The last thing you need is a drug that will drive CoQ10 levels down even further.

Statin Drugs

Again, I've been sounding the warning bell on these dangerous drugs for years. Lipitor, Zocor, Mevacor, Crestor and the like are great at driving your LDL cholesterol levels through the floor; unfortunately, they do the same thing to CoQ10 levels. Here are just a few of the risks you face if you're taking statins:

- Inability to concentrate;
- Depression;
- Confusion;
- Impotence;
- Amnesia;
- Lowered sex drive;
- Disorientation;
- Weakened immune system;
- Shortness of breath;
- Liver damage;
- Fatigue;
- Kidney failure;
- Nerve pain;
- Muscle weakness;
- Rhabdomyolysis (painful bursting of muscle cells);
- Death.

These drugs are hardly worth the risks. And most don't need to lower their cholesterol in the first place. It's more about paying attention to your real risk factors such as homocysteine, triglycerides, and C-reactive protein.

Blood Pressure Drugs

Sixty-seven million Americans have high blood pressure according to the American Heart Association. If all of them were to take some of the most common drugs to treat hypertension, they'd also be deficient in vitamin B6 and CoQ10.

Diuretics

There are two kinds of diuretics: thiazides and loop diuretics. They're great at lowering blood pressure. Doctors also prescribe them for diseases of the kidney and liver, as well as for heart health.

While they help to fight these health conditions, they can also cause serious health problems. Hydrochlorothiazide lowers levels of zinc, magnesium, and potassium. Loop diuretics like furosemide and bumetanide also deplete calcium, and vitamins B6 and C.

Don't Wait For These Health Problems to Crop Up

To sum it all up, here's a list of prescription drug classes and their effects. (I've included information on two more kinds of medication: antibiotics and anticonvulsants. Anticonvulsants work for people suffering from epilepsy, but they're also widely prescribed to treat bipolar disorder.)

Prescription drugs: Categories and Nutrient Depletion	
Estrogen/progestin (hormone replacement)	Vitamin B2, B6, B12, C, folic acid, zinc, magnesium
Statins	CoQ10
Acid blockers	CoQ10, B12, folic acid, iron, vitamin D, beta- carotene, zinc

Corticosteroids	Calcium, magnesium, potassium, zinc, copper, selenium, vitamin C, D
Aspirin	Vitamin C, iron, folic acid
Blood pressure drugs	Vitamin B6, CoQ10
Diuretics	Vitamin B1, B6, C, potassium, magnesium, calcium, zinc
Antibiotics	B vitamins, K, magnesium, potassium, calcium, zinc, iron
Anti-diabetics	Vitamin B12, folic acid, CoQ10
Anti-convulsants	Vitamin B1, B7, B12, folic acid, CoQ10, vitamin D, vitamin K, calcium, carnitine

If you're on any one of these drugs, talk to your doctor about taking supplements to counter their adverse effects on your nutrition and overall health. Be sure to keep him or her "in the loop" about the amounts you're taking and any effects you notice over time.

Here's a list I've put together of signs to watch out for. They may mean you're missing an important nutrient:

Medical Malnourishment: Nutrients and Signs to Watch Out For	
B1 (Thiamine)	Depression, memory loss, weight loss, fatigue, numbness
B2 (Riboflavin)	Dermatitis, lesions at the corners of the mouth, swollen tongue, vision loss
B3 (Niacin)	Skin lesions, insomnia, depression, aggression, swelling, diarrhea, weakness, "brain fog," balding
B5 (Pantothenic Acid)	Fatigue, numbness, foot pain
B6 (Pyridoxine)	Depression, fatigue, dermatitis, anemia, glucose intolerance
B7 (Biotin)	Balding, depression, dermatitis, nausea, anorexia
B9 (Folate)	Anemia, fatigue, cervical dysplasia, diarrhea, gingivitis, depression, irritability, insomnia

B12 (Cobalamin)	Anemia, fatigue, poor nerve function, diarrhea, loss of memory
Vitamin C	age spots, bleeding at the gums, fatigue
Calcium	Weakened bones and fractures, muscle spasms
Magnesium	Fatigue, irritability, weakness, muscle cramps, insomnia, anorexia
Potassium	Fatigue, irregular heartbeat, irritability, confusion, reduced nerve function.
Iron	Anemia, weakness, fatigue, poor immune function
Zinc	Slow wound healing, decreased immunity, loss of taste and smell, balding, skin disorders, sexual dysfunction
Selenium	Poor immune function, heart disease
CoQ10	Hypertension, fatigue, cardiovascular diseases
Carnitine	Muscle weakness, inability to digest fat, stunted growth in children, poor athletic performance

If you're not taking supplements and wonder if you should, here are the basics that I recommend to most of my patients.

- Vitamin C: 1,500 mg. to 4,000 mg. per day.
- B Complex: B6 – 150 mg; Folic Acid – 1,600 mcg.; B12 – 800 mcg. per day.
- CoQ10: 200 mg. (or 50 mg. of my Accel) per day.
- Cod Liver Oil: one to two tablespoons a day.

---

[1] Das, et al. "Vitamin C aspirin interaction in laboratory animals." *Journal of Clinical Pharmacology and Therapeutics.* 1992. 17(6):343-6.

[2] Lawrence, et al. "Aspirin and folate binding: in vivo and in vitro studies of serum binding and urinary excretion of endogenous folate." *Journal of Laboratory and Clinical Medicine.* 1984. 103(6):944-8.

[3] Webb, J. "Nutritional effects of oral contraceptive use: a review." *Journal of Reproductive Medicine.* 1980. 25(4):150-6.

[4] Bielenberg J. "Folic acid and vitamin deficiency caused by oral contraceptives." *Medizinische Monatsschrift für Pharmazeuten.* 1991. 14(8):244-7.

[5] Sturniolo, et al. "Inhibition of gastric acid secretion reduces zinc absorption in man." *Journal of the American College of Nutrition.* 1991. 10(4):372-5.

[6] Aymard, et al. "Haematological adverse effects of histamine H2-receptor antagonists." *Medical Toxicology and Adverse Drug Experience.* 1988. 3(6):430-48.

[7] Tang, et al. "Gastric acidity influences blood response to a beta-carotene dose in humans." *American Journal of Clinical Nutrition.* 1996. 64(4):622-6.

Chapter 8

Why Cholesterol Will Make You Live Better, Longer

Is everyone still telling you that cholesterol will kill you? Every time you see your doctor does he tell you to drive your cholesterol lower? And all those TV commercials that tell you how important it is to get your cholesterol lower.

But I've got a stack of studies on my desk proving that people with the highest cholesterol live the longest!

Your body needs a good supply of cholesterol. Even LDL, which you've been told is "bad cholesterol," is needed by your body. I can prove that LDL is critical for fighting infection in your body. And there's proof that people with low LDL are more vulnerable to infection. This sometimes can be fatal.

The truth is that if you follow modern medicine's advice on cholesterol, you may as well be playing Russian roulette with a loaded gun. Drive your cholesterol levels down and you put yourself at greater risk for cancer, major depression, chronic illness, fatigue, low sex drive, broken bones and weakened muscles, and brain disorders.

Not only should you quit obsessing over cholesterol — you want to keep levels high for a number of health benefits, including:

- Gain protection from heart attack;
- Ward off infectious disease and help destroy life-threatening microbial invaders;
- Boost mood and brainpower;

- Maintain optimal functioning of your nervous system;
- Strengthen muscles;
- Prevent cancer;
- Help your body to absorb vital nutrients;
- Regulate proper hormone production, including the sex hormones testosterone and estrogen, and optimize reproductive health and fertility;
- Shorten your body's recovery time from injury;
- Optimize metabolism.

High cholesterol is not the demon that everyone makes it out to be. Now I am going to show you why. Plus I will tell you what you need to know to keep heart disease off your list of things to worry about and build an indestructible heart — safely and naturally.

Forget What You've Been Told

Here's the first thing your doctor never told you: people with high cholesterol live longer. This is fact.

In fact it's old news. The media and the mainstream medical establishment simply haven't gotten the message. As incredible as it may sound, there's literally a library's worth of research proving just how beneficial *high* cholesterol is.

Not only is the data connecting cholesterol and heart disease weak to non-existent, but the opposite is true: the evidence is overwhelming that people with high cholesterol levels not only suffer fewer heart attacks — they're also **less likely to die from all causes than people with low cholesterol.**

The first hint emerged almost two decades ago, when a researcher at the Yale Department of Cardiovascular Medicine was surprised to find that people over 70 with very low cholesterol levels were *twice as likely* to die from heart failure.[1]

Then a "meta-study" came along and took a wrecking ball to the cholesterol myth. Published in the internationally prestigious *Quarterly Journal of Medicine*, it extensively surveyed results from decades of research on heart disease involving hundreds of thousands of individuals.

The conclusion? ***Absolutely no correlation exists between cholesterol and heart attack risk.***[2] People with high cholesterol had a lower overall mortality rate than those with low cholesterol, period. In fact the study showed that cholesterol protects *against* hardening of the arteries — and wards off infectious disease.

This gets at another important fact about cholesterol you won't hear from most doctors: it's a powerful immune booster. It helps your body guard against cold, flu, and even more serious illnesses like staph infection.

For instance, LDL cholesterol — the so-called "bad kind" — binds to dangerous bacterial toxins and helps your body eliminate them. If your cholesterol levels are too low — from taking a statin drug like Lipitor, for instance — you're putting your health in jeopardy.

The science proves it. In 19 studies of more than 68,000 deaths, people with the lowest cholesterol numbers had the highest mortality rate from gastrointestinal and respiratory diseases.

A similar look at the health profiles of 100,000 people over 15 years found that those most frequently admitted to the hospital with an infectious disease had the lowest cholesterol levels from the beginning of the study onwards.[3]

Even individuals who already suffer from serious health problems benefit from cholesterol. One study of patients on dialysis showed that those with higher cholesterol levels had a significantly higher survival rate than the low cholesterol group.[4]

So what's the real deal on cholesterol?

It's a critical component of every cell membrane in your body. It serves as your cells' "skin," preventing bad stuff from getting in and maintaining their internal strength. Your body also uses cholesterol to repair itself. In fact, you'll find high concentrations of cholesterol — in scar tissue.

Your brain's rich in cholesterol; it's one of the main compounds that keep it functioning properly. It's critical to boosting memory and brainpower. Your entire nervous system needs it to function normally.

It helps your brain absorb serotonin, the "feel-good" neurotransmitter, which is why abnormally low cholesterol levels can often lead to memory loss, depression, "brain fog," and lowered sex drive (again, commonly reported side effects of statin drugs like Lipitor and Mevacor).

Cholesterol's also one of the basic building blocks for a number of critical hormones. Your adrenal glands need loads of it to produce the hormones that enable your body to metabolize and regulate blood sugar and mineral absorption. You also wouldn't be able to make testosterone or estrogen without it.

This means that cholesterol lies at the core of healthy metabolism, muscle strength and power, optimum organ function, sex drive, and virility.

Cholesterol plays a critical role in enabling your body to absorb fat-soluble vitamins, including A, D, E, and K. Taken together, these nutrients are responsible for the optimal health and functioning of nearly every system in your body.

Vitamin D is one of nature's most potent cancer fighters and the key to strong bones, balanced insulin levels, good mood — and a healthy heart. Vitamin A is a powerful antioxidant, and vitamin E is crucial to preserving your eyesight as you age.

And you already know about its immune-strengthening benefits.

Bottom line: people with low cholesterol are in serious danger for a wide variety of health threats, including heart attack.

So what's really the main culprit behind most kinds of heart disease?

What You Should *Really* Watch Out For

Now you know that contrary to everything you've ever heard, cholesterol has nothing to do with heart disease risk.

The fact is that serious heart disease isn't caused by any one *substance*, but rather by a *condition*. I can sum up this dangerous condition in a single word: inflammation. And almost all the heart drugs on the market today don't do anything to treat it.

Chronic inflammation is your heart's worst enemy. The good news is it's easy to monitor and even easier to control — safely and naturally, without drugs.

Here's why when it comes to heart disease, it's the real "Enemy Number One":

We've known for years that inflammation of the tissue that lines your arteries (the "endothelium") is the main cause of atherosclerosis, or hardening of the arteries. Endothelial damage leads to the buildup of arterial plaque — a substance made up of bad stuff that gets trapped in damaged tissue, including triglycerides, waste from cellular metabolism, and calcium.

As plaque builds up over time, it blocks the flow of vital nutrients and oxygen to the rest of your body, including your heart. Starve your heart of oxygen and pretty soon you'll have a heart attack.

Plaque buildup around damaged arterial tissue can also cause small ruptures that lead to blood clots. These clots can eventually starve the heart of oxygen by blocking blood flow. And if they break free, they can do damage elsewhere, interfering with your heart's pumping action — or going to your brain and causing a stroke.

So the main thing you want to keep an eye on is not your cholesterol levels. You want to have your doctor check for signs of an inflammatory response in your body.

Inflammation of the arterial linings happens for two main reasons. The first may surprise you. It's infectious disease.

You know that your body responds to foreign invaders by unleashing an army of white blood cells to surround and destroy them. As they attack harmful bacteria and other microorganisms, white blood cells also release a class of hormones called "cytokines."

Cytokines kick your immune system into high alert, signaling for "reinforcements" of white blood cells to help combat diseases. Unfortunately, they also cause an inflammatory response across your entire body — including the delicate linings of your arteries.

This is why people who don't floss regularly are at greater risk for atherosclerosis and heart attack. The bacteria that colonize the area below your gum line unleash a continuous, low-level flow of toxins into your bloodstream. If they're not cleared out, your immune system responds, causing the inflammation that can eventually lead to arterial damage.

It turns out that the presence of cytokines is directly linked to the risk of fatal heart attack. German researchers looked at over 150 patients suffering from chronic heart failure. They found that high concentrations of cytokines in the bloodstream were the strongest predictor of death.[6]

Another major cause of chronic inflammation is free-radical damage. You already know about the power of antioxidants—they neutralize these breakaway molecules that would otherwise attach themselves to healthy cells and do "radical" harm by disrupting proper function, even damaging DNA.

When this happens, it's called "oxidative stress." With enough free radicals running rampant through your body, your arterial walls suffer damage.

Not only that — free radicals are what turn otherwise harmless substances into plaque. This is one of the most important facts about cholesterol and fat that most doctors still don't get. These natural compounds by themselves are not only harmless. They're essential to good health.

But when free radicals get a hold of them, it's a different story. Cholesterol doesn't build up in your blood vessels. It's *oxidized* cholesterol that binds to damaged arterial tissue and becomes part of the plaque that leads to heart attack.

A final marker of heart disease risk is an amino acid called homocysteine. This is a natural byproduct of cellular metabolism that most doctors don't usually mention. Every cell in your body makes it as the cell turns fuel into energy. It gets dumped into your bloodstream afterwards. Think of it as "cellular waste."

It just so happens that homocysteine irritates the lining of your blood vessels. Excess homocysteine leads to a chronic inflammatory response that will keep your blood vessels from opening up, or "dilating," properly. Over time, it can cause atherosclerosis.

Four Factors for True Heart Health

So here's what I recommend you do to ensure *real* heart health and a long, healthy life:

Keep your cholesterol test results in perspective. The bottom line is your total cholesterol levels aren't much use in predicting your risk of heart disease. What *does* matter is that your HDL level — the "good" kind of cholesterol — is high enough. If it's around 85, then it doesn't matter if your total cholesterol is 150 or 350. Boosting HDL is a cinch. A combination of regular exercise and dietary changes are all you need. Eating more lean meats (either red or white) is a great way to raise your HDL naturally.

Stop inflammation. C-reactive protein (CRP) is a good indicator of inflammation and an excellent predictor of heart disease. A simple blood test can measure your levels. The good news is that if you have elevated levels there are simple things you can do to lower them.

The best thing you can do to keep levels low is exercise. Studies show that just moderate exercise lowers CRP levels. In people who just exercised a small amount five times a week CRP levels were cut by 30%.[7]

I also recommend some heart-saving supplements to my patients such as L-arginine, folic acid, and antioxidants such as vitamin E and vitamin C.

500 milligrams of L-arginine daily will help improve blood flow and dilate blood vessels in the lining of the heart, and support heart and

muscle growth. You can also get L-arginine in food sources such as red meat, fish, chicken, beans, nuts, and dark chocolate.

Get your antioxidants. With free-radical damage as a major cause of inflammation, you need to prevent it by boosting your immune strength and fighting off free radicals with a daily dose of antioxidants.

Here are six powerhouses that I recommend to my patients (amounts are daily):

Vitamin C — 3,000 mg. (in divided doses).
Carotenoids — 2,500 IUs.
Vitamin E — 400 mg. of mixed tocopherols and tocotrienols.
CoQ10 — 200 mg., or 50 mg. of reduced CoQ10 (Accel).
Alpha-lipoic acid (ALA) — 100 mg.
Lutein — 20 mg.
Lycopene — 20 mg.

Unfortunately, when your antioxidant system fails homocysteine levels build in your blood. And, homocysteine is the biggest risk factor for heart attack and stroke. So it is critical that you…

Keep your homocysteine levels in check. A simple blood test will give you an accurate reading, although your doctor probably won't run it unless you ask. A level above 10.4 mM/L is abnormally high. I generally shoot for a goal of below seven with my patients.

Lowering your homocysteine is also a simple matter of getting the right supplements. Here's what I give my patients (amounts are daily):

- **Vitamin B12** — 500 mcg.
- **Folic Acid** — 800 mcg.
- **Vitamin B6** — 25 mg.
- **Riboflavin (B2)** — 25 mg.
- **TMG (trimethylglycine)** — 500 mg.

---

[1] Krumholz, et al. "Lack of association between cholesterol and coronary artery

disease mortality and morbidity and all-cause mortality in persons older than 70 years." *Journal of the American Medical Association.* 1990. 272:1335-1340.

[2] Ravnskov U. "High cholesterol may protect against infections and atherosclerosis." *Quarterly Journal of Medicine.* 2003. 96:927-34.

[3] Jacobs, et al. "Report of the conference on low blood cholesterol: Mortality associations." *Circulation.* 1992. 86:1046-1060.

[4] Irribaren, et al. "Serum total cholesterol and risk of hospitalization, and death from respiratory disease. *International Journal of Epidemiology.* 1997. 26:1191-1202; and Irribaren, et al. "Cohort study of serum total cholesterol and in-hospital incidence of infectious diseases." *Epidemiology and Infection.* 1998. 121:335-347.

[5] Liu, et al. "Association Between Cholesterol Level and Mortality in Dialysis Patients: Role of Inflammation and Malnutrition." *Journal of the American Medical Association.* 2004. 291:451-459.

[6] Rauchhaus, et al. "Plasma cytokine parameters and mortality in patients with chronic heart failure." *Circulation.* 2000. 102:3060-3067.

[7] Church T, Barlow CE, Earnest CP, et al. "Assocation between cardiorespiratory fitness and C-reative protein in men."*Arteriosclerosis and Thrombosis: Journal of Vascular Biology.* 2002 Nov 1; 22(11):1869-1879.

Chapter 9

Doctor Kickbacks Leading to Children Drugged

More children are being prescribed antipsychotic drugs for behavioral problems than ever before. In 2007, 500,000 children were prescribed at least one antipsychotic drug. And get this — over 20,000 of those children were under age six! Meanwhile, the doctors prescribing them are getting huge kickbacks from the drug companies.

For example, from 2001 to 2007, child psychiatrists Dr. Joseph Biederman and Dr. Timothy Wilens, each received at least $1.6 million in "consulting" fees from various drug makers, and a third Harvard doctor was paid over $1 million from drug makers.

At the same time, Dr. Biederman's drug company-sponsored research led to an overall 40-fold increase in the diagnosis of pediatric bipolar disorder.

Children are now the fastest-growing segment of an $11.5 billion antipsychotic drug industry, fueled by the growing popularity in diagnosing bipolar disorder in children.

The *New York Times* found that financial relationships between doctors and drug companies leads to more children being prescribed antipsychotic drugs and that psychiatrists who received at least $5,000 from drug makers wrote three times as many antipsychotic prescriptions for children as psychiatrists who received less or no money.

Behavioral Drugs for Children — More Risk than Benefit

Many studies show the dangers of antipsychotic drugs to control behavior including increased risk of:

- Diabetes;
- Metabolic syndrome;
- Irregular heart beat;
- Tachycardia;
- Heart attack.

Canadian researchers found antipsychotic drugs contribute to "significant weight gain," leading to metabolic syndrome and diabetes.[1] And the journal *Drug Safety* reports, "...cardiovascular adverse effects from antipsychotic drugs are extremely common."[2]

Even more telling is the fact that the Drug Enforcement Administration classifies stimulant drugs (commonly used to treat ADHD) in the same category as cocaine and methamphetamines.

In 2006, an FDA advisory panel voted to place a black-box warning on all ADHD drugs such as Ritalin, Concerta, and Adderall because of their risk of death and serious cardiovascular problems. But the FDA's Pediatric Advisory Committee voted against it and won.[3]

Skip the Drugs for Baby

While the causes of many of these behavioral problems are not known for certain, research suggests that our modern diet and environment play a key role. Specifically, food additives and preservatives are linked to poor behavior.

A recent study published in the *Lancet* found that common food additives and colorings can increase hyperactivity in children.[4]

Most behavioral problems are linked to the brain and central nervous system. That's why environmental toxins that affect the central nervous system — like heavy metals, industrial solvents, and chemicals — are thought to be a cause.

And a direct link between these toxins and behavior was shown in a study where monkeys that were exposed to lead and polychlorinated biphenyls (PCBs) developed clear symptoms of ADHD.[5]

Here are four natural and safer alternatives you can begin implementing immediately:

Diet — What children eat has a huge impact on their behavior and well-being.

At Central Alternative High School in Appleton, Wisconsin, students had serious behavioral problems. In response, the school implemented a five-year "healthy eating" program consisting of non-chemically processed foods, that were free of additives and preservatives.

Behavioral problems vanished and students' academics improved significantly.[6]

Make sure your child avoids junk foods and instead give him/her a diet rich in vegetables, fruits, nuts, and lean meats. Avoid processed foods as much as possible (this means anything out of a box or wrapper). Also, eliminate sugary drinks like sodas and artificially flavored fruit juices. Substitute with purified water instead.

Supplements — Because most children's diets are lacking, it's important to supplement with nutrients proven to improve behavior.

Most children with behavioral problems are seriously deficient in omega-3s.

A study done at the University of Adelaide in Australia proves supplementing with omega-3s yields better results than the popular ADHD drug Ritalin![7]

Cod liver and flax seed oils deliver the two kinds of omega-3s the body needs. You can also get your child to eat more lean meats, eggs, and nuts, preferably free-range, grass-fed and organic. These are all great sources of omega-3.

Pine bark extract is another natural supplement that works. One European study using pycnogenol, an organic compound found in the bark of the French maritime pine tree, showed that after only one month, children's behavior improved significantly on as little as 1 mg. per day.[8]

Finally, 5-HTP, a compound produced in the body naturally, is effective at calming a hyper child. It's a precursor to serotonin, one of the chemicals in the brain that relieves anxiety and depression. I recommend 50 mg. with meals.

Good Old-Fashioned Discipline — Many child psychologists find that when there's a behavioral problem, usually there's also a discipline problem.

Behavioral pediatrician Lawrence Diller suggests using the advice found in Dr. Thomas Phelan's book *1-2-3 Magic*. Simply, it involves counting to three and then placing the child in "timeout."

Also, let your child know the rules, and what the consequences are for not following them. If your child fails to clean his room, for example, let him know that he'll be placed in timeout and won't be able to play with his toys for the rest of the day.

Even more important, follow through and be consistent with what you say you are going to do. By the same token, don't forget to reward exceptionally good behaviors.

Nurturing — Paying attention to your child, giving him/her responsibilities, and building his self-esteem is another key to eliminating behavior problems.

You can do this a number of ways. Assign chores that need to be completed each and every week. Pay attention by listening, and by nurturing any special interests. Build self-esteem by offering praise when appropriate and letting your child figure things out on his own.

---

[1] Roger S McIntyre, et al. , "Antipsychotic Metabolic Effects: Weight Gain, Diabetes Mellitus, and Lipid Abnormalities" *Can J Psychiatry* 2001;46:273-281

[2] Buckley, N Sanders, Prashanthan. "Cardiovascular Adverse Effects of Antipsy-

chotic Drugs." *Drug Safety.* 23(3):215-228, 2000.

[3] "Pediatric panel says black box warning not necessary for ADHD medications." *American Association of Pediatrics News.*2006; 27: 1-7.

[4] McCann D, et al. "Food additives and hyperactive behaviour in 3-year-old and 8/9-year-old children in the community: a randomised, double-blinded, placebo-controlled trial." *The Lancet.* 3 Nov. 2007; (370) 9598:1560-1567.

[5] Rice D. "Parallels Between Attention Deficit Hyperactivity Disorder and Behavioral Deficits Produced by Neurotoxic Exposure in Monkeys." *Environmental Health Perspectives Supplements.* Volume 108, Number S3, June 2000.

[6] "Impact of Fresh, Healthy Foods on Learning and Behavior", *Natural Press*, 2004.

[7] Macrae F "Fish oil 'calms children better than Ritalin'" *Daily Mail.* http://www.dailymail.co.uk/health/article-391503/Fish-oil-calms-children-better-Ritalin.html

[8] Trebatická, et. al "Treatment of ADHD with French maritime pine bark extract, Pycnogenol." *European Child and Adolescent Psychiatry.* 2006. 15(6):329-35.

Chapter 10

Should You Have Access to the Secrets of Your Genetic Code?

Some Doctors Don't Trust You to Make the Right Decisions

The *Journal of the American Medical Association* (*JAMA*) recently published their concerns about direct-to-consumer personal genome testing. This test gives you the ability to see a map of your own genome — and the chronic diseases you may be prone to develop later in life.[1]

So what has them so concerned? Information. Yes, they're afraid information may be dangerous.

The doctors writing for *JAMA* fear you might waste your doctor's valuable time and put a strain on the health care system by asking them to interpret the results of your personal genome test. They even imply these test results will put you at greater risk by exposing you to unneeded tests or therapies.

This is both ironic and disturbing. It appears we have a medical system that says drugs are safe and information is dangerous.

Over 100,000 Americans die from prescription drugs *every year*.

But they claim *information* is dangerous?

Isn't it clear that risky prescription drugs — not information — might drain your resources and put you at greater risk?

The information you get from a genome test is open to interpretation.

And some people may jump to the wrong conclusion. But you have the right to information that impacts your health and your future — and you certainly have the right to talk to your doctor without fearing that you're wasting his or her time.

Let's take a closer look at personal genome testing. If you decide it is right for you, I'll show you who to talk to and where to go. All the resources you need are right here.

Your Genes Are the Blueprint of Your Future

The function of genes is to create proteins that are used for almost every function of your cells. Proteins are also critical to the function of the body's organs and tissues.

Nearly every cell in your body depends on thousands of proteins to do their jobs in the right places at the right times. But sometimes a mutation in a gene prevents these proteins from working properly.

A mutated gene changes the instructions for making a protein, which causes it to malfunction or to be missing entirely. When this happens to a protein that has a critical role in the body, it can cause a medical condition.

It's helpful to understand that genes don't cause disease. In other words, you don't have a "cancer gene." But you may have a mutation in a gene that makes proteins function in a way that creates cancer.

Does Genome Testing Make Sense for You?

Genome testing can tell you if your DNA has a gene mutation. This can give you a sense of relief from uncertainty. It can also help you make informed decisions about managing your own health care.

But it can also scare you senseless. If you discover you have a predisposition to heart disease or breast cancer, you may jump to the wrong conclusion.

I want to stress to you that interpreting the results of personal genome testing should be done carefully. It's counterproductive if you run screaming for your life because your results show that you share a genetic trait with others known to get cancer.

Consider this: **Just because you share a trait doesn't mean you have a disease. And it doesn't necessarily mean you'll develop that disease in the future.**

There are many factors that determine gene transcription. You have more control than you think. You can influence which genes get turned on and off. Diet, exercise, and nutritional supplements play a big role.

If you and your doctor determine that your test results correlate to an increased risk of a particular disease, you can take preventative measures. That might mean running diagnostic tests, taking herbs or nutritional supplements known to support your body's natural defenses to that disease, or specific diet choices to keep it from getting a foothold.

If you decide to go ahead with testing, here are a few options…

Contact These Three Companies and Discover Your Personal Genetic Map

23andMe:

Recently mentioned in *Time* magazine, 23 And Me offers genetic testing to the general public for $399. When you order, the company sends you a kit. You send back a saliva sample and within eight to ten weeks you can log onto its website and view your results. Its scan includes a full list of diseases, traits and conditions.

Website: www.23andme.com

deCODEme:

DeCODEme's technique is similar but more expensive, $985 for a full scan. However, you can order a cardiac risk test for $195 or a cancer risk test for $225. These last two are less expensive but won't give you as much information as the full scan.

Website: www.decodeme.com
Contact: _info@decode.is_

GeneDx:

This company specializes in helping families with rare disorders and may not be your first choice if you're looking for a basic scan. But if you're concerned about specific diseases you inherited or diseases that run in your family, this might be a good option.

Costs vary per test and range from $500 to $6,000, but GeneDx works with your insurance company, so your cost may be lower than the genetic testing offered to the public. The testing is not provided directly to consumers. You need to order it through a health care provider or genetic counselor.

Website: www.genedx.com
Contact: 301-519-2100 genedx@genedx.com

---

[1] McGuire A, Burke W. "An Unwelcome Side Effect of Direct-to-Consumer Personal Genome Testing." *JAMA*, Dec 10, 2008.Vol 300, No. 22.

Chapter 11

Why Would a Harvard Medical School Professor Have 47 Ties to Big Drug Companies?

Have you ever watched a TV ad with supposed "everyday people" telling you how taking a pill transformed their lives, and they tell you to "ask your doctor" about getting a prescription at your next appointment? When you don't even have osteoporosis, "high" cholesterol, or the inability to produce tears?

Well, those slick, engaging drug ads you see on TV are just the tip of the iceberg.

Doctors on the take, expensive and impressive sounding studies, and other "underground" marketing sell you more drugs than any TV commercial ever will.

You see, big drug companies regularly fund the sources you trust for so-called "honest and unbiased" information.

- By giving perks and special gifts to doctors who prescribe more of their drugs;

- By awarding multi-million-dollar "research" grants to universities;

- And by bankrolling journalists, radio talk-show hosts, and scientists… all designed to "educate" you on the safety of their drug.

Make no mistake. This is an investment. A big investment.

I'm going to show you the tricks Big Pharma uses to continue to sell you drugs with known deadly side effects.

But wait. It's not all bad news. You'll also get three easy ways to avoid becoming a victim of these deceptive plots.

Big Pharma Goes to College

What do Dr. Charles Nemeroff of Emory College, Dr. Alan Schatzberg of Stanford, and Dr. Joseph Biederman of Harvard all have in common?

They are all influential members of highly respected colleges in the U.S. *And they've all been paid millions through their financial ties with drug manufacturers.* They're also responsible for teaching thousands of future doctors how to cure what ails you.

If Big Pharma is lining their pockets, what do you think these "educators" are teaching the next generation of doctors?

Listen, most medical schools in America are merely pumping out drug salesmen, NOT producing quality doctors who actually know how to cure disease.

Most of these students truly want to learn how to cure people. Instead they are slowly and intentionally being indoctrinated into believing drugs are the only way.

However, don't take my word for it. Just look at the grade that the *New York Times* gave to Harvard.[1]

Harvard Gets an 'F'

Let's look at some of the facts of the story:

- Drug companies contributed $8.6 million last year for basic science research and another $3 million for continuing education classes.

- 1,600 out of 8,900 professors and lecturers admit that either they or a family member have had some kind of financial interest in a business related to their teaching, research, or clinical care. (Former dean Dr. Joseph Martin supplemented his university salary with up to $197,000 a year from drug maker Baxter.)

- 17 industry-owned teaching hospitals and research facilities dot the Harvard campus. (Take Dr. Laurie Glimcher for example, who runs the immunology lab at the campus and made $270,000 from Bristol-Myers Squibb in 2007.)

- Sleep researchers donated $8 million for three industry-endowed chairs. Any coincidence that it seems like every patient in my practice thinks they need a "sleep study"?

- Various "prizes" can be won by the faculty. (One is a $50,000 award named after Bristol-Myers Squibb. Another is a $1 million subsidy from Pfizer for MD students.)

With all this money from the drug industry free for the taking at Harvard, no wonder one professor had 47 ties to the industry!

One faculty member, who is also the former editor in chief of the *New England Journal of Medicine*, even acknowledged that too many medical schools have struck a 'deal with the devil' when it comes to pharmaceutical companies.

Of course it doesn't stop there. The scientific community is on the take as well.

Pfizer's Prolific Pain Researcher

So far we've just talked about Big Pharma's influence on the doctors you trust for advice to get you well.

But Big Pharma uses secret tactics to hook you on drugs way before you need to visit your doctor's office.

Let's take those drug ads, for example.

Have you ever noticed how prescription drugs are always "proven" safe and effective in clinical studies? Do you know who pays for these studies?

Big Pharma does. And when BILLIONS in profits are on the line, the facts get pushed under the rug.

Take the case of Dr. Scott Reuben. Many of his clinical trials found that Celebrex and Lyrica (both Pfizer drugs) were effective against postoperative pain. However, when it was revealed that Dr. Reuben fabricated data in 21 medical journals, the drugs had already been sold for 13 years.[2]

How many Pfizer advertisements used the "proof" of Dr. Reuben's clinical trials to sell more Celebrex and Lyrica pills? Nobody can know for sure.

Public Radio's 'Most Honored and Listened to Health and Science Program' Sponsored by Big Pharma?

Then there's the case of psychiatrist and radio talk show host Dr. Frederick Goodwin. From 2001 to 2007 he earned at least $1.3 million from various drug companies.

His NPR program "The Infinite Mind" reached over one million listeners daily. And won 60 journalism awards in the 10 years it was on the air.

Dr. Goodwin frequently discussed subjects important to the commercial interests of the companies he was on the payroll for. In a Sept. 20, 2005, broadcast, he stated, "Modern treatments — mood stabilizers in particular — have been proven both safe and effective in bipolar children."

That year he was paid $329,000 by GlaxoSmithKline for promoting Lamictal, a mood stabilizer.[3] Public radio is supposed to be "listener supported" not bought and paid for by Big Pharma.

These cases highlight a huge conflict of interest. Big Pharma aggressively pays sources that you trust for honest, unbiased health advice to promote their supposedly safe drugs.

But it goes even deeper. Even when Big Pharma knows their drugs are not safe, they suppress the evidence and continue to sell you drugs that they know could have serious adverse effects on your health.

They're Gambling with Your Life

Donald Schell had been taking Paxil for just 48 hours when he shot and killed his wife, his daughter, his granddaughter and himself.

On June 7, 2001, a jury found SmithKline Beecham (now GlaxoSmithKline, makers of Paxil) liable and ordered them to pay $6.4 million to relatives of Donald Schell.

Why? Because the jury believed honest disclosure of research data by the drug maker could have prevented the slaughter.

The fact is GlaxoSmithKline suppressed the evidence for years that its own research showed Paxil caused suicidal behavior.

Stories like this are tragic. But they highlight Big Pharma's willingness to ignore the dangers of their own drugs to make a profit. Barely a month goes by without another record-setting fine imposed against drug makers.

The following chart shows you a few fines imposed against drug companies in just the past few years:

	Multiple Drugs	Multiple Drugs	Oxycontin	Zyprex	Bextra
Cephalon	$443M				
Schering		$435M			
Purdue Farms			$630M		
Eli Lily				$1.4B	
Pfizer					$2.3B

Now, you'd think that these fines may cause Big Pharma to start walking the straight and narrow, but I doubt it. A $2.3 billion fine doesn't mean much to Pfizer when you consider they took in over $48 billion in 2007 alone.

In fact, it was Pfizer that decided to continue selling Celebrex despite the evidence of the risk of deadly heart attack and stroke.

The cold, hard fact is that the only person who will really safeguard your health is you.

Three Ways to Make Sure You're Not a Victim of Big Pharma's Deceptive Marketing Practices

First, don't blindly trust your doctor's advice.

My Last Free Viagra Booze Cruise

Picture me on a bus chock-full of half-baked doctors all talking about Viagra. Scary, isn't it?

I was younger and greener than I am now, but here's what happened that day...

We were all at Joe Robbie Stadium... enjoying a Miami Dolphins game and getting wined and dined by several Viagra drug reps.

I'm telling you, they pulled out all the stops.

There was catered food and an open bar waiting for us when we arrived at the stadium. We watched the game from high-priced, air-conditioned box seats. All the while we had our fill of food and drink, brought to us by very attractive waitresses.

What did we have to do in return? Just listen to a presentation on the benefits of Viagra by the drug reps on the bus ride home. (After we were all liquored up, of course!)

They even passed out pads with Viagra prescriptions already written on them. All we had to do was sign on the dotted line.

What a racket!

Since then I've refused even so much as a free pen from those pill-pushing drug reps.

Sadly, that's not the case with most doctors. Drug samples, fancy dinners, and extravagant trips have long been free for the taking.

But only as long as the doctor plays by their rules. And that's not something I'm willing to do.

When my patients ask why they have never seen a single drug rep in my office, I just give them one of my newsletter articles like this one.

At best, they've only been taught to treat your condition by throwing pills at it. At worst, they could be telling you to take a certain drug solely because they know they'll get a fat commission check.

The best way to test their knowledge is to ask plenty of questions. And don't walk away until you're satisfied with the answers.

- Why are you prescribing this drug for me?
- How does it work?
- Are there any side effects?
- Does it interact with other drugs, supplements, food, etc?
- Are there any natural alternatives to this drug?

Next, research any prescription drug before you take it.

The simple way to do this is just to type the drug name in Google. This will yield tons of information on side effects, lawsuits against the drug maker, and fines levied against them for illegal marketing.

And even though I'm not a big fan of the FDA, it's still a good idea to check the FDA website (at http://www.fda.gov/medwatch/) to see if the drug is under investigation.

(Word of caution here: It takes the FDA a long time to investigate a drug and have it pulled from the shelves. So this isn't entirely reliable.)

You can also find information about side effects and reactions to drugs and treatments at these websites:

- www.drugs.com
- www.Rxlist.com

Finally, the best way to avoid Big Pharma's tricks is to not put yourself in a position to need drugs in the first place. Ben Franklin's famous quote "An ounce of prevention is worth a pound of cure" is worth repeating.

If you're not taking supplements and wondering where to start, here are the basics that I recommend to most of my patients.

- Vitamin C: 1,500 mg. to 4,000 mg. per day.
- B Complex: B6 — 150 mg.; Folic Acid — 1,600 mcg.; B12 — 800 mcg. per day.
- CoQ10: 200 mg. (or 50 mg. of my Accel) per day.
- Cod Liver Oil: 1 to 2 tablespoons a day.

The right type of exercise also works wonders for your health. I say the right type because much of the fitness advice passed off today does more harm than good.

In fact, that's why I developed the PACE™ exercise program for all of my patients to use. It burns fat, reverses heart disease, and adds years of healthy living to your life... without cardio, lifting weights, or giving up the foods you love.

---

[1] "Harvard Medical School in Ethics Quandary." *New York Times,* March 2, 2009

[2] "Mass. doctor accused of fraud by faking research." Boston.com. January 14, 2010.

[3] "Drugmakers Paid Radio Host $1.3 Million for Lectures." *New York Times.* 11/22/2008.

Chapter 12

What Doctors Are Reading May Put Your Health at Risk

Most doctors rely on a handful of medical journals as a main source for information.

But drug companies are influencing what these journals publish.

And more importantly, what they don't publish.

Many unfavorable facts and trials about new drugs don't make it into these journals.

Why?

A recent study showed that between two thirds and three quarters of the trials published in the major journals — *Annals of Internal Medicine, Journal of the American Medical Association (JAMA), Lancet,* and *New England Journal of Medicine* — are funded by the pharmaceutical industry.[1]

Drug company ads made up 72% of all advertisements in the top five medical journals in 2006 and 2007.

Plus, journals with the most pharmaceutical ads were significantly more likely to publish articles concluding that dietary supplements were unsafe, than the journals with fewer pharma ads.[2]

Studies concluded pharmaceutical advertising biased these medical journals against non-drug therapies.

As a result, they often only publish stories that favor the drug companies.

Here's what I'm talking about…

The *JAMA* once published a positive story about Celebrex. It was based on the clinical trial funded by its inventor, Pharmacia.

Later on, they discovered that researchers had omitted some side effects. They had failed to include six months of results from the trial and concealed that the drug caused ulcers.

By then, Pharmacia had already distributed 30,000 copies of *JAMA* article to doctors.

The Good News Is They're Now Being Exposed

Finally, even those in the industry are fed up.

Dr. Drummond Rennie, a deputy editor of *JAMA*, said, "Drug companies try to bury negative results from clinical trials of new drugs well before publication.

To prevent publication of unfavorable results, companies have threatened researchers, stopped trials, and blocked publication. The consequence is biased reporting, resulting in biased treatments."[3]

Dr. Richard Horton, editor of the *Lancet*, wrote, "Journals have devolved into information-laundering operations for the pharmaceutical industry."[4]

Marcia Angell, former editor of the *New England Journal of Medicine*, called these publications "primarily a marketing machine" for big drug companies "co-opting every institution that might stand in [their] way."

You may be taking the advice of a doctor whose primary source of medical information is one of these journals.

That could be dangerous.

Many doctors are being lied to by a source they have relied on for dozens of years.

"Journals have devolved into information-laundering operations for the pharmaceutical industry."

– Dr. Richard Horton, Editor, *The Lancet*

Think about this…

How many drugs that were used 50 years ago are still around today?

I bet you can't name more than one or two.

We hardly use any of the drugs today that we used 50 years ago.

Where have they gone?

They've all been exposed for what they are. And were quietly withdrawn from the market.

Today there's Vioxx, Bextra, Zelnorm, Rezulin, just to name a few that have been taken off the market since 2000.

Drugs Withdrawn From the Market Since 2005		
Drug	**Year**	**Reason(s) Withdrawn**
Rezulin	2000	Withdrawn because of risk of liver damage.
Lotronex	2000	Withdrawn because risk of fatal complications from constipation was so severe.
Propulsid	2000s	Withdrawn due to risk of irregular heartbeat.
Survector	2000	Withdrawn because of liver damage and side effects to the skin.
Propagest	2000	Withdrawn due to risk of stroke in women under 50 when taken at high doses for weight-reduction.
Trovan	2001	Withdrawn because of risk of liver damage.
Baycol	2001	Withdrawn due to risk of muscle breakdown leading to kidney damage.

Raplon	2001	Withdrawn in many countries due to risk of fatal asthma and bronchitis.
Vioxx	2004	Withdrawn because of risk of heart attack.
Adderall	2005	Withdrawn in Canada due to risk of stroke.
Palladone	2005	Withdrawn because of a high risk of accidental overdose when taken with alcohol.
Cylert	2005	Withdrawn from U.S. market because of liver damage.
Tysabri	2005-06	Voluntarily withdrawn from U.S. market due to risk of brain damage.
Exanta	2006	Withdrawn because of risk of liver damage.
Permax	2007	Voluntarily withdrawn from the U.S. due to risk of heart valve damage.
Zelnorm	2007	Withdrawn due to risk of heart attack and stroke.
Trasylol	2007	Withdrawn due to increased risk of complications or death.
Accomplia	2008	Withdrawn due to risk of severe depression and suicide.
Raptiva	2009	Withdrawn due to increased risk of brain damage.
Reductil	2010	Withdrawn in Europe due to risk of heart disease.

That's why it's critical for you to stay informed.

It's important you learn everything you can about a drug before using it. Don't trust drug labels, package inserts, or even doctors to give you the full story.

Many of them get their information on new drugs from these medical journals, sexy sales reps, and the drug companies. None of which have your best interests in mind.

Here's a suggestion to help you get the information you need.

The next time a doctor wants to write you a prescription, ask him these three questions before rushing to your local pharmacy:

1. Are there any natural alternatives?

2. What are the side effects of this drug?

3. How long have you been recommending this drug?

It's also a good idea to ask your doctor to explain why he thinks this drug is a good choice. And remember: It's your body, and you have a right to refuse any prescription.

---

[1] Egger M, Bartlett C, Juni P. "Are randomised controlled trials in the BMJ different?"2001. *BMJ* 323: 1253.

[2] Fugh-Berman A, Alladin K, Chow J. "Advertising in Medical Journals: Should Current Practices Change?" 2006. *PLoS* Med 3(6): 130.

[3] Wilson,D. "Many New Drugs Have Strong Dose of Media Hype." March 16, 2010. *Seattle Times.*

[4] Horton R. (2004) "The dawn of McScience." 2004. *New York Rev Books.* 51(4): 7–9.

[5] Adapted from Wikipedia, *List of Withdrawn Drugs* and Worstpills.org

Chapter 13

100,000 Prescription Deaths and Counting

Last year, over half a million Americans were hurt by prescription drugs. *And 100,000 of them died.*[1,2]

How did that happen? If some prescription drugs are that dangerous, how are they getting approved?

The answer is not simple. There are good people involved in the process. But the incentive in the system has become distorted.

Here's how it happened…

The FDA now regulates $2.5 *trillion* worth of food, drugs, and medical devices. That's 25% of all U.S. consumer spending.[3]

Plus, over the last two decades, America's appetite for prescription drugs exploded. The FDA, struggling to keep up, needed to get drugs approved faster.

But the bureaucracy has grown so big that it's not very efficient. So the FDA tried to shortcut the time for drug approval by getting the drug companies themselves to pay for the research.

In 1992, Congress passed the *Prescription Drug User Fee Act* to give the FDA more desperately needed funds. The law allows drug companies to pay the FDA to approve their drugs.

This funding is called "user fees," which this year will equal nearly one-third — $920 million — of the FDA's budget.[4]

The fees make sense for the drug companies because delayed drug approval means millions in lost revenue. So, paying "user fees" to the FDA gets drugs approved fast. In fact, this funding boost has made the FDA the fastest drug approval agency in the world.

But that turned out to make a bad situation worse. Now you have government employees and supervisors very sensitive to what the drug companies think of them because they're dependent on the companies for funding.

The FDA's own scientists even admit to this. Scientists like David Graham. He's played a key role in getting 12 drugs removed from the market, including Vioxx. Take a look at what he said after the FDA made Merck pull Vioxx from the market because of the risk of heart attacks:

"As currently configured, the FDA is not able to adequately protect the American public. It's more interested in protecting the interests of industry. It views industry as its client, and the client is someone whose interest you represent. Unfortunately, that's the way the FDA is currently structured."[5]

How does this affect you? Because as a result of this current structure, more than 20 approved drugs have been recalled since 1992.

Before the *Prescription Drug User Fee Act* — when the FDA received no funding from pharmaceutical companies — only eight drugs were withdrawn from the 1950s through 1992.[6]

But withdrawn drugs are just scratching the surface. There are countless dangerous — even deadly — drugs that remain on the market. Drugs like statins and powerful NSAIDs. Not to mention recalls due to contamination and other manufacturing problems.

A few potentially deadly drugs that were approved for prescription include:

- **Avandia**: 83,000 heart attacks, 304 deaths, and thousands of reports to the FDA, and 10 separate studies say it increases the risk of heart attack by up to 80% ... and it's still being prescribed to thousands of diabetes patients.[7,8]

- **Baycol**: This statin drug caused a rare but sometimes fatal muscle ailment. There were 31 reported deaths directly linked to it before Baycol was pulled from the market.

- **Vioxx:** Prescribed 105 million times... it killed 57,000 people before its maker finally stopped selling it.

That in no way means there aren't lifesaving drugs developed by responsible people that have helped millions of Americans. But one brand new study by the American Sociological Association found that 85% of new drugs cause more harm than good.[9] And Celebrex, a pain reliever similar to Vioxx, has caused hundreds of heart attacks, but is still prescribed.[10]

That can certainly make you wonder if we don't need to slow down a little bit, and take a closer look at what drugs get approved, and how fast.

Whether that happens or not, there's good news.

You Have the Power to Make Your Own Decisions

There are forces out there that aren't working to your advantage. Despite the smart people doing hard work and all the helpful science, not everyone's incentive is your health. But don't worry. You have plenty of help, and you can make your own choices.

You'd never hear that from a big company because showing you how to keep yourself well isn't half as profitable as treating symptoms with drugs. But there are natural remedies and preventatives that can keep you away from the pharmacy for good.

My 100%-Natural Plan: Nine Keys for Avoiding Chronic Illnesses and the Dangerous Drugs That Treat Them

1. Eat like our ancestors. Cavemen ate what they could hunt and gather. And that was natural meats and eggs, veggies, unmodified fruits and nuts, and olives. They ate a lot more protein and fats than most modern Americans. And they ate a lot fewer carbs — and no processed foods or food cooked with vegetable oils. As a result, their archaeological records show virtually *no* heart disease, diabetes, osteoarthritis or obesity.

2. Enjoy the food you were born to eat. I'm talking about fat. Eating fat does not make you fat and unhealthy. But eating the wrong kinds of fat will. Our bodies need fat to absorb vitamins. In fact, vitamins A, D, E, K, and CoQ10 can't even be absorbed without fat. What's more, when you deprive yourself of fat, you eat more carbs. And an excess of them can put you at risk of weight gain, heart problems, diabetes and stroke. The best fat sources are foods loaded with Omega-3s (such as walnuts, almonds, cod liver oil, and wild-caught salmon). But stay away from bad fats, like processed foods and vegetable oils. And don't even go near potato chips, cookies, and salad dressing. They're loaded with the very worst fats — trans fats.

3. Power up your body with protein. It's critical to the health of every cell in your body. It's the one food you can truly indulge in — because overeating protein actually puts your body in fat-burning mode. Always choose grass-fed beef, free-range poultry, and cage-free eggs.

4. Stay away from starches and grains. Starchy, high-carb foods spike your blood sugar. And that triggers the release of insulin. Over time, this can put you at risk of insulin resistance. And when that happens, you'll be on the fast track to obesity, diabetes, and heart disease. Always eat foods with a low glycemic index (GI) and glycemic load (GL).

5. Throw away your jogging shoes. Aerobics, cardio, and marathon running do *not* make you healthy. They downside your heart, shrink your lungpower, and encourage your body to make more fat. That's because your heart and lungs were designed for short bursts of intense exertion. A broad variety of exercise, intensity and progressivity — like my PACE program — will give you the daily exercise you need to strengthen your muscles and bones. Without treadmills, trainers or gyms.

6. Go organic whenever possible. Pesticides and insecticides can harm the nervous system, immune system and major organs, like the liver and kidneys. They also can cause problems with growth and neurological development in children. Organic farmers don't use these chemicals. And that makes organic food much safer and healthier.

7. Rid your body of toxins. The world we were designed to live in millions of years ago has changed drastically. And our bodies haven't adapted quickly enough to flush out the countless pollutants that are now a big part of our everyday lives. The easiest way to rid your system of toxins is to drink plenty of filtered water, and to eat fruit and fibrous vegetables. Getting rid of chemicals and heavy metals in your body will help you live a longer, disease-free life.

8. Don't fear the sun. Your body needs exposure to the sun to produce vitamin D — which helps you maintain strong, healthy bones and fight disease. Contrary to what you've been told, the sun isn't bad for you — it's nature's cancer fighter. Just by getting a little sunlight every day (about 20 minutes for fair-skinned people and two to four times that much for those with dark skin) could reduce your risk of 16 types of cancer.[11] Of course, I'm not telling you to go outside without sunscreen — just make sure it's chemical-free.

9. Supplement your diet (if necessary). The best way to get the nutrients you need is through a healthy organic diet. But if you don't feel like you're taking in enough, you can also safely supplement. And I emphasize "safely" because unlike prescription drugs, people are not dropping dead from dietary supplements (vitamins, amino acids, herbals and homeopathics).[12]

Here are the vitamins and nutrients I recommend taking daily:

Vitamin/ Nutrient	Food Source	Daily Supplement Dosage	Benefits
B2	milk, cheese, leafy green vegetables, liver, kidneys, legumes, tomatoes, yeast, mushrooms, and almonds	40 mg.	Good for blood cell formation and cataract prevention.
B6	roast beef, salmon, peanut butter, lima beans, chicken, sunflower seeds, spinach	50 mg.	Boosts brain and immune function. Helps prevent cancer.
B12	milk, eggs, grass-fed beef, chicken, yogurt, trout, salmon, haddock, clams, ham	500 mcg.	Helps digestion and prevents anemia and nerve damage.
Folic Acid	green leafy veggies, calf liver	800 mcg.	Helps cell production and prevents dementia.
Vitamin C	citrus fruits, green pepper, broccoli, kale, Brussels sprouts	At least 500 mg. twice a day	Boosts immunity.
Zinc	steak, oysters	30 mg.	Maintains healthy immune system.
Vitamin D	cod liver oil, eggs, milk and orange juice fortified with vitamin D, sardines, tuna, beef liver, Swiss cheese, ham	2,000 IU If your levels test low, take 5,000-10,000 IU from a variety of sources.	Calcium absorption for healthy, strong bones. Prevents osteoporosis, hypertension, cancer and several autoimmune diseases.

Vitamin/ Nutrient	Food Source	Daily Supplement Dosage	Benefits
Ubiquinol form of CoQ10	pork, beef, chicken	50 mg. (increase your dosage to 100 mg. per day if you have high blood pressure, heart disease, high cholesterol, gingivitis, age-related memory loss, chronic fatigue or are a vegetarian)	Destroys free radicals in the cell membranes. Treats heart disease, high-blood pressure and high cholesterol.
Ome-ga-3s	wild-caught salmon, grass-fed beef, sacha inchi oil, nuts, leafy green veggies, eggs, avocados	18-24 grams	Prevents heart disease, cancer — even strokes. Lowers blood pressure and triglycerides (blood fat). Boosts memory and brain power.

[1] "Quarter Watch 2009," *Inst. For Safe Med Prc*. June 17, 2010; Retrieved Sept. 30, 2010 from Internet.

[2] Moore, T, Cohen, M, Furberg, C. "Serious Adverse Drug Events Reported to the Food and Drug Admin." *Arch Intern Med*. 2007; 167(16): 1752-1759

[3] Gardiner H "The Safety Gap," *New York Times Magazine* Nov. 2, 2008

[4] Zajac, Andrew, "Freeze? What Freeze? FDA in Line for Another Budget Boost," *Los Angeles Times* Feb. 2, 2010

[5] Loudon, Manette, "The FDA Exposed: An Interview With Dr. David Graham, the Vioxx Whistleblower," *Organic Consumers Association*. Aug. 30, 2005.

[6] Center for Drug Evaluation and Research Report to the Nation 2005: http://www.fda.gov/downloads/AboutFDA/CentersOffices/CDER/WhatWeDo/UCM078935.pdf

[7,8] Rosen, C.- "Revisiting the Rosiglitazone Story — Lessons Learned." *N Engl J Med*. 2010; 363:803-806

[9] "Pharmaceuticals: A Market for Producing 'Lemons' and Serious Harm, Analysis Finds." American Sociological Association. August 17, 2010.

[10] Henderson, Diedtra, "How safe is Celebrex?" *Boston Globe* Feb. 25, 2007; Retrieved August 25, 2010 from Internet.

[11] Grant, W et al. "The Association of Solar Ultraviolet B (UVB) with Reducing

Risk of Cancer: Multifactorial Ecologic Analysis of Geographic Variation in Age-adjusted Cancer Mortality Rates." *Anticancer Research.* 2006; 26: 2687-2700.

[12] "No Deaths from Vitamins, Minerals, Amino Acids or Herbs." *Orthomolecular Medicine News Service.* Jan. 19, 2010.

Chapter 14

One More Flew Over the Cuckoo's Nest

Remember *One Flew Over the Cuckoo's Nest*? You know the way Jack Nicholson was docile and apathetic at the end? That's because he got a frontal lobotomy. Doctors don't do surgical frontal lobotomies any more, but they did perform them on mental patients up until the 1950s.

In 1949, Henri-Marie Laborit, a French army surgeon, was using a certain kind of anesthetic during operations. He noticed that patients who were extremely anxious became relaxed and indifferent to the surroundings.

These patients were so subdued and cooperative it was as if they had gotten what he called a "pharmacological lobotomy."[1]

In 1950, researchers added chlorine to Laborit's anesthetic called promethazine and invented chlorpromazine. This new drug seemed to slow the involuntary movements of mental patients and make them indifferent to their environment.

You might know chlorpromazine better as Thorazine, and it was the first antipsychotic medication.

More than 50 years later, doctors aren't doing surgical lobotomies any more. But they're prescribing antipsychotics more than any other drug.

Let me explain.

Anti-psychotic drugs were originally created and sold only to treat schizophrenia and extreme manic depressive disorder.

But now they're no longer just being prescribed for mental illnesses that incapacitate people. And that's how the drug companies have managed to make this the number-one selling class of drugs.

In fact, if you've been diagnosed with chronic depression, dementia, autism, ADHD, post-traumatic stress disorder (PTSD), or even Tourette's syndrome, you're probably getting your own "pharmacological lobotomy."

So Just How Did Antipsychotics Become America's Biggest Selling Drug?

In 1990, the now-giant pharmaceutical companies reintroduced them as "atypical antipsychotics." At first, they were still seen as drugs used to treat serious mental illness. But that all changed when drug makers began to use clever marketing tactics to promote broad, off-label uses of the drugs and downplay the dangers.

As of 1999, 70% of antipsychotics have been used for off-label reasons.[2] The most common are dementia, depression, obsessive-compulsive disorder, PTSD, personality disorders, Tourette's syndrome and autism.[3] But some are even used for eating disorders (Risperidone), cocaine dependence and restless leg syndrome (Aripiprazole), agitation and imsomnia (Quetiapine) and stuttering (Olazapine).[4]

What are some of the tactics Big Pharma used to make these drugs so popular? Gifts, meals, money, and vacations for doctors and researchers who promote the drugs. And that's just scratching the surface.[5]

Cracking Down on Off-label
Uses of Antipsychotics

Drug makers such as AstraZeneca, Johnson & Johnson, Bristol-Myers Squibb, Eli Lilly, and Pfizer have either settled health care fraud lawsuits filed against them for the fraudulent marketing of antipsychotics, or they're currently under investigation for health care fraud.

There are still more than 1,000 of these suits, many focused on the deceitful promotion of anti-psychotics.

In fact, many of the "scholarly" studies about the safety and effectiveness of antipsychotics were really ghostwritten by pharmaceutical marketing execs. These studies then became the basis of even more research that reaffirmed the "safety" of antipsychotics. And that's because many of the researchers didn't know the previous studies were erroneous to begin with.[6]

What's more, drug makers found clever ways to get around regulations aimed at reining in their marketing practices. For example, drug companies can't promote off-label uses of drugs. But they can hire researchers, consultants and others to do it for them. And that's just what Pharma giants like AstraZeneca, Johnson & Johnson, Bristol-Myers Squibb, Eli Lilly, and Pfizer — have been doing for years.[7]

Case in point: Harvard professor Joseph Biederman. A 2008 Senate investigation revealed that he received more than $1.6 million from makers of antipsychotics for children. According to the *Archives of General Psychiatry*, his studies on bipolar disorder led to a forty-fold increase in children being diagnosed with the condition. And some of his studies were published during the same time he was getting paid by Big Pharma.[8]

Drug makers also took advantage of the loose definition of "psychiatric problems,"[9] which can range from depressed mood to anxiety disorder to schizophrenia, and everything in between.

That's because they know doctors can legally prescribe any approved drug to patients — even if it's for a condition other than what the drug has been approved to treat.

But...

All Too Often These Drugs Cause More Harm than Good

Antipsychotics are some of the most dangerous drugs on the market.

That's because they've been linked to pneumonia, high blood pressure, heart disease, weight gain, stroke and diabetes.

And they're being prescribed to two of the most vulnerable groups: children and the elderly.

Did you know that 25% of all nursing home residents have taken these drugs?[10] And according to a survey by the Alzheimer's Society, 25% of nurses said they'd seen antipsychotics used inappropriately on dementia patients.[11]

Meanwhile, antipsychotics carry black-box warnings about the increased risk of death in elderly patients.[12]

A study published by *Lancet Neurology* examined 165 Alzheimer patients. One group took antipsychotics, and the other took a placebo during this period. After three years, less than a third of those who took anti-psychotics were still alive compared to nearly two-thirds who took the placebo. And those who did survive experienced mental decline and an increase in Parkinson's disease, sedation, edema, chest infections and stroke.[13]

But many elderly people in nursing homes — who don't even have dementia — are also being given these drugs. Drug maker Eli-Lilly even went as far as to promote what they called "5 at 5" treatments in nursing homes — 5 mg. of their antipsychotic Zyprexa each day — to zonk out disruptive residents.

A recent University of Massachusetts Medical School study assessed the use of antipsychotics among 16,586 residents newly admitted to 1,257 nursing homes in 2006. They found that about 30% (4,818) of new residents in the study received at least one antipsychotic medication in 2006. But 32% of those who received the meds didn't even have dementia, psychosis or any other clinical reason to be using them.[14]

But the elderly aren't the only group at risk. Children are, too. In fact, a new study published in *Health Affairs* reveals children ages 2-5 are being treated with antipsychotics twice as much as they were 10 years ago. And they're not being used to treat schizophrenia and bipolar disorder. They're being prescribed for disruptive behavior, hyperactivity and developmental disabilities — as a first, not last, resort.[15] Less than 50% of the children studied who were taking the antipsychotics had ever received therapy, let alone an evaluation from a mental health professional.[16]

The effects of these drugs on the developing brains of children are unknown. In fact, there have NEVER been any long-term studies of antipsychotic use in children.[17]

But in adults their effects are known all too well. A recent study that examined the effects of antipsychotic drugs like aripiprazole, olanzapine, quetiapine, risperidone, or ziprasidone found that any adult who takes these drugs has a 225% risk of suffering a stroke.[18] Antipsychotics have also been linked to significant weight gain and diabetes.

If Your Doctor Recommends Antipsychotic Drugs for You or Someone You Love, Consider These Alternatives

1. Know the risks. Always read drug labels. You can find them online. The label clearly indicates the approved use of the drugs, side effects, and FDA warnings. If your doctor has prescribed a drug for anything other than its approved use, ask questions, seek a second, third or fourth medical opinion, and be sure to seek counsel from an alternative health doctor. Also, do your own homework. I'd recommend these two websites for information about side effects and reactions to drugs and treatments.

- www.drugs.com
- www.rxlist.com

2. Make sure your doctor is looking for the underlying causes of your behavior and not just writing a prescription. Many times a condition can be resolved once the underlying cause is treated. The best doctors will prescribe a combination of therapy to treat your condition — such as natural foods and vitamin and herbal supplements — along with behavioral or developmental therapies. If any doctor prescribes an antipsychotic to you as a first — and not last — resort, run in the other direction.

3. Eat foods that will lift your spirits. That means natural foods high in protein, vitamin B1, and vitamin C. Proteins contain amino acids which help to regulate emotions. Also, foods rich in vitamin B1 — such as asparagus, romaine lettuce, mushrooms, spinach, green peas, tomatoes, eggplant and Brussels sprouts — help to metabolize carbs that give your body energy and improve your mood.

I also recommend a daily dose of vitamin C. A new double-blind study published in *Nutrition* shows that it's not just one of nature's best immune boosters.[19] It's also an effective antidepressant.[19] The best way to get your dosage of vitamin C is to eat citrus fruits, green pepper, broccoli, kale, Brussels sprouts, steak and oysters. Or you can supplement with 500 mg. twice a day.

4. Get your omega-3s. Omega-3s fight chronic illnesses and ease symptoms of mental and developmental disabilities. That's because they play a critical role in brain development and functioning. A deficiency in omega-3 can affect the levels and functioning of dopamine and serotonin — your body's feel-good hormones, which play an important role in your mood and behavior.

A new study published in the *Archives of General Psychiatry* examined 81 people at high risk of psychosis. Half of the participants received fish oil supplements for 12 weeks, and the other half took a placebo. After 12 weeks, only two people in the fish-oil group developed a psychosis compared to 11 in the placebo group.

The best omega-3 sources are wild-caught salmon, grass-fed beef, sacha inchi oil, nuts, leafy green veggies, eggs and avocados. Or you can supplement. I recommend 18-24 grams a day.

5. Consider this natural amino acid. Amino acids such as 5-HTP increase levels of chemicals in the brain connected to mood and concentration. These are natural and safe alternatives to antidepressants, antipsychotics and ADHD drugs I use in my medical practice. They aren't harmful or addictive, and they actually work. They're easy to find at health food stores. I recommend 50 to 100 mg. of 5-HTP three times per day with meals.

6. Sleep. Inability to sleep is one of the most common symptoms of psychiatric problems, but not sleeping can throw your whole body out of whack. One of the most powerful sleep aids I recommend is melatonin. Look for drops, or a sublingual that melts under your tongue. It's easier to absorb and works fast. Start with 0.5 mg. and work your way up to 3 mg. max. Take it 20 minutes before you want to fall asleep.

7. Avoid stress. This underlies many behaviors — from anxiety, agitation, frustration and outbursts of anger — to difficulty sleeping, eating and getting through each day. You can get your life back in balance by identifying what's stressing you and taking action to get rid of the stress in your life. Often this alone can "cure" many behavior problems and struggles with depression.

8. Limit sugars and grains. Eating starchy carbs can cause too much insulin to build up in the blood. When this happens, your body will release insulin to try to bring your blood sugar down. But if your blood sugar gets too low, you become hypoglycemic. And hypoglycemia can spike glutamate to levels that can cause everything from agitation and depression to anger and panic attacks.

9. Exercise at least three or four days a week. It'll boost your body's feel-good chemicals. One of the most important is serotonin. Your brain needs balanced levels of this hormone to maintain a good mood. Short duration, high-intensity workouts, like my PACE™ program, are all you need to increase your serotonin levels. It only takes 12 minutes a day.

If you are making the decision to put your elder relative in a nursing home...

Make sure there are plenty of staff around who can provide daily compassionate care and hands-on psychosocial therapy. Many nursing homes resort to using antipsychotics because they lack the personnel to deal with aggression and outbursts from dementia patients. They're also forbidden by law to use physical restraints on residents. So they use less visible "drug restraints."

In addition to making sure there's adequate staff trained to use intervention strategies — such as therapy — be sure the environment is stimulating for your loved one. Look for nursing homes that offer strategies to reduce boredom and agitation, such as exercise, music and intellectually stimulating games.

And finally, visit the nursing home as much as you can — without making an appointment — to see if your loved one and other residents seem doped up. If they do, don't hesitate to get them out of there.

If Your Pediatrician Has Prescribed an Antipsychotic Drug for Your Child...

Just say NO — point blank. There have been no studies to indicate the long-term consequences of antipsychotics for children. But countless studies show their dangerous effects on adults. Seek the approaches above as alternatives.

---

[1] Ramachandraiah C, Subramaniam N, Tancer, M. "The story of antipsychotics: Past and present." *Indian J Psychiatry*. Oct.-Dec. 2009; 51(4): 324–326

[2] Glick, I. "Treatment with atypical antipsychotics: new indications and new populations." *Journal of Psychiatric Research*. May-June 2001; Vol. 35, Issue 3, pgs. 187-191.

[3,4,5,6,7,18] Shekelle Paul, et al. "Efficacy and Comparative Effectiveness of Off-Label Use of Atypical Antipsychotics." *Comparative Effectiveness Reviews*. No. Agency for Healthcare Research and Quality (US); January 2007.

[8,9] Archives of General Psychiatry, 2007.

[10] Douglas, I, Smeeth, L. "Exposure to antipsychotics and risk of stroke: self-controlled case series study." *British Medical Journal*. Aug. 28, 2008.

[11] A.U. "77% of nurses say people with dementia in hospital given dangerous drugs." *Alzheimer Society*. Oct. 2009

[12] Yan Jun. "FDA Extends Black-Box Warning to All Antipsychotics." *Psychiatric News*. American Psychiatric Association. July. 18, 2008; 43,14:1.

[13] Ballard Clive, et al. "The dementia antipsychotic withdrawal trial (DART-AD)." *The Lancet Neurology*, Feb. 2009; 8,2: 151-157.

[14] Chen Y, Briesacher Becky, FieldT, et al. "Unexplained Variation Across US Nursing Homes in Antipsychotic Prescribing Rates." *Arch Intern Med*. 2010; 170 (1): 89-95.

[15,16] Olfson Mark, et al. "Trends in Antipsychotic Drug Use by Very Young, Privately Insured Children." *Jour. Am. Acad. Child & Adol. Psych*. Jan. 2010; 49,1: 13-23.

[17] Wilson, D. "Side Effects May Include Lawsuits." *New York Times.* Oct. 2, 2010

[19] Zhang, M, et al. "Vitamin C provision improves mood in acutely hospitalized patients." *Nutrition.* Aug. 4, 2010.

Chapter 15

Why You Never Have to Worry about Heart Disease

We really shouldn't be spending all of this time worrying about heart disease. In fact, it only takes us in the wrong direction.

Truth is, you need to do the opposite. Get rid of that worry once and for all. I'll show you rock-solid evidence that what you really need to do is easy and just feels right.

But first, let's get one thing straight — there's no real proof cholesterol causes heart disease. ***You actually need cholesterol to avoid heart attacks and heart disease.*** And I'll show you how easy it is to boost your HDL. You don't need drugs or doctor's prescriptions. And you don't need to follow a crazy diet.

Your cholesterol blood level can tell you useful information about your health and fitness, but it's not the great predictor of heart disease that conventional medicine leads us to believe. In fact, these numbers make very poor crystal balls, as I learned from experience.

Years ago, I began inheriting a group of patients who "dropped out" with other doctors because they refused to lower their cholesterol levels. These cantankerous old men didn't trust doctors and weren't willing to change their lifestyles in ways that seemed to contradict their instincts.

Over the years, I noticed that these cranky rebels with high cholesterol rarely had heart problems. The University Hospital in Switzerland announced that cholesterol fails to demonstrate an important (statistically significant) connection with coronary artery disease.

Clearly, cholesterol isn't the ultimate heart-attack warning it was made out to be.

When you get past the medical mythology and look directly at the evidence, the literature points out that nearly *75% of people who have heart attacks have normal cholesterol levels.*[1]

Cholesterol is Essential for Life, Health and Sex

Although cholesterol has a bad reputation for clogging the arteries, it's not the enemy. Cholesterol is essential for life and health. It provides energy to cells, helps make cell membranes, and assists in the formation of sheaths around nerves. Plus, it plays a vital role in the production of the sex hormones testosterone, estrogen and progesterone, and other adrenal hormones like DHEA and cortisol.

While cholesterol is in some foods we eat, the liver manufactures most of it. In fact, each day our bodies churn out about 1,000 milligrams of cholesterol, compared to the average dietary intake of about 325 milligrams for men or 220 milligrams for women.

No matter whether it comes from the liver or our diet, cholesterol and other dietary fats must move from the digestive system and into the cells to perform these terrific tasks. Fat must be packaged into protein-covered particles that allow the fat to mix with the blood. These tiny particles are lipoproteins (lipid — or fat — plus protein).

The two most well-known lipids are HDL and LDL. And don't be fooled by LDL's "bad cholesterol" label. Your body needs both to stay healthy.

Turns out, the maverick patients were right not to take everything their doctors said as Gospel. We now know that total blood cholesterol levels do not give us a clear picture of heart-attack risk. Still, most doctors continue to turn to conventional cholesterol screening as the best predictor of heart attacks.

Cholesterol Levels Can't Predict Heart Attacks

Doctors and drug companies often refer to the famous Framingham

Study when talking about cardiovascular risk. Framingham is a small town near Boston, where for more than 50 years, researchers followed the population and tracked risk factors for heart disease. Government organizations often cite it as a reason to beat cholesterol into submission, using potent prescription drugs if necessary. But what does the study really reveal?

Amazingly, Framingham researchers themselves reported that *"80% of heart attack patients had similar lipid levels* [i.e., fat levels in the blood] *to those who did not have heart attacks."*[2]

In other words, **cholesterol levels do not predict heart attacks in the vast majority of patients.** The link between cholesterol and women was essentially zero: Women with low cholesterol died just as often as women with high cholesterol. Furthermore, according to data from the Framingham study, almost half of the people in the study who had a heart attack had **low cholesterol.**

Ironically, as the study participants grew older, the association between cholesterol and heart disease became weaker, not stronger. In fact, according to the data, for men above age 47, cholesterol levels made *no difference* in cardiovascular mortality.[3]

Since 95% of all heart attacks occur in people over age 48 — and those who have heart attacks at an earlier age are usually diabetics or have a rare genetic problem — then, most people don't have to worry about their cholesterol levels!

Even if we could show an association between cholesterol blood levels and heart disease, it would not prove that cholesterol caused heart disease.

The Protective Effects of High Cholesterol

Now here's another fact to make you wonder what the "experts" were thinking: High cholesterol seems to have a protective effect in the elderly. According to research done at the Department of Cardiovascular Medicine at Yale University, nearly *twice as many people* with low cholesterol had a heart attack — compared to those with high cholesterol levels.[4]

Data from the Framingham Study also support the finding that when blood cholesterol decreases, the risk of dying actually *increases*.

There is no question that blood cholesterol is involved in the accumulation of plaque in the arteries. Plaque buildup narrows the arteries and restricts blood flow. This can lead to heart attacks and strokes. Yet the conventional approach continues to miss the most important point: The plaque buildup is dangerous, not the presence of cholesterol itself.

Big Pharma Reaps Windfall Profits by Promoting the Cholesterol Lie

Pharmaceutical companies continue to milk billions of dollars annually from the American public as long as they promote the myth that cholesterol causes heart disease. As the previous evidence shows, elevated cholesterol levels don't cause heart attacks. Therefore, it's unnecessary to take drugs to lower cholesterol.

Results from numerous independent drug trials also don't support the connection between cholesterol and heart disease. The National Heart, Lung and Blood Institute conducted the Lipid Research Clinics Coronary Primary Prevention Trial to test the effectiveness of *cholestryramine*, a drug known to lower cholesterol.

Seven years later, researchers analyzed the data and found that the cholesterol levels decreased by 8%, but there were no important (statistically significant) differences in heart-attack rates.[5]

Researchers have summarized all drug trials published before 1994 (the year drug companies introduced statin drugs). These studies found that the number of deaths from heart attack was equal in the treatment and control groups. And the total number of deaths was actually greater in the treatment groups. None of the trials showed any important (statistically significant) decrease in the death rate from coronary disease.[6]

What it all boils down to is that these cholesterol-lowering drugs lowered cholesterol — but they didn't decrease deaths from heart attack.

Generating Over $30 Billion a Year, Statins Are the Most Profitable Drug in History

In 1994, drug companies introduced a new class of cholesterol-lowering drugs known as statins. These drugs interfere with the body's production of cholesterol. They also block the production of other essential nutrients, including CoQ10.

These drugs not only lower blood cholesterol levels but also, for the first time, some studies showed a slightly lowered risk of heart attack. But before we reach the conclusion that the lowering of cholesterol caused the modestly lowered heart attack rate, we run into a problem.

There was no relationship between the amount of the cholesterol reduction and the amount of the risk reduction. We call this phenomenon "lack of exposure response." What this usually means is that the factor being investigated — in this case cholesterol — isn't the true cause, but is secondary to or merely associated with the true cause.

Stated another way, statins may reduce heart-attack risk, but they do so in some way other than reducing cholesterol.

The drug companies that sponsor these studies are very slick at directing attention away from this failure. Only very recently has it come to light that statins do other things more directly related to heart disease risk. They lower the inflammatory marker, C-reactive protein.

The "lack of exposure response" may be because statins help by reducing inflammation — not cholesterol.

But there is more to the story. Statins are expensive. A typical dose costs about $1,000 to $1,500 per year. And, more significantly, statins block an antioxidant system important to your cardiovascular health and rob your organs of a crucial nutrient.

Statins can make you chronically fatigued and cause muscles aches. They also stimulate cancer growth in rodents. In human studies, breast cancer was more common in women who took the drug than those in the control group.

Additionally, it's wise to cautiously review information from drug studies that pharmaceutical companies fund. These corporations benefit remarkably when research results recommend a new drug. Statins are the most profitable drugs in history to date.

Those profits buy a lot of propaganda, such as lobbyists in Washington, direct-to-consumer advertising and marketing to doctors, including free continuing medical education about how to prescribe the drugs! This is the fox overseeing the hen house — and the consequences involve your health.

Good Cholesterol is Your "Trump Card" When Fighting Heart Disease

Maybe you've heard about the two types of cholesterol: low-density lipoproteins (LDLs) and high-density lipoproteins (HDLs). LDLs help lay down the plaque deposits in the arteries (that's why they call these "bad"), and HDLs help *remove plaque* from the arteries (that's why they call these "good").

HDL is the single most important cholesterol factor in determining your risk of developing heart disease. Don't worry about lowering your total cholesterol level or your LDL level. *Just raise your HDL cholesterol.*

The Framingham Study shows that high levels of HDL are directly related to lower risk of heart disease. In fact, it showed that increased HDL could reduce coronary disease independent of LDL cholesterol.[7]

This is the real eye-opener: If your HDL is above 85, you are at no greater risk of heart disease if your total cholesterol is 350 than if it's 150.

High HDL trumps other cholesterol concerns. Why isn't this simple and powerful advice getting through? For one reason, there is no drug to boost HDL. What's the best way to increase HDL cholesterol?

You have several options.

One of the easiest is taking niacin (vitamin B3) as a supplement. I've been prescribing niacin for years. I have tested its effectiveness in thousands of patients in my 30 years practicing medicine.

And in study after study, niacin has proven itself to be a heart-healthy warrior.[8,9] In one study from the prestigious journal *Atherosclerosis*, researchers showed how niacin raised HDL by a remarkable 24%.

In a group with low HDL, niacin improved heart-healthy markers across the board, including:[10]

- A 24% increase in HDL—the heart-healthy "good" cholesterol;
- A 35% increase in adiponectin, the hormone that melts fat away;
- A 38% decrease in LDL;
- A 12% decrease in triglycerides, the real culprit behind clogged arteries.

First, start with a diet that boosts your intake of vitamin B3. Foods rich in niacin include liver, chicken, beef, avocados, tomatoes and nuts. As always, stick with grass-fed meat, free-range chicken and organic produce and nuts.

Second, supplements are a great way to go. In this case, it's crucial you take the right dose — and limit how much is in your body at any given time. I recommend taking 500 mg. of "sustained release" niacin.

Taking a bit too much can lead to "flushing." So you may want to start with every other day and slowly work up. In my clinic, I often gradually increase to up to 2 grams per day.

Aside from niacin, here are seven easy and effective ways to boost your HDL:

1. Restore omega-3s to your diet. Wild-caught fish, grass-fed beef, free-farmed, organic poultry, nuts, olive, eggs and avocados are all rich in "good" fats. And cod liver oil — the best omega-3 supplement — will boost your HDL levels naturally.

2. Get more of this cholesterol. Be sure to focus on your HDL level. If it's below 35, you should take steps to increase it. Steps like increasing your exercise, taking niacin and eating garlic.

3. Eat a low-carb diet. This will help to balance your HDL and reduce your LDL.

4. Practice my PACE™ program. My exercise alternative to aerobics and cardio boosts reserve capacity in your heart — critical for avoiding heart attacks — and raises HDL.

5. Consume alcohol in moderation. A glass of wine can help raise your HDL. Moderation is the key.

6. Stop smoking. It sounds obvious, but if you smoke, you should stop. Not only does smoking lower your HDL, it constricts your blood vessels and raises your risk of heart attack in many other ways as well.

7. Drop the excess weight. Carrying excess pounds increases your risk of heart disease. Even a little weight reduction will raise your HDL levels.

---

[1] Castelli, W. "Cholesterol and lipids in the risk of coronary artery disease-- the Framingham Heart Study." *Canadian Journal of Cardiology.* July 1998;A:5A-10A.

[2] Gordon T, Castelli, W, Hjortland, M, et al. "High density lipoprotein as a positive factor against coronary heart disease." *The Framingham Study, American Journal of Medicine.* May 1997; 62(5):707-714.

[3] Ravnskov, U., *Cholesterol Myths*, pg. 56.

[4] Krumholz, H, Seeman T, MerrillS, et al. "Lack of association between cholesterol and coronary heart disease mortality and morbidity and all-cause mortality in persons older than 70 years." *Journal of the American Medical Association.* Nov.

1994; 272(17):1335-1340.

[5] A.U. "The Lipid Research Clinics Coronary Primary Prevention Trial results. I. Reduction in incidence of coronary heart disease." *Journal of the American Medical Association.* Jan. 20, 1984; 251(3):351-64.

[6] Ravnskov U. "Cholesterol-lowering trials in coronary heart disease: frequency of citation and outcome" *British Journal of Medicine.* July 4, 1991; 305(6844):15-19.

[7] Castiglioni A, Neuman W. "HDL Cholesterol: What is its true clinical significance?" *Emergency Medicine.* Jan. 2003; 30-42.

[8] Carlson L. "Nicotinic acid: the broad-spectrum lipid drug. A 50th anniversary review." *Journal of Internal Medicine.* 2005; 258(2):94–114.

[9] McKenney J. "New perspectives on the use of niacin in the treatment of lipid disorders." *Archives of Internal Medicine.* 2004;164(7):697–705.

[10] Linke, et al. "Effects of extended-release niacin on lipid profile and adipocyte biology in patients with impaired glucose tolerance." *Atherosclerosis.* 2008.

Chapter 16

A Shocking New Treatment

"Deep brain stimulation" is what they're calling it.

It almost sounds soothing and nice.

Did you hear about this? Scientists use electrodes to "stimulate" the brains of depressed people.

The whole thing works through surgically implanted probes in your brain that are connected to an electrical device sewn into your chest.

They say it's like a pacemaker for your brain.

I call it the new shock therapy.

People with Parkinson's disease use similar things to improve their mobility. But when the devices are turned on, *the patients can't talk.* The flow of electricity interrupts other brain functions.

I don't believe anything that invasive can be good for you.

And it's just another in a long line of "treatments" for depression that the modern medical industry has come up with over the last 30 years.

First there were the original drugs used to treat depression like Prozac and Zoloft.

They can be helpful for those with severe depressive conditions, and millions of people have benefited from their use.

But recently, doctors have taken it upon themselves to go beyond the intended use of some newer medications. There's a growing list of pharmaceutical drugs being prescribed "off-label" to people who are depressed.

Off-label means a drug was approved to treat one condition, but is being prescribed for a different use — without FDA approval.

For example, the drugs Seroquel and Risperdal are powerful antipsychotic medications. They're intended to be given only to people who have schizophrenia or manic episodes or autism. But doctors are giving them to patients who are depressed, even though the drugs are not approved to treat those patients.

Not only that, but the drug companies have been hiding the side effects of their drugs for years. One of the most common problems hidden from you over these last 30 years is that many if not all of these drugs are addictive.

Drug companies have gone out of their way to prove that their medications are not addicting. They back up the claims with their own scientific studies, or don't reveal the studies at all if they show the wrong result.

Now that we've seen non-drug-company-sponsored studies, we know that patients do develop problems, both physical and mental, from stopping some prescription drugs.

This is because if you use them for long enough, stopping can cause a response where your body creates more of the original symptom so it can receive a larger dose of drugs.

The medical industry likes to call this "discontinuation syndrome." But it sounds a lot like withdrawal because of addiction to me.

And even though the symptoms aren't usually life threatening, they can be distressing to people going through them. People sometimes mistake them as signs of heart problems. This has led patients to go to the emergency room, spending hours getting diagnostic tests that frighten them even more.

Now modern medicine is trying something even more frightening. A surgically implanted electrical device that might help you be in a better mood, but impairs speech and other brain functions.

I believe you should have the choice as to whether or not you continue to take a medication. And having surgery should not be a choice between being happy and being able to talk.

That's why I prefer using natural remedies in my practice. They're completely safe and effective, and have no dangerous side effects.

Try my natural four-step prescription for a better mood, more confidence and a happy outlook on life:

Step 1: Get some exercise. Regular physical exertion releases serotonin — the "feel-good hormone" — in your brain. I recommend an invigorating 10 to 15 minutes of exertion at a time. Exercising for long periods is a waste of time, and leads to overuse injuries.

Instead, try doing 10 minutes of calisthenics using your own body weight. That's short enough not to wreck your body, and long enough to leave you feeling energized. That's because exercise also gives you a psychological boost — a release of endorphins. They're the brain's natural morphine-like pain relievers. They also cause a sense of pleasure.

Step 2: Get some sunshine. There's a reason we describe someone who is happy as having a "sunny disposition." Sunshine enhances your health and well-being. You were designed to live under the sun. Sunshine also releases serotonin in your brain.

And here's something most people don't know. Many depressed people have trouble sleeping because they don't make enough serotonin. Your body uses serotonin to make melatonin, the sleep-inducing hormone.

This is why it's easy to fall asleep in the warm sunshine. It's also why exercise and going outdoors are two of the best ways to avoid becoming depressed. And the feel-good effect is multiplied if you can exercise outside.

Step 3: Eat foods that are native to you. Processed foods are filled with chemicals that affect hormones, brain function and mood. Choose fresh and natural instead. Protein contains amino acids, which feed the brain and regulate emotions.

Stay away from stimulants, including caffeine and alcohol. They cause mood swings, anxiety, depression and insomnia.

Step 4: Get some extra help if you need it. If you're still not feeling enough relief, there are a few nutrients you should take a look at.

• The first is **vitamin B6**. Depressed people usually have a deficiency of this vitamin. It's vital to regulation of mental function and mood. Meanwhile government surveys suggest that only a third of adults get enough vitamin B6. Two of the best sources are chickpeas and chestnuts. Other foods rich in B6 include bananas, tuna, turkey, eggs and spinach. I recommend 40 mg. a day.

• Another important nutrient is **magnesium**. It plays a role in the transmission of nerve impulses in your brain and helps relax you. In fact, the signs of magnesium deficiency are depression, anxiety, irritability and brain fog. If you need to supplement, start with 300 mg. a day, but you might need to take as much as 400 mg, twice a day.

• Also, make sure you get enough **omega-3s**. Your body needs fat to make brain and nerve cells. What's more, fat can actually put a smile on your face. It helps the membranes of your brain cells absorb serotonin to put you in a good mood, and keep you there. The fat that your brain craves most is omega-3.

In one study, participants took a pure omega-3 supplement, and their brains started growing. In fact, the parts of their brains that grew were directly responsible for happiness.[1] In other studies, researchers found that people suffering from major depression had very low levels of omega-3 in the areas of the brain that help with mood.[2]

You can easily start boosting your omega-3 intake today. For the full antidepressant benefit, take 4 grams per day. Two great sources are cod liver oil, which gives you 4.5 grams of omega-3 in just a teaspoon full, and Sacha Inchi oil. It has almost 7 grams in every tablespoon full.

• One little-known nutrient for treating depression is **5-HTP** (5-hy-doxytryptophan). It's a naturally occurring amino acid that converts to serotonin in the brain. Start by taking the minimum dose and work up slowly, 20 to 50 mg. a day.[3]

---

[1] Conklin et al., "Long-chain omega-3 fatty acid intake is associated positively with corticolimbic gray matter volume in healthy adults," *Neuroscience Letters* 2007; 421(3):209-12

[2] McNamara et al., "Selective deficits in the omega-3 fatty acid docosahexaenoic acid in the postmortem orbitofrontal cortex of patients with major depressive disorder," *Biological Psychiatry* Dec. 21, 2006

[3] Shaw, K., Turner, J., Del Mar, C., "Tryptophan and 5-hydroxytryptophan for depression," *Cochrane Database Syst. Rev.* 2002;(1):CD003198

Chapter 17

I'm Proud of My High Cholesterol

Cholesterol does not cause heart disease. Cholesterol is what heart disease acts upon.

Cholesterol is a good thing. The more you have, the longer you'll live.

In fact, the prestigious medical journal the *Lancet* did a study that looked at 724 people and followed them for 10 years. Researchers found that higher cholesterol meant a lower chance of dying from *any* cause.[1]

Cholesterol is a part of your body, and it's a bad idea to declare war on a part of your body.

Unfortunately, many people who rely on mainstream medicine for health information haven't gotten the message.

The way modern medicine treats cholesterol is the same as saying, "You have Alzheimer's disease, let's cut off your head." It's like if you come to me to have your bone mineral density measured, and I say, "We've found a problem with your bones. We have to take them out."

You treat the problem, not the part of your anatomy that the problem is affecting. But that's what we've done with cholesterol. Because it's diseased doesn't mean you want to get rid of it. You want to get rid of the disease.

All things being equal, the more cholesterol you have the better. A study from the Department of Cardiovascular Medicine at Yale University found that seniors **with low cholesterol died twice as often** from a heart attack as did elders with high cholesterol.[2]

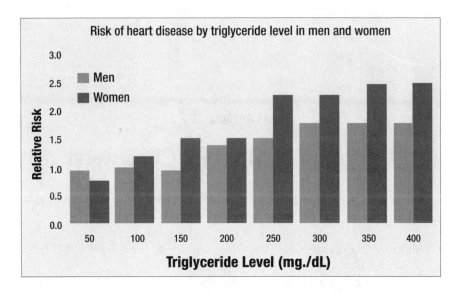

Cholesterol is a normal and important part of your anatomy. You need your cholesterol. It becomes diseased because there are unnatural inflammatory and oxidative pressures that are distorting it and causing it to be diseased.

Cholesterol isn't the bad guy. It's the oxidation and inflammation that are the bad guys.

And you don't remove the part of your body that the bad guys are acting on.

The solution I use with my patients who have inflammation is to try and get their HDL to be as high as half of their triglycerides.

There's no evidence that high cholesterol increases heart risk if your HDL is at least half your triglycerides.

If you can make your HDL higher than your triglycerides, that's even better.

My HDL is twice as high as my triglycerides, and I'm proud of my high cholesterol.

A pretty good HDL level is about 45. And we want your triglycerides to be below 150, normally. But if you can get your triglycerides down to 100, and your HDL up to 50, then it doesn't matter what your total cholesterol is. There is no risk.

In my case, I actually had my HDL at *twice* my triglycerides.

Here's how I got my triglycerides down to 50 and I got my HDL up to 105, and you can, too:

Step 1) Use my four secrets and be proud of your high cholesterol

- **I ate a whole bunch of garlic.** A decade worth of studies prove garlic significantly lowers triglycerides while raising HDL. With so much evidence, you'd think modern medicine would stop ignoring garlic's benefits and start recommending at least two cloves a day.

I ate even more. I put it in my omelet for breakfast. I used garlic and olive oil dressing on a chicken salad or fish salad I would have for lunch most days. In the evening I would use garlic in a side dish like stir-fry vegetables.

And you know the odor that garlic produces? Your body tends to handle it better with time. It comes from the sulfur, but your body gets better at processing it. I only noticed a garlic odor at the beginning and after a few days it went away.

- **I took two grams of niacin every day.** Niacin can raise HDL by 15% to 35%. This makes niacin, a simple B vitamin, more effective than any cholesterol drug ever invented.

- **I took one tablespoon of cod liver oil a day.** It's one of the richest sources of omega-3 on earth, and the more omega-3 you get, the lower your triglycerides will be. A new study gave people 3 grams of omega-3 a day, and lowered their triglycerides by 27%.[3] There are 15 grams of omega-3 in a tablespoon of cod liver oil.

Studies also show that triglycerides weaken HDL, and stop it from having its full protective effect on your heart.[4] That makes omega-3 HDL's best friend. And taking it is simple and easy. It doesn't have the fishy taste it did when your grandmother may have forced you to take it years ago. My cod liver oil has a clean lemon-lime flavor.

- **I worked out with PACE™**, because intense, short periods of exertion like I describe in my PACE™ program will reliably boost HDL. For example, one study looked at Navy personnel going through intense training and after only 5 days, their HDL had increased 31%.[5]

Step 2) Eat low-glycemic foods to drive down your triglycerides

A good idea I use with my patients — and it's the way I eat, too — is to stick with low-glycemic foods, which can really get your triglycerides way under 150.

Here's how it works.

Usually, insulin helps you convert triglycerides into energy. When you constantly eat starchy grains or sugary food, your body produces *lots* of insulin to try to process all the blood sugar. Over time, you become resistant to the effects of all that insulin, and you don't convert triglycerides into energy. They stay in your blood.

A new review from the Framingham Heart Study followed almost 3,000 people for 14 years. Those who were more insulin resistant had higher triglycerides and lower HDL.[6]

To raise HDL and lower triglycerides, I have my patients stay away from carbs that come from grains, refined sugars and processed foods. I also have them avoid trans fats, caffeine and high fructose corn syrup, which all increase insulin resistance.

Instead, I have them eat mostly protein from animals. Animal protein has zero effect on your blood sugar. It also raises your insulin sensitivity and lowers your triglyceride levels.

One incredible study on the effect of eating protein instead of carbs is from the *Southern Medical Journal*. They gave people foods consisting mostly of beef and beef fat. They ate no sugars, milk, or grains. Their triglyceride levels dropped 35%, while their percentage of HDL jumped 50%.[7]

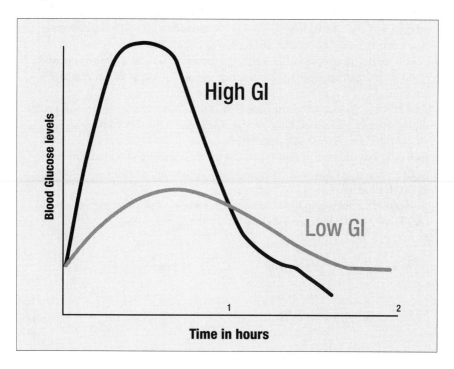

Please turn to the back of the book for my glycemic index that shows you which foods spike your blood sugar and cause you to make waves of insulin.

As you can see from the chart to the right, high-glycemic-index foods make your blood sugar go wild, and can even cause you to have a low blood sugar "crash."

Eating low-GI foods stabilizes your blood sugar. This makes your insulin work better, keeping your triglycerides low, and your HDL high.

[1] Weverling-Rijnsburger AW, Blauw GJ, Lagaay AM, Knook DL, Meinders AE, Westendorp RG. "Total cholesterol and risk of mortality in the oldest old." *Lan-*

cet. 1997 Oct 18;350(9085):1119-23.

[2] Krumholz HM et al. "Lack of association between cholesterol and coronary heart disease mortality and morbidity and all-cause mortality in persons older than 70 years." *JAMA* 1990; 272, 1335-1340.

[3] Skulas-Ray AC, Kris-Etherton PM, Harris WS, Vanden Heuvel JP, Wagner PR, West SG. "Dose-response effects of omega-3 fatty acids on triglycerides, inflammation, and endothelial function in healthy persons with moderate hypertriglyceridemia." *Am J Clin Nutr.* 2011 Feb;93(2):243-52.

[4] Li Tian, et al. "The impact of plasma triglyceride and apolipoproteins concentrations on high-density lipoprotein subclasses distribution." *Lipids Health Dis.* 2011; 10: 17.

[5] Smoak, B.L., Norton, J.P., Ferguson, E.W., et al., "Changes in lipoprotein profiles during intense military training," *J. Am. Coll. Nutr.* Dec. 1990;9(6):567-72

[6] Sander J. Robins; Asya Lyass; Justin P. Zachariah; Joseph M. Massaro; Ramachandran S. Vasan. "Insulin Resistance and the Relationship of a Dyslipidemia to Coronary Heart Disease." *Arteriosclerosis, Thrombosis, and Vascular Biology.* 2011;31:1208-1214.

[7] Newbold HL. "Reducing the serum cholesterol level with a diet high in animal fat." *South Med J.* 1988 Jan;81(1):61-3.

Chapter 18

I'm Not Done Yet

I've been saying that cholesterol is not the bad guy, that it doesn't cause heart disease, for 20 years.

But I'm not done yet.

The reason I can't let go of this is because the problem has actually gotten much worse, not better.

Seventy-five percent of the patients who come to me with heart disease are *already* on a statin drug when I see them.

My first job is to try and talk them out of taking them. They're usually scared and think they're going to die if they stop taking it.

The big drug makers love to run slick TV ads trying to convince you that lowering your LDL will protect you from heart disease. Doctors often further misinterpret the science and lead patients to believe that they have to lower their cholesterol with drugs or die of heart disease.

Because of this, statin drug use has increased over the last 15 years. Since I've been saying you shouldn't take them:

- There are 10 times as many people using statin drugs as there were in 1994.

- Spending on statin medications increased by another $160 million in 2010.

- The cholesterol-lowering drug Lipitor was the biggest seller of any drug last year. It brought in $7.2 billion for Pfizer.

Crestor, another statin, was also high on the bestseller list. It grossed $3.8 billion.

- Statin use grew by 2.3% last year alone. Doctors wrote 255 million prescriptions for these drugs in 2010 — more than any other class of drug. That's up from 210 million in 2006.[1]

- Almost half the men in the U.S. who are over 65 have been put on a statin drug. And almost 40% of women. Here's the chart from the government's "Health 2010" report:

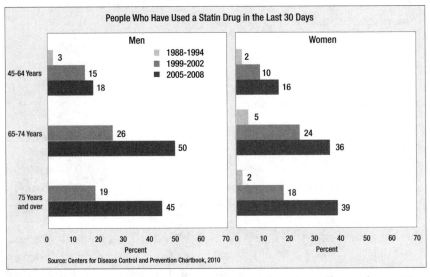

People Who Have Used a Statin Drug in the Last 30 Days

Source: Centers for Disease Control and Prevention Chartbook, 2010

If you've gone to a cardiologist, you know what I'm talking about. Virtually every cardiologist in the country is putting virtually every one of their heart patients on a statin drug.

And it's about to get worse. The FDA has given the okay for statin makers to market their drugs to completely healthy folks.

The companies are now allowed to try and get you to take a statin drug if you're a man over 50 or a woman over 60 and you have one heart risk factor. *Even if you are currently healthy with no history of heart problems.*

Never mind that a comprehensive review of studies by the non-partisan Cochrane group found that doctors should not prescribe a statin to you if you fall into that group.[2]

Never mind that another review by the prestigious medical journal the *Lancet* found that statins increase the risk of diabetes by almost 10%.[3]

What makes that study so important is that no one was ever told statins could cause diabetes. The *Lancet* only found out because their review looked at most of the major clinical studies of statins, and *also unpublished study results*. They included the secret results of the Crestor study that the FDA reviewed but were never made public.

The FDA and doctors have also closed their eyes to other dangerous side effects of these drugs. The list is long and frightening. Here are just a few:

Inability to concentrate	Confusion or Disorientation
Amnesia	Rhabdomolysis (painful busting of muscle cells)
Shortness of breath	Fatigue
Nerve pain	Muscle weakness
Depression and other mood disorders	Impotence
Lowered sex drive	Weakened immune system
Liver damage	Death

It seems like they don't even try and find out what's causing your problem anymore. That's not part of the diagnosis process. They just do this pattern of choices that's from a differential diagnosis that they learned in a class. Someone has this symptom, this is how you sort through which diagnosis to make, and this is what you do.

And what you do always ends in a drug therapy or an operation. Those are the only things they consider. Anything else is not worthy of consideration. Not what someone might be eating… not what they might be doing. The process doesn't have any faith in nature or your body.

Your body needs lots of cholesterol. Far from being the enemy that modern medicine claims, it's really a building block essential for life. It makes your memory work, helps make your sex hormones, and functions as a powerful antioxidant protecting you from cancer and aging.

Artificially lowering your cholesterol with a statin drug interferes with your body's essential functions. Instead, what you want and need is high cholesterol. Specifically, you want is to get your HDL cholesterol as high as you can get it. Then it doesn't matter what your LDL is.

In fact, high HDL trumps other cholesterol concerns. Why isn't this simple and powerful knowledge getting through? For one reason, there is no drug to boost HDL. What's the best way to increase HDL cholesterol? With four simple steps:

Step 1) Eat More Fat. Fat is also an essential nutrient, just like cholesterol. The diet dictocrats are trying to ban all fat from your food. It's only making Americans fatter and sicker. The truth is that healthy fats raise your HDL.

The first healthy fat to get more of is monounsaturated fat. One study found that people who ate the most monounsaturated fats had significantly higher HDL compared to people who ate the least. The same study also found that monounsaturated fats increase the effectiveness of the other things you do to raise your HDL.[4] The fats you find in nuts, olive oil, avocados and beef fat are all monounsaturated fats.

The second kind of fat that will raise your HDL is a group called polyunsaturated fatty acids (PUFAs). You might know them better as the essential fatty acids omega-3s and omega-6s. To get more PUFAs, eating fish is your best bet. But I just read a study where they added plant based PUFAs like those in Sacha Inchi oil to fish oil and gave it people to help raise their HDL. The plant nutrients increased the effectiveness of the fish oil to raise HDL even more.[5]

You want to get more omega-3s than omega-6s. Eat high-quality wild-caught fish, and stay away from farm-raised fish that have too many omega-6s and not enough omega-3s. Cod liver oil and Sacha Inchi oil are your best supplement sources for PUFAs.

Step 2) Eat More Meat. Here's one of my favorite stories that shows how wrong modern science is when it comes to its attitude toward cholesterol. "Educators" were looking to prove that you shouldn't eat meat because it raises LDL cholesterol. They believe the modern myth that meat is bad for you.

So these people from The National Cholesterol Education Program did a study. I would have loved to be a part of this one. They had people eat almost a half pound of lean red meat or lean white meat every day for two 36-week periods. In between, the people could eat whatever kinds of meat they wanted.

The researchers were surprised to find that eating meat raises HDL and lowers total cholesterol. And it doesn't matter if it's white or red meat.[6] It was no surprise to me. I've been basing all my meals around protein as long as I can remember and my HDL is 105.

But here's the kicker. Stay away from grain-fed meats.

Stick with meat from grass-fed animals. Grass-fed beef has more healthy fats like omega-3 and fewer calories than grain-fed. It also has more B vitamins, CoQ10, zinc, vitamin E, and beta-carotene.

Step 3) Take the Vitamin E You've Never Heard Of. Vitamin E is actually a group of eight nutrients, four tocopherols, and four tocotrienols. The vitamin E you can buy at the store is usually only the alpha-tocopherol. But the alpha, beta, gamma and delta tocotrienols have powerful heart benefits.

A new study that shows tocotrienols raise HDL and also lower two other heart risk markers, triglycerides and C-reactive protein.[7] Plus, tocotrienols have more antioxidant activity than tocopherols and are anti-inflammatory.

Cranberries, coconuts, chicken and palm oil have tocotrienols, but not much. Personally, my favorite source is annatto. I first encountered it in the Andes Mountains. The natives there recognize annatto oil as a powerful health tonic.

You can find annatto and palm oil at your local health food store or specialty grocery store. You can also use a tocotrienols supplement. Look for one that has as much gamma and delta tocotrienols as you can get, because those are the two that seem to have the most benefit.

Step 4) There's one more thing you should do to keep your HDL high. Use my PACE™ program. My alternative to aerobics and cardio reliably boosts HDL because you focus on slightly increasing the intensity of your exertion with each workout, not on making them longer.

One study looked at the effects of shorter periods of intense training on HDL, and found that intense training raised HDL by 15%.[8] And remember, that study was simply looking at higher intensity for short periods vs. lower intensity for longer periods. If they had tested for PACE™, there would have been even more dramatic differences.

I often prescribe PACE™ to my patients who need to raise their HDL. All it takes is 12 minutes a day, three times a week.

---

[1] A.U. "The Use of Medicines in the United States: Review of 2010" A.U. "The Use of Medicines in the United States: Review of 2010" IMS Institute for Healthcare Informatics. April 2011.

[2] Taylor F, Ward K, Moore, T, et al. "Statins for the primary prevention of cardiovascular disease." *Cochrane Database of Systematic Reviews* 2011; 1.

[3] Sattar N, et al. "Statins and risk of incident diabetes: a collaborative meta-analysis of randomised statin trials." *Lancet.* Feb 27, 2010;375(9716):735-42.

[4] JenkinsD. "Adding monounsaturated fatty acids to a dietary portfolio of cholesterol-lowering foods in hypercholesterolemia." *CMAJ.* Dec. 14,2010;182(18):1961-7.

[5] Micallef M, Garg M. "The lipid-lowering effects of phytosterols and (n-3) polyunsaturated fatty acids are synergistic and complementary in hyperlipidemic men and women." *J. Nutr.* June 2008;138(6):1086-90.

[6] Hunninghake, et al. "Incorporation of lean red meat into a National Cholesterol Education Program Step I Diet." *Journal of the American College of Nutrition* 2000;19(3):351-360.

[7] PrasadK. "Tocotrienols and Cardiovascular Health." *Curr Pharm Des.* Jul 21, 2011.

[8] Musa D, Adeniran S, Dikko A, Sayers S. "The effect of a high-intensity interval training program on high-density lipoprotein cholesterol..." *J. Strength Cond Res.* Mar. 2009;23(2):587-92.

PART 2
A PLATE FULL OF LIES

Chapter 1

How Agribusiness Turned 12 of Your Favorite Fruits and Vegetables into Toxic Threats

What You Need to Know to Stay Safe

I love the taste of a fresh strawberry. I'm lucky that I live in Florida and I can go out in my yard and pick them. But if you buy them from a store, there's something you need to know.

The food industry puts poisons on your food, and they stay in your body even after you eat them.

During one test, there were 30 different pesticides found on the strawberries sold as ready for you to eat.[1]

Some of these chemicals rob you of the nutrients you need. Many have unpredictable effects in your body that we know very little about.

And it's not just strawberries. Spinach is another example of something I love, but another test revealed 10 different pesticides on a single commercial sample of spinach.

The good news is, you can avoid most of these chemicals if you follow the few rules of thumb I give my patients. I'll tell you about those in a moment.

But first, you should know that even low doses of common pesticides that big agricultural companies use, like organochlorine (OC) pesticides, have been strongly linked to various chronic diseases including diabetes and heart diseases.

The pesticide *endosulfan* is an important example. It turns up both in your food and on other crops like cotton.[2] Despite evidence that this chemical was harmful, the FDA insisted it was safe.

But one study says these pesticides may be a major reason why Americans are often deficient in one of the most powerful disease and cancer-preventive nutrients we know of, vitamin D.

The prestigious medical journal *PLoS One* did a review of a study that measured people for 13 different OC pesticides. They found high levels of 7 different OC pesticides in 1,275 people, including the pesticide DDT, which was banned 40 years ago.

The study revealed that those with the most pesticides in their bodies had the lowest levels of vitamin D.[2]

What you may not know is that the FDA allows the practice of — and even defends — using the chemicals. Not only that, but they've participated in the practice. They've made it difficult for other people to be able to put products in front of you other than what comes from Big Agribusiness.

They are friends with Agribusiness, they're paid by Agribusiness, and the politicians are elected by and in some cases come from the ranks of Agribusiness.

And the FDA only moved to stop the use of endosulfan because of the danger to agricultural employees, not because of the danger to you who are consuming the crops. And they're supposed to be in charge of regulating our food safety.

In fact, the FDA hasn't banned endosulfan so much as it's being phased out. Agriculture companies will still be able to use it until 2016.[3] That means it's going to be around in our environment for a long time.

That concerns me because these pesticides only add to the environmental chemical burden that wreaks havoc on your hormones. When these chemicals get into your blood, your body mistakes them for real hormones. For men, this means the gradual loss of masculine characteristics and development of feminine features and abnormal growth of the prostate. In women, it means a rise in breast and ovarian cancers and a dramatic worsening of symptoms of menopause.

These industrial pesticides might also have other effects we don't even know about yet. How could anyone know what decades of consuming pesticides and other hormone-disrupting chemicals will do? In terms of human evolution, it's a brand-new problem, and we have no way of knowing what all the effects will be.

This is why, to help protect you and your family, I recommend you follow these three general guidelines:

1. The first rule of thumb I give my patients is that while it may not be economically practical for you to always buy everything organic, it may make sense to buy organic for the worst offenders.

Here's how the best and the worst stack up:[4]

The Dirty Dozen
Buy These Organic

1. Apples
2. Celery
3. Strawberries
4. Peaches
5. Spinach
6. Nectarines – imported
7. Grapes – imported
8. Sweet bell peppers
9. Potatoes
10. Blueberries – domestic

11. Lettuce

12. Kale/collard greens

The 15 Lowest in Pesticides

1. Onions

2. Sweet corn

3. Pineapples

4. Avocado

5. Asparagus

6. Sweet peas

7. Mangoes

8. Eggplant

9. Cantaloupe – domestic

10. Kiwi

11. Cabbage

12. Watermelon

13. Sweet potatoes

14. Grapefruit

15. Mushrooms

After you buy produce, you may wash your fruits and vegetables to get rid of the dirt, bugs, wax and pesticides. It may help, but many of today's pesticides are designed to bind to the surface and don't easily wash off.

Surprisingly, the food checked by the government in the test I mentioned above was washed and prepared for normal consumption before it was tested. Even if you rinse with water, you could still get chemical contamination.

2. So my second rule of thumb is to take these additional steps to prepare your produce:

- Peel your fruits and vegetables and remove outer leaves on cabbage, lettuce, garlic and onions.

- For the produce you don't peel, soak them in a mixture of vinegar and water (equal parts). After 10 or 15 minutes, rinse them with cold water.

- Alternatively, soak your produce in a weak mixture of dish-washing liquid. Then rinse well with cold water.

- If you don't have time to soak, you can fill a spray bottle with 1 cup of water, 1 tablespoon of lemon juice and 2 tablespoons of baking soda. Spray on, let sit and rinse with cold water.

- Or try the old-fashioned way: Fill your sink with water. Add a capful of bleach. After 10 to 15 minutes, remove and let the produce soak in fresh water, then rinse well.

- Avoid commercial produce that's bruised. They're more likely to have concentrations of pesticides deep within the fruit.

3. My third rule of thumb is that if you grow your own produce like I do, it's a good idea to use a soap-and-water solution to get rid of aphids.

However, stay away from products that claim to be "eco-friendly" or "natural" when they clearly are not.

For example, avoid synthetic pyrethroids. They're similar to pyrethrins, which are natural insect-killing extracts from the flower chrysanthe-mum. But pyrethroids are created in a lab. Permethrin is one of those synthetics to avoid.

Also, stay away from "geraniol." It's billed as natural because it's made from roses, lemons and geraniums, but it's been banned in Europe be-cause of its toxicity to humans.

In my garden, I use **neem oil** to keep out pests. This extract from the fruit of the neem tree has been used for pest control in parts of Asia and India for over 2,500 years. It's completely nontoxic. When the En-vironmental Protection Agency went to test neem for toxicity, it found zero reactions, even at the highest exposure.

In fact, you can use any part of the tree for pest control — the twigs, the leaves or the berries. The tree will grow in Florida. In other places and colder climates, I've seen it grown indoors in pots. Even sitting in a pot, it'll serve to keep the bugs out. You can take a couple leaves and put them in your cabinets to keep cockroaches out. Or you can fray up the ends of the stems (so that the twigs are like brushes) and leave those around, and they'll work the same as the leaves do.

As more and more people understand the hazards of chemicals on our food and in the home, market pressure will encourage the introduction of even more of these safer products.

---

[1] "Report Card: Pesticides in Produce." Environmental Working Group. Retrieved March 25, 2012.

[2] Yang J, Lee Y, Bae S, Jacobs D Jr, Lee D. "Associations between Organochlorine Pesticides and Vitamin D Deficiency in the U.S. Population." *PLoS ONE* 2012; 7(1): e30093.

[3] "Endosulphan Memorandum of Agreement." Environmental Protection Agency, July 2010. www.epa.gov. Retrieved March 25, 2012.

[4] "Shopper's Guide to Pesticides and Produce." Environmental Working Group. Retrieved March 25, 2012.

Chapter 2

Can Bagels Make You Go Blind?

Have you noticed your vision getting worse yet?

It happens to most of us as we grow older. It's often the initial effects of age-related macular degeneration, the leading cause of blindness among people over 65. It has now become more common than cataracts and glaucoma combined. The macula is an area at the back of the retina. As people grow older, it can begin to degenerate leading to blurred vision and eventually blindness.

Fortunately, there's something you can do about it. I'll review the latest research on the cause of this disease. I'll tell you what I know about how you can keep your eyes healthy and working as best as they can for years to come.

Starchy Carbohydrates Linked to Risk of Blindness

A recent study published in the *American Journal of Clinical Nutrition* revealed a strong link between dietary carbohydrates and AMD.[1]

Researchers at the Laboratory for Nutrition and Vision Research at Tufts University looked at the quality of vision and diet among 4,099 people ages 55 to 80. Specifically, they measured not only the amount of carbohydrate participants consumed but the *type* of dietary carbohydrate most common in their diets.

They found that participants who ate starchy carbohydrates were *40% more likely to develop AMD*. Those who ate carbs ranking in the top 20% of the glycemic index — which measures sugar-ready carbs — were most at risk.

For my regular readers, this additional warning about dietary carbo-hydrate will come as no surprise. As I've written for years, a new and unnatural change in carbohydrate is the root cause responsible for a wide range of serious health problems, including obesity, heart disease, and diabetes.

In study after study, this dietary change, although ignored by medi-cine, has been found to be the culprit behind the biggest diseases of our time. Now we can add AMD to the list.

So what can you do about it? Do you have to avoid carbs altogether?

The answer is no. You just have to eat the **right kind** of carbohydrates.

Here's the Best Tool to Improve Your Carbohydrate

The body converts all carbohydrates into glucose, or blood sugar. In order to digest blood sugar, the pancreas kicks into gear, producing the hormone insulin to make the sugar available to cells for metabolism.

Carbohydrates vary in how fast they turn into sugar in the body. The faster they breakdown, the higher the glycemic index (GI) score. Please see the glycemic index (GI) and glycemic load (GL) charts at the back of the book.

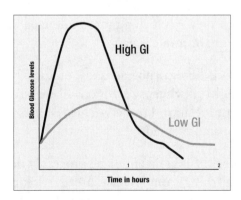

As you can see from the graph above, foods with a high GI spike your blood sugar very quickly — usually within the first 30 to 45 minutes after eating them. But the drop off is equally rapid and dramatic. That's why you'll feel tired and slow after the buzz of a high-carb meal wears off.

Here's a table ranking some of the most common carbohydrates in the American diet:

Common Food Glycemic Index
High
95% Cornbread

80-90% Corn flakes, maltose, honey, white potatoes

70-79% Whole-grain bread, millet, white rice, new potatoes
Moderate
60-69% White bread, shredded wheat, bananas, raisins, Mars Bars

50-59% Spaghetti, corn, whole cereals, peas, yams, potato chips

40-49% Oatmeal, sweet potatoes, navy beans, oranges, orange juice
Low
30-39% Peaches, cherries, blueberries, apples, ice cream, milk

20-29% Kidney beans, lentils, fructose

10-19% Soybeans, peanuts

0-10% Most green vegetables

As you can see, starches are the chief culprits. They not only produce more blood sugar; they result in a more prolonged elevation in blood sugar and insulin than simple sugars.

The starchiest foods, like cornbread and potatoes, have glycemic ratings close to 100. Meanwhile, sweet foods like cherries only score 22. In other words, the relationship between sweetness and the glycemic rating has been misrepresented.

How does this work? All grains must be processed before humans can digest them. Everything from lasagna, bread, cookies, pizza, spaghetti, crackers and chips are heavy in starches. These foods cause an unnatural surge in insulin levels into the blood. This is what ultimately does the most harm. Too much insulin leads to inflammation, heart disease and excess fat deposition. And ultimately, it paradoxically robs you of energy.

Now we know it is also associated with age-related vision loss by contributing to the onset of AMD.

Here are a few simple tips to bear in mind before you dig into a high-carb meal:

- Don't eat grains, period. This includes "healthy whole grains." Cereals are no more natural to your diet than the cardboard box with all that natural Mother Nature's goodness pasted all over it.

- Avoid potatoes and other tubers that grow below ground, like parsnips and sweet potatoes.

- Eat vegetables that grow above ground.

- Don't eat corn. You are best not to classify it as a vegetable — it's a grain.

- Skip "low-fat" processed foods altogether.

- Avoid container foods with added sweeteners, especially high-fructose corn syrup. You'll find it in many foods and drinks and it's the absolute worst.

- Focus on high-fiber foods. Fiber slows digestion, so the sugar in fiber-rich foods enters you bloodstream more slowly. You don't need grains for fiber. The fiber in fruits and vegetables is best.

Two Great Tips for Healthy, Powerful, Lifelong Vision

Several recent studies have suggested very concrete ways you can modify your diet to avoid AMD: Eat a diet rich in the right kinds of fat, and get enough vitamin D.

One study at the National Institutes of Health looked closely at the link between nutrition and AMD on its connection on 4,519 people aged 60 to 80 between 1992 and 1998.[2]

They were first assessed for signs of macular degeneration. If they had it, the researchers then determined how far it had progressed. Patients also completed a food questionnaire that measured intake of certain vitamins, minerals and other essential nutrients such as fatty acids.

Of the total, 1,115 patients had no symptoms of disease at the outset, while 658 people had a severe form of the disease. When their diets were evaluated, the researchers found that people who ate more fish — more than two medium servings per week or more than one serving of broiled or baked fish — were least likely to have the disease.

Fish is rich in omega-3 fatty acids. This is the so-called "good" fat. It's found in abundance in grass-fed beef, wild-caught fish, eggs, poultry, nuts, seeds, and certain vegetables. Omega-3s boost heart health, strengthen the mind, and raise your "good" (HDL) cholesterol levels.

Now we know that they also prevent AMD.

You want to eat a diet high in protein and rich in omega-3s. Be sure to choose organic, free-range, or wild-caught meats whenever possible. These contain the proper balance of protein and fat for optimal eyesight and overall good health.

Another important dietary supplement that's good for your eyes is vitamin D. In fact, a study recently published in the *Archives of Ophthalmology* concluded that vitamin D will actually prevent the onset of AMD.[3]

Researchers looked at the dietary intake of vitamin D among 7,752 people taking part in a large national study between 1988 and 1994 — 11% of the patients had AMD. The researchers found that vitamin D was associated with reduced risk of early AMD, but not advanced AMD.

The people were split into five groups based on level of vitamin D in the blood. Those in the highest group had a 40% lower risk of early AMD than those in the lowest group.

Researchers suggested vitamin D may cut the risk of early age-related macular degeneration by reducing inflammation or preventing blood vessel growth in the retina (the same effect that omega-3s have on the body).

You'll need about 1,000 IUs of vitamin D daily to get its eye-strengthening benefit.

Three Natural Nutrients to Preserve Your Eyesight

My grandma used to tell me to eat my carrots because they're good for the eyes. Turns out she was right.

The substances contained in carrots, called "carotenoids," are essential to good eyesight. You can get these critical substances into your diet by taking vitamin supplements.

A word of warning: Not all supplements containing "carotenoids" are the same. You want to be sure that you're getting "mixed" carotenoids. These are most effective in preserving eyesight, but vitamin manufacturers often cut corners by including only one type of carotenoid.

The two carotenoids to look for are lutein and zeaxanthin. In combination, they're the most potent treatment of AMD available. They're naturally present in the retina and concentrated in the macula.

Another nutrient proven to enhance eye health: tocopherols. These are forms of vitamin E that are potent free-radical destroyers. *JAMA* published a study which proved that increased intake of these nutrients lowered the risk of AMD.

The bottom line is that there is a lot you can do to prevent age-related macular degeneration from happening to you — safely and *naturally*.

---

[1] Chung-Jung C, et al. Association between dietary glycemic index and AMD.

American Journal of Clinical Nutrition, 86(2007):180-188.

[2] Risk Factors Associated with AMD. *Ophthalmology.* 2000, 107(12): 2224–2232.

[3] Ravinder A, et al. The Relationship of Dietary Lipid Intake and AMD. *Archives of Ophthalmology* 125(2007):671-679.

Chapter 3

When Bagels Attack — What You Need to Know about Gluten and How It Affects Your Body

Your body has two "brains."

You know about the one in your head, of course, but there's also one in your gut. This one decides what's considered food and what isn't. It knows what you need for nutrition.

Your "gut brain" processes the antigens (molecules recognized by your system) and has a memory of what it's supposed to digest, what should just pass through, and what needs to be destroyed.

Problems start when you eat something foreign to your gut.

You see, the food industry tells you that processed foods, grain, wheat, and bread are "good" for you. Even the national food pyramid says most of your daily intake should come from grains.

But what the food industry doesn't know (or doesn't tell you) is that your gut doesn't know what to do with the grain products you eat. And sometimes your body rejects them.

More and more people are showing signs of intolerance to grains and processed foods. And they all have something in common — gluten.

I'm going to tell you how gluten affects your body and what you can do to keep your body strong.

What Is Gluten Anyway?

Gluten is a sticky, gluey protein found in grains like wheat, barley, rice, and rye.

This gooey protein is commonly used in baked goods. Gluten holds on to the carbon dioxide made from yeast and expands. It's what makes dough stretchy, holds cookies together, makes cake rise, and makes bagels doughy.

You can also find gluten in some unlikely places, like pasta, beer, soy sauce, certain medications, toothpaste, and even lipstick.

Who Is Affected by Gluten?

Gluten intolerance was once very rare. But it's become much more common in modern times.

Where Gluten Can Hide...

- **Sausage:** Most brands of sausage use breadcrumbs as fillers.
- **Hamburgers:** Bread or wheat products are often mixed in for texture.
- **Ketchup, Ice Cream, and Mayonnaise:** Some brands mix in wheat flour for thickness.
- **Prepackaged Grated Cheese:** It's coated in flour to prevent sticking.
- **Beer and Whisky:** These alcoholic drinks are made from grains.

Something has changed in our environment to make gluten intolerance more prevalent. It's directly related to what we put in our bodies.

Gluten isn't part of our native diet. So it's natural that our bodies reject it.

Here's the thing…

Your "gut brain" thinks gluten is a foreign substance. It doesn't know that it's meant to be a source of nutrition. So, when gluten reaches your gut, your gut panics.

Your gut reacts by sending antibodies to attack the unknown substance. This causes your immune system to become hyper alert with autoimmune components. And it can cause your body to attack its own tissue.

When your immune system attacks, it damages the villi (small "fingers" in your small intestine that absorb nutrients from your food), so they can't absorb what your body needs to live. This can cause your body to destroy its own tissues and shut down. Leaky gut syndrome, malabsorption, and malnutrition are some common outcomes.

The longer gluten intolerance is left untreated, the worse the outcome can be. Unfortunately, it's one of the most misdiagnosed conditions out there. The symptoms are very similar to other digestive problems like irritable bowel syndrome and vary from patient to patient.

Common Symptoms of Gluten Intolerance

- Abdominal pain;
- Bloating;
- Cramping;
- Weight Gain or Loss;
- Constipation;
- Diarrhea;
- Alternating Constipation and Diarrhea.

If left untreated, gluten intolerance can cause:

- Cancer;[1]
- Reduced blood flow to the brain (cerebral hypo perfusion);[2]
- Vitamin D deficiency;[3]
- Miscarriage;[4]
- Low birth weight;[5]
- ED;[6]
- Thyroid disease.[7]

Getting Back to Basics

Although gluten-free diets are prescribed to people who are gluten intolerant, everyone can benefit from eating less grains and processed food.

When you cut out grains and processed foods, you're getting back to your native way of eating. This will boost your energy, improve focus, improve digestion, and aid with the absorption of nutrients.

Remember, gluten is found in wheat, rye, barley, bran, wheat germ, buckwheat, millet, and other grains. If you see ANY reference to these types of grains on a food label, steer clear.

Not only that, but here's a list of some additives and ingredients you'll want to stay away from if you're eating gluten-free:

- Distilled grain vinegar;
- Malt;
- Hydrolyzed protein;
- Instant dry yeast or yeast extract;
- Food starch;
- Maltodextrin;
- Grain alcohol;
- Rennet;
- Semolina.

Many food manufacturers now put "gluten-free" on their packaging.

Coconut flour and almond flour are excellent choices. If you can't find these, rice flour makes a good gluten-free alternative.

---

[1] Freeman HJ. "Adult celiac disease and its malignant complications." *Gut Liver* 2009. 3(4):237-46.

[2] Addolorato G, Di Giuda D, De Rossi G, et al. "Regional cerebral hypoperfusion in patients with celiac disease." *Am J Med* 2004. 116(5):312-7.

[3] Eid WE. "Osteodystrophy in celiac disease: ultimate complications and possible

treatment." *S D Med* 2009. 62(11):429-31.

[4] Molteni N, Bardella MT, Bianchi PA. "Obstetric and gynecological problems in women with untreated celiac sprue." *J Clin Gastroenterol* 1990. 12(1):37-9.

[5] Pellicano R, Astegiano M, Bruno M, Fagoonee S, Rizzetto M. "Men and celiac disease: association with unexplained infertility." *Minerva Med* 2007. 98(3):217-9.

[6] Farthing MJ, Rees LH, Dawson AM. "Male gonadal function in coeliac disease: III. Pituitary regulation." *Clin Endocrinol* (Oxf). 19(6):661-71.

[7] Sategna-Guidetti C, Volta U, Ciacci C, Usai P, Carlino A, et al. "Prevalence of thyroid disorders in untreated adult celiac disease patients and effect of gluten withdrawal: an Italian multicenter study." *Am J Gastroenterol* 2001. 96(3):751-7.

Chapter 4

Before You Switch to Soy — Try Real Raw Milk

While recent campaigns have tried to blame milk as a cause of asthma, arthritis, allergy and gastrointestinal distress among other ailments, you can use milk as part of a healthy diet.

Most of the links between these problems and milk are with *processed* milk products. That may be key because like all foods, how good it is greatly depends on the source.

You'll learn:

The benefits of whole milk vs. skim.

The harmful effects and denaturalization of milk through pasteurization and homogenization.

How to separate fact from fiction about whole milk and raw milk.

The healing power and great taste of raw milk.

How to make the healthiest milk choice.

Where to buy raw milk.

The Untold Story of Pasteurization and Homogenization

During the early 1800s, Robert M. Hartley, an accomplished zoologist, proclaimed in praise of cows, *"It is scarcely necessary to say, that they supply us with the most truly precious of our earthly gifts.* [Without cows], *how different would be the social, commercial and political condition of the most civilized of the human race!"*[1]

Mr. Hartley had no idea how prophetic his enthusiastic statement was. As New York City and other major cites rapidly grew in the 1800s, city families were unable to keep a family cow for their dairy needs. As demand for milk was just as great, milk was sold in mass quantity through dairy farmers.

To deal with the problems of delivery and freshness, industrialists came up with new ways of processing milk. Unfortunately, processed milk can be dangerous for both the cow and the consumer.[2]

Homogenization Leads to Chronic Disease

Whole milk most closely resembles actual cow's milk after pasteurization. Skim milk is another story. Aside from having all of its natural nutrients destroyed during processing, nonfat *dried* milk is added as a protein and vitamin additive.

Production of nonfat dried milk involves forcing skim milk out of a tiny hole at high temperature and pressures, a process that not only destroys nutrients but also causes the production of nitrates — which are potent carcinogens. Furthermore, the process causes oxidation of the cholesterol in milk.[3]

What's more, skim or fat-free milk is full of milk sugar (lactose). When you remove the fat, all you're left with is sugar. So much so, farmers often feed their pigs fat-free milk in order to fatten them up.

When you look at the following chart, it all becomes clear:

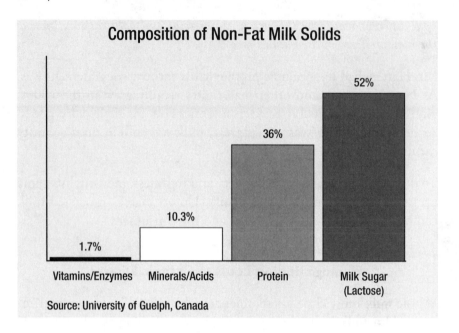

While I have mentioned in the past that cholesterol in food poses no danger, *"**oxidized** cholesterol has been shown to initiate the process of injury and pathological plaque build-up in the arteries."*[4]

Thus the unknowing consumer who drinks reduced-fat milk in order to prevent heart disease and cancer may actually increase his risk of chronic disease.[5]

Health Ailments Associated with Pasteurized Milk[6]	
Symptoms/Minor Ailments	Life Threatening or Altering Diseases
Diarrhea Cramps Bloating Gas Gastrointestinal bleeding Iron-deficiency anemia Colic in infants Allergies Skin rashes Increased tooth decay Recurrent ear infections in children Acne Infertility Growth problems in children	Arthritis Atherosclerosis Autism Cancer Heart Disease Leukemia Osteoporosis Rheumatoid Arthritis Type 1 Diabetes Type 2 Diabetes

Nature's Healthiest Option: Raw Milk

Raw Milk has a creamier texture and is full of essential nutrients and vitamins unadulterated by the processing that brings commercial milk to your grocery store. It is without a doubt your healthiest option.

Most farmers drink raw milk because of taste and the knowledge that it is healthier for you. There is not a huge market for raw milk and in some states it is illegal to sell raw milk. Raw milk sales average around 20% for those who are able to sell it. More typically, the farmer drinks the raw milk and sells processed milk. But you have the power to change this.

You too can enjoy nutrient rich raw milk. It may not be readily available at your grocery store, but your local dairy farmer and some natural food markets do provide this choice. If you live in areas where that this is not possible, read on as I will tell you how to work around this government roadblock.

Raw Milk: Fact vs. Fiction	
FICTION	**FACT**
Raw milk has too much harmful bacteria to safely drink.	If bottled correctly and safely, risk for infection is almost zero.
Raw milk is too fattening and high in cholesterol for human consumption.	Nonsense. Raw milk is an excellent source of CLA* and good fat. Your body responds better to unadulterated fat with healthier skin, hair, nails, digestion among other critical organ functions.
Raw milk causes heart disease.	No way. Pasteurization and homogenization are the contributing culprits of heart disease.
Pasteurization makes milk safe to drink.	Wrong again. While pasteurization minimizes bacteria contamination it does not ensure safety.
Raw milk causes allergies.	Pasteurized milk is the culprit. Many lactose intolerant or allergic drinkers are able to enjoy raw milk even years after abstaining from pasteurized milk.

*CLA (Conjugated Linoleic Acid) a heart healthy and beneficial fatty acid.[7]

Milk from grass-fed cows has a beneficial fatty acid known as CLA, short for Conjugated Linoleic Acid. Countless studies have shown that CLA has many potential health benefits. For comparison, grain-fed cows have as little as one fifth the CLA in their milk as grass-fed.[8]

Where to Find Raw Milk

While raw milk is not readily available at your chain supermarket it can be found at natural food supermarkets and through your local dairy farmer. In the event that it is illegal to purchase raw milk in your state there are some clever options available to sidestep this law. One of which is to buy part ownership of a cow with your local dairy farmer in order to "purchase" raw milk. It may be the cheapest way to "own" a dairy cow.

The best source for information on where to purchase raw milk and how to get around governmental restrictions is http://www.realmilk.com

---

[1] Schmid, Ron. ND. "The Untold Story of Milk: Green Pastures, Contented Cows and Raw Dairy Foods, New Trends Publishing, Inc. Washington DC, 2003: p. 228-229, 2003.

[2] Ibid.

[3] "Home: The Facts About Real Raw Milk - A Campaign for Real Milk." Real Milk Finder, last modified February 3, 2015.

[4] Ibid.

[5] Ibid.

[6] Mercola, Joseph, MD. "The Real Reasons Raw Milk is becoming more popular." Mercola.com. April 24, 2004.

[7] "Not All Milk Is The Same!" Raw-Milk-Facts.com, last updated June 21, 2012.

[8] Ibid.

Chapter 5

The Truth about Soy — This Modern "Health Food" Could Be Making You Sick

Would you knowingly eat something that causes nausea, gas pains and indigestion? That leads to hormonal imbalance, thyroid problems, gout and even cancer? That contains "bad" fats and other unhealthy substances? Something that has no positive effect on your heart whatsoever?

I certainly wouldn't. And neither should you.

For years now, you've been hearing about the "miraculous" benefits of soy-based products. In 1999, the FDA endorsed soy protein as a way to lower saturated fats and cholesterol in the American diet, leading to an explosion in the food industry's use of soy-based products.

But beneath all the soy-health hoopla, I've found studies strongly suggesting that many of these products pose a number of serious health risks.

I'm going to tell you which soy-based products to avoid — and why. I'll also give you a few simple guidelines for eliminating them from your diet and replacing them with healthy alternatives.

The Dangerous Realities behind the "Soy Revolution"

In the January 2006 issue of the journal *Circulation*, the American Heart Association announced that soy has little effect on cholesterol and is unlikely to prevent heart disease.[1]

This doesn't mean that all types of soy are unhealthy. But it proves that soy isn't the "miracle food" the FDA and the food industry would have you believe.

Soy-based products are everywhere. And that's a problem. You may not realize it, but soy crops up in unexpected places. It's in your fridge and cupboard — from ice cream and yogurt to pasta and cereal. Not to mention the frying oil used in fast food.

How did this happen?

After FDA approval, the food industry jumped on the soy bandwagon in a big way. By 2004, 80% of all vegetable oils were derived from soy, and nearly all processed foods now contain some form of it.

Here are five surprising facts about soy:

1. Soy and Indigestion:

The problems start with the soybean itself. In raw form, it's poisonous to the human body. In fact, eating raw soy can cause stomachaches, nausea, cramping, and gas.

Other soy ingredients prevent the body from absorbing essential minerals. Ironically, soy also makes it more difficult for the body to digest protein, the very thing soy was supposed to provide as an alternative to meat protein.

2. Soy and Hormonal Imbalance:

Even more serious, soybeans contain substances called "isoflavones" that mimic estrogen, the female hormone. Eating enough soy can disrupt a woman's menstrual cycle. One researcher calculated that, based on body weight, feeding your baby exclusively on soy formula is like giving it *five birth control pills a day!* [2]

3. Soy, Gout, and Thyroid Problems:

As if that weren't enough, there's a chemical in soy that can cause gout and thyroid enlargement. Eating as little as 45 grams of soy products a day can cause thyroid malfunction within 3 months in healthy adult men and women.[3]

4. Soy, Cancer, and Harmful Fats:

Soy causes cancer in animal studies.[4] (By the way, soy makes its way into most industrial animal feed, which means it's also making its way to your table.) It's also high in omega-6 fatty acids — up to 18% of the whole bean. This is the kind of fat you're supposed to *reduce* in your diet.

5. Soy and Blood Clotting:

Another chemical in soy makes red blood cells cluster together. Among other dangers, this prevents the body from absorbing oxygen.

How to Tell the Difference between Good Soy and Bad Soy

The Asian diet is famous for its heavy use of soy-based products like tofu and soy sauce. So why aren't the Japanese suffering from these ill effects? The answer lies in the way soy in Asian countries is traditionally processed.

For thousands of years, ancient farmers used soy as a fertilizer, not as food. They recognized that you would never want to eat raw soy.

The Chinese introduced soy into the human diet only after discovering that the natural fermentation processes rendered it edible. <u>Fermented soy-derived foods like tempeh, miso, and natto do not contain significant amounts of soy's toxins</u>. In fact, they're very healthy.

Tofu, also a staple in traditional Asian cuisine, is not a fermented soy product. But the process of making tofu removes most of the harmful toxins in a different way.

Like some cheeses, tofu is made from the pressed "curds" of the bean. The "whey," or liquid left over after the pressing, is thrown out — and most of the toxins along with it.

Compare this with the modern industrial processing soy undergoes in the West to produce soy oil, flour, and other soy byproducts contained in most processed foods:

- Washing in alkaline;
- Boiling in petroleum-based solvents;
- Bleaching;
- Deodorizing;
- Adding chemicals;
- Heat-blasting;
- Crushing into flakes.

Does that sound appetizing to you?

What's more, soy in this country is genetically modified. The jury is out on how this may affect human health. What we do know is that some industrial processing techniques leave trace amounts of aluminum in soy products. Dietary aluminum leads to dementia according to some studies.

Four Simple Steps to Avoid Harmful Soy By-Products and Boost Your Health

1. Avoid processed foods whenever possible. This should go without saying, but I always recommend eating whole foods, grass-fed beef, and other minimally processed food products, across the board. These energize your body and result in vigor, strength, and long-term health.

2. Check the label. Soy byproducts are everywhere, and they go by many (FDA-approved) names. Here are the ones to look out for:

- Lecithin;
- Vegetable protein;
- Soy protein isolate;

- Soy flour;
- Protein concentrate;
- Textured vegetable protein;
- Vegetable oil;
- Plant sterols.

I'm not saying small amounts of this stuff will kill you, but it's best to be aware of how much you're consuming, given the potential health hazards. If you find these ingredients on the label, try to find substitutes without them.

3. Limit your overall soy intake to a maximum of 25 grams per day. This isn't as easy as calorie counting, but again, it's worth watching how much soy and soy-based products are finding their way into your diet.

4. Stick to traditional soy foods. Tofu (in moderation), tempeh, miso, natto, and soy sauce are all fine. Other kinds of foods that substitute soy for meat, like soy-based hot dogs, are not healthy alternatives.

---

1 Sacks FM, Lichtenstein A, et al. Soy Protein, Isoflavones, and Cardiovascular Health. An American Heart Association Science Advisory for Professionals From the Nutrition Committee. *Circulation* 2006, 113:1034.

[2] Michael Fitzpatrick, MD as quoted in Lawrence, Felicity, "Should we worry about soya in our food?, *Guardian,* July 25, 2006.

[3] Kaayla Daniel as quoted in Nestor, James, "Too Much of a Good Thing? Controversy rages over the world's most regaled legume," *SFGate.com*, August 13, 2006.

[4] Rackis J, et al. The USDA trypsin inhibitor study, Background, objectives and procedural details. *Qualification of Plant Foods in Human Nutrition.* 1985, vol 35.

Chapter 6

Frankenstein Lurking in Your Pantry

Exposing the Lies about Soy and Genetically Modified "Frank-en-Foods"

The world's biggest, most powerful agriculture companies are experimenting with your life. You never agreed to take part in it. But it's triggering infertility, tumors, kidney and liver disease and more.

Big-Agra giants like Monsanto are helping to put untested mutations on your dinner table. These Franken-food experiments are better known as GMOs, or genetically modified organisms.

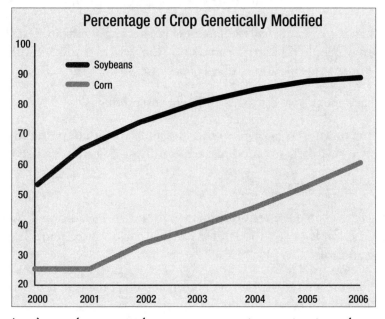

Big-Agra's number one cash crop — soy — is creeping into thousands of products you eat every day, whether you know it or not. Sixty to seventy percent of ALL processed foods contain some soy.

And, almost all soy crops are genetically modified. This "mutant soy" is clinically documented to cause depression, fatigue, infections, brain fog, nausea… *even cancer.*

Genetically modified foods have a shaky track record and have never been proven safe. And the test results that reveal the real dangers never see the light of day. When you eat them, you're taking part in a global Franken-foods experiment.

I'll show you how and why this horror show is unfolding and what you can do to avoid the crippling side effects.

I'll also uncover the compelling studies showing soy is no "miracle food," and give you eight simple steps to avoid the hidden soy in your diet and how to get these Franken-foods off your dinner table.

The "Soy" in Your Food Isn't Nature's Soy

You may have heard that the Japanese are among the healthiest, longest-lived people on earth. There's no sure way to know why this is true, but the speculation is that it's because of what they eat.

And Japanese people eat many different soy products.

Food manufacturers have taken this idea and run with it, trying to convince you that their soy products are healthy — but there's a problem.

It's not the same soy.

You see, the Japanese ferment their soybeans in a traditional way to make the kinds of soy foods they eat like natto, miso, tempeh, edamame and tofu.

But those are a far cry from soy foods made from the genetically modified, heavily processed soy that's in nearly every product you can buy at your local grocery store.

First, Japanese soy products are made with soybeans from conventional breeding programs and are *not genetically modified*. The Japanese don't allow franken-soy.

Second, their soy products are produced through natural fermentation processes.

Natto is made by simply:

1. Soaking soybeans in water, until the beans stop swelling.

2. Steaming them so the beans become soft but don't lose their skin.

3. Laying the cooked beans on cooked rice straw and tying the package shut to let a little heat and oxygen ferment it naturally.

That's it. Three steps. Soak, steam, ferment.

The Chinese have been doing this for thousands of years. And they discovered that mashing up soybeans and mixing them with certain minerals would make a sort of curd... now known as tofu.

And the Chinese and Japanese have known for centuries what food manufacturers don't want you to know: you don't eat unfermented soybeans.

They have huge amounts of natural toxins that block food digestion and also absorption of essential vitamins and minerals. Modern research has discovered that non-fermented soy has elements that can depress thyroid function, stunt growth, and cause red blood cells to clump together.

Producers Are Lying to You about Their Soy

But food manufacturers have spent billions to blind us to these effects, and instead tell you how "nutritious" their soy products are.

Vegetarians have latched on to the soybean as a wonder food, using the food manufacturers' own propaganda. They claim it's high in protein, low in calories, carbohydrates and fats, has no cholesterol, is high in vitamins, and is easy to digest.

This is the language they use to demonize the traditional foods that nourished our ancestors for thousands of years: butter, raw milk, meat and eggs.

The truth is, the soy you find in processed food is genetically modified, oxidized, nutritionally worthless at best, and dangerous at its worst. It's simply a chemically extracted fraction of the bean.

Instead of "soak, steam, ferment," here's how they process soy industrially:

- Industrial crushing processes called "cracking" breaks down the raw, genetically modified bean into thin flakes.

- They are then "defatted" by percolating them like coffee.

- Instead of water the flakes are cooked in a petroleum-based hexane solvent to extract the soy oil.

- The remains of the flakes are toasted and ground into meal.

- For soy flour, the oil then goes through a process of:

  1. Cleaning;

  2. Bleaching;

  3. Degumming;

  4. And deodorizing — all to remove the solvent, and soy's horrible smell.

The sludge that forms in the oil during storage used to be a waste product. Now you know it as soy lecithin.[1]

In other words, the part of the soy that's left over as garbage after the petroleum processing and bleaching is the heart-destroying oil that makes up the trans fats in every kind of junk food you can think of.

And do you know how they make the soy protein isolate used in fake meat and dairy products that vegetarians and food manufacturers claim is so good for you?

It goes something like this:

- A slurry of soy beans is first mixed with an alkaline solution to remove fiber.

- The mix is then separated using an acid wash (this is done in aluminum tanks that can suffuse the toxic metal into the soy).

- It's then neutralized in an alkaline solution.

- The curds are spray-dried at high temperatures to produce the soy isolate protein powder.

- Then they use a high-temperature, high-pressure process to squeeze out a vegetable protein (textured vegetable protein, or TVP) used for other foods — like kids' meals at public schools.

Does that sound nutritious, or even natural?

In fact, it's unhealthy, and downright dangerous.

1. The high-temperature processing makes any protein completely worthless.

2. The spray drying forms nitrites, which are known carcinogens.

3. A toxin called lysinoalanine forms during application of the alkaline solution.[2]

This is what's in store for you when you eat so-called "health" foods made with soy.

When you process *any* food:

- It strips out most if not all of the minerals and natural co-factors.

- It destroys phytonutrients.

- It alters the physical properties of the food itself (think "trans fats" and high- fructose corn syrup).

And, as if the processing isn't bad enough, the actual soybeans forced on growers by companies like Monsanto could be the most frightening part of it all.

Government Steps In to Hide the Danger of GMOs

When giant agricultural corporations wanted to flood the market with genetically modified seeds, there was a problem. What about safety? What were the effects of eating an ear of corn laced with pesticide? What would happen if someone ate soybeans designed to survive the potent weed killer called Roundup?

"Not a problem," announced the federal government.

As long as these "Franken-foods" are "substantially equivalent" to the real thing, the GMO products would be deemed safe — and made available for sale.

> *"Monsanto should not have to vouchsafe the safety of bio-tech food. Our interest is in selling as much of it as possible. Assuring its safety is the FDA's job."*
>
> Phil Angell, Director of Corporate Communications for Monsanto

So, if a GMO food — or other plant — is "substantially equivalent" in composition and nutritional characteristics, *it doesn't have to be tested for safety.*

Responsible scientists were quick to point out the problems with substantial equivalence.

In 1998, Geneva's Center for Environmental Law argued against the World Trade Organization accepting "substantial equivalence" as a standard for GMO safety.

They said it was inadequate to prove safety, would undermine meaningful standards in those countries, and that it ignored scientific research that showed "substantially equivalent" GMO foods had significant negative health impacts.[3]

For example, in 1989, Showa Denko (a Japanese chemical engineering company) genetically engineered bacteria that would produce the food supplement tryptophan.

This unexpectedly also produced trace amounts of a toxin that caused 37 people to die and 1,500 to become permanently disabled. Several hundred more have since died. And this genetically modified product was a purified single chemical that had passed the required substantial equivalence testing.[4]

Plus, there's no such thing as "substantial equivalency." If you change even one gene of a natural food, you're changing the physical nature of the entire food. So how can you say that's even close to equivalent? Who knows what consequences it will have? How could anyone know?

Unfortunately for all of us, commercial interests won out over science, and substantial equivalency is allowed. And now you're part of the biggest food experiment ever conducted — and you never gave your okay.

The American Academy of Environmental Medicine points out that GMO foods have been linked to:

- Infertility;

- Weakened immune system;

- Accelerated aging;

- Genetic problems with cholesterol, insulin control, cell signaling, and protein formation;

- Changes in the liver, kidney, spleen and gastrointestinal system.[5]

These Franken-foods may be considered "substantially equivalent," but the research shows they're substantially more dangerous, too.

There's plenty of solid evidence. Take a look at some of the studies I've found.

Eighty-Five Percent of the Foods on Store Shelves Contain GMOs

In the rush to please the Big-Agra giants, our government has sold us out. Today, as many as 85% of the processed foods on store shelves contain genetically modified ingredients.[6]

And that's not good, if the few studies on GM foods can be believed.

In 2008, Italian researchers found that GM foods had a negative impact on the immune systems of mice.[7] Turkish scientists found evidence of liver and kidney disease in rats fed genetically modified corn.[8] And Danish researchers found enough differences in rats fed genetically modified rice to question its safety.[9]

So where are the studies? A medical researcher in Spain found that there's an almost complete lack of proof that GM foods are safe.[10] And there's a good reason why.

No One Is Allowed to Test GMO Crops

So where is all the research on genetically modified crops? It's hard to come by.

And there's a good reason for that. *The manufacturers won't allow it.*

That's right. Monsanto — and the handful of other big producers of genetically modified crops — *don't allow scientific testing.*

If you want to get your hands on GMO seeds, you have to sign an "end-user agreement," just as if you were buying software. And these end-user agreements ban testing and comparisons to other products. The only testing that happens is testing that the manufacturers approve.

As *Scientific American* points out, the only tests approved are those that the manufacturers decide are "friendly."[11]

So, are genetically modified foods safe for you to eat? Sorry... That's on a need-to-know basis. And the manufacturers have decided that *you* don't need to know.

And in the case of soy, what you don't know *can* hurt you.

Soy is one of the most widespread and successful GMOs in history. All soy is genetically modified and it's in thousands of products you eat every day.

Soy-based products are everywhere in today's American diet. You may not realize it, but soy crops up in unexpected places in your fridge and cupboard, from ice cream and yogurt to pasta and cereal. Not to mention the frying oil used in fast food.

How did this happen?

Because the FDA endorsed it, the food industry jumped on the soy bandwagon in a big way. By 2004, 80% of all vegetable oils were derived from soy, and nearly all processed foods now contain some form of it.

Big-Agra Connections in the White House

Monsanto and other Big-Agra fat cats are at the highest levels of power. Just look at Obama's choices to head the USDA and the FDA: Tom Vilsack and Michael Taylor.

Mr. Vilsack is a long-time supporter of genetically modified foods. And Michael Taylor, the "food-safety czar," is the proverbial fox guarding the henhouse.

The Fox Guarding the Henhouse:
Monsanto Rules Over Obama Administration

Failing on his campaign promise to rid the government of Big-Agra special interests, Obama littered his administration with former Monsanto executives and researchers.

Aside from Tom Vilsack and Michael Taylor taking top positions in Obama's White House, here's just a partial list of other Big-Agra thugs making key decisions about YOUR health:

Roger Beachy: Director of the USDA National Institute of Food and Agriculture, Beachy is former director of the Monsanto-funded Danforth Plant Science Center.

Islam Siddiqui: Now the Agriculture Negotiator for the U.S. Trade Representative, he is also Vice President of the Monsanto-funded pesticide-promoting lobbying group, CropLife.

Rajiv Shah: Former agricultural director for the pro-biotech and frequent Monsanto partner Gates Foundation, he was USDA Under Secretary and now head of USAID, spreading Big-Agra influence overseas, mostly to third-world countries.

Elena Kagan: As Obama's Solicitor General, she took Monsanto's side on a case against organic farmers. She now sits on the Supreme Court.

Ramona Romero: Corporate counsel to chemical giant DuPont, Romero was nominated by Obama and confirmed by the Senate to serve as General Counsel to the USDA.

Taylor has a long history of lobbying for, and being employed by, Big-Agra companies with a vested interest in GMOs. Not only was Taylor a vice president at Monsanto, he was one of the FDA officials who signed off on an FDA policy stating that GMOs don't need safety testing.

Monsanto's Long Arm of Corruption
Reaches around the Globe

Back in 2000, Monsanto wanted to plant over 49,000 acres of genetically modified cotton in Indonesia. But hours before the agreement with Indonesia's government was to be signed, it was shot down by the Ministers of Economy and Environment. There had been no environmental assessment, as required by Indonesian law.

But just five months later, the Minister of Agriculture signed the agreement with Monsanto, *without the required environmental assessment.*

Why? As it turns out, it was a $50,000 bribe from a Monsanto employee that did the trick.

But that $50,000 was just the tip of the iceberg. As it turned out in U.S. court, Monsanto had paid some $700,000 in bribes to Indonesian officials, and wound up slapped with a $1.5 million fine.[12]

According to a report in the *Asia Times*, 140 Indonesian officials received bribes from Monsanto over the deal, including a former Minister of Agriculture, whose wife received a house worth $373,990.

Now, I realize that Indonesia was known at the time for official corruption. But if the genetically modified crop was really safe, wouldn't it be easier to simply prepare the required assessment?

Even more disturbing is an earlier U.S. government policy that cleared the way for us to become unwilling lab rats.

The Great Soy Hoax: "Miracle Food" Exposed as Toxic Burden

For years now, you've been hearing about the miraculous benefits of soy-based products as a "healthy" meat substitute.

In 1999, the FDA endorsed soy protein as a way to lower saturated fats and cholesterol in the American diet, leading to an explosion in the food industry's use of soy-based products.

But let me ask you a question: Would you willingly eat something that causes nausea, gas pains, and indigestion? That leads to hormonal imbalance, thyroid problems, gout, and even cancer? That contains "bad" fats and other unhealthy substances? That has no positive effect whatsoever on heart health?

Of course, you wouldn't.

But beneath all the soy-health hoopla, I've found studies strongly suggesting that many of these products pose a number of serious health risks.

REVEALED: the Five Big Dangers of Soy

In the journal *Circulation*, the American Heart Association announced that soy has little effect on cholesterol and is unlikely to prevent heart disease.[13]

This isn't meant to suggest that all types of soy are unhealthy. But it proves that soy isn't the "miracle food" the FDA and the food industry would have you believe.

Here are five reasons why that's bad news for your health.

1. Indigestion and Blockage of Key Nutrients:

The problems start with the soybean itself. In raw form, it's poisonous to the human body. In fact, eating raw soy can cause stomachaches, nausea, cramping, and gas. Other soy ingredients prevent the body from absorbing essential minerals. Ironically, soy also makes it more difficult for the body to digest protein, the very thing soy was supposed to provide as an alternative to meat protein.

2. Boost of Feminizing Estrogen:

Even more serious, soybeans contain substances called "isoflavones" that mimic estrogen, the female hormone. Eating enough soy can disrupt a woman's menstrual cycle. One researcher calculated that, based on body weight, feeding your baby exclusively on soy formula is like giving it *five birth control pills a day*![14]

3. Gout and Thyroid Disruption:

As if that weren't enough, there's a chemical in soy that can cause gout and thyroid enlargement. Eating as little as 45 grams of soy products a day (about three-quarters of a cup of tofu, for instance) can cause thyroid malfunction within three months in healthy adult men and women.[15]

4. Cancer and Harmful Fats:

Soy causes cancer in animal studies.[16] (By the way, soy makes its way into most industrial animal feed, which means it's also making its way to your table.) It's also high in omega-6 fatty acids — up to 18% of the whole bean. This is the kind of fat we're supposed to reduce in our diet.

5. Dangerous Clotting of Red Blood Cells:

Another chemical in soy makes red blood cells cluster together. Among other dangers, this prevents the body from absorbing oxygen.

There's Only One Safe Way to Eat Soy

The Asian diet is famous for its heavy use of soy-based products like tofu and soy sauce. So why aren't the Japanese suffering from the ill effects of soy?

Their soy is not genetically modified, and they don't process it industrially.

Fermented soy-derived foods like tempeh, miso, and natto do not contain significant amounts of soy's toxins.

Tofu, also a staple in traditional Asian cuisine, is not a fermented soy product. But the process of making tofu removes most of the harmful toxins in a different way.

Like some cheeses, tofu is made from the pressed "curds" of the bean, while the "whey," or liquid left over after the pressing, is thrown out — and most of the toxins along with it.

How to Avoid the Franken-Food Monster

- **Avoid processed foods whenever possible.** I always recommend eating whole foods, grass-fed beef, and other minimally processed food products, across the board. These energize your body and give you vigor, strength, and long-term health.

- **Check the label**. Soy byproducts are everywhere, and they go by many (FDA-approved) names. Here are the ones to look out for:

1. Vegetable protein;

2. Soy protein isolate;

3. Soy flour;

4. Protein concentrate;

5. Textured vegetable protein;

6. Vegetable oil;

7. Plant sterols.

Now I'm not saying small amounts of this stuff will kill you, but it's best to be aware of how much you're consuming, given the potential health hazards. If you find these ingredients on the label, try to find substitutes without them.

- **Limit your overall soy intake to a maximum of 25 grams per day**. This isn't as easy as calorie counting, but again, it's worth watching how much soy and soy-based products are finding their way into your diet.

- **Stick to traditional soy foods**. Tofu (in moderation), tempeh, miso, natto, and soy sauce are all fine. Other kinds of foods that substitute soy for meat, like soy-based hot dogs, aren't healthy alternatives.

- **Buy organic whenever you can**. The safest foods are certified-organic foods. If your grocer doesn't carry organic foods, let them know you'll shop elsewhere if they don't begin stocking them.

- **Stick with "non-GMO" labeled dairy products and other packaged foods**. This can be tricky, because the manufacturers of genetically modified foods are lobbying hard to get "non-GMO" labels banned. But for now, they're still legal. And, in my opinion, a good sign that these foods are safer.

- **Grow your own, when you can**. Non-GMO seed companies have moved much of their seed production to Europe and Asia, where contamination is less likely. American agribusiness giants have less clout in these countries, and untainted seeds are still available. Also, you may be able to get seeds from farms in places like North Carolina that grow non-GMO soybeans for the Japanese market.

- **Let your members of Congress and the Senate know you're concerned** about this issue and demand that genetically modified crops be banned until proven safe.

---

[1] Lawrence, F. "Should we worry about soya in our food?" The Guardian. July 25, 2006

[2] Rackis, et al."Evaluation of the Health Aspects of Soy Protein Isolates as Food Ingredients." prepared for FDA by Life Sciences Research Office, Federation of American Societies for Experimental Biology1979, pg 22.

[3] Stilwell M, Van Dyke B. "Codex, Substantial Equivalence and WTO Threats to National GMO Labeling Schemes." CIEL. 1998.

[4] A) "Tryptophan produced by Showa Denko and epidemic eosinophilia-myalgia syndrome." National Center for Biotechnology Information. October 1996.
   B) Fagan, John B. "Tryptophan Summary." Holistic Medicine Web Page. November 1997.
   C) "Toxic L-tryptophan: Shedding Light on a Mysterious Epidemic." Seeds of Deception "Genetically Modified Foods." American Academy of Environmental Medicine.

[5] "Genetically Modified Foods." American Academy of Environmental Medicine. 2015.

[6] Harlander S. "Safety Assessments and Public Concern for Genetically Modified Food Products: The American View." *Toxicologic Pathology.* 2002;30(1):132-134

[7] FinamoreA, et al. "Intestinal and Peripheral Immune Response to MON810 Maize Ingestion in Weaning and Old Mice." *J. Agric. Food Chem.* 2008;56(23):11533–11539.

[8] Kiliç A, Akay M. "A three generation study with genetically modified Bt corn in

rats: Biochemical and histopathological investigation." *Food Chem Toxicol.* Mar. 2008;46(3):1164-70.

9 Poulsen, M., et al., "A 90-day safety study in Wistar rats fed genetically modified rice expressing snowdrop lectin Galanthus nivalis (GNA)." *Food Chem Toxicol.* Mar. 2007;45(3):350-63.

10 Domingo, J.L., "Toxicity studies of genetically modified plants: a review of the published literature." *Crit. Rev. Food Sci. Nutr.* 2007;47(8):721-33.

11 "Do Seed Companies Control GM Crop Research?" *Scientific American.* July 20, 2009.

12 "The seeds of bribery scandal in Indonesia." *Asia Times Online.* January 20, 2005.

13 Sacks Frank, et al. "Soy Protein, Isoflavones, and Cardiovascular Health. An American Heart Association Science Advisory for Professionals From the Nutrition Committee." *Circulation.* 2006, 113:1034.

14 Lawrence, F. "Should we worry about soy in our food? *The Guardian.* July 25, 2006.

15 Nestor J. "Too Much of a Good Thing? Controversy rages over the world's most regaled legume." SFGate.com, August 13, 2006.

16 Rackis J, et al. "The USDA trypsin inhibitor study, Background, objectives and procedural details." *Qualification of Plant Foods in Human Nutrition.* 1985;35.

Chapter 7

Is Frankenbug in Your Food?

Frankenbug is loose on the farm, and no one knows what will happen next.

A brand-new microscopic bug that never existed before in nature is now in animal feed that comes from genetically engineered crops. And this Frankenbug has been clearly linked to infertility and miscarriage in cattle, horses, pigs, sheep, and poultry.[1]

A letter by a respected professor at Purdue University, written to agriculture secretary Tom Vilsack, warned of a "microscopic pathogen that appears to significantly impact the health of plants, animals, and probably human beings."

Prof. Don M. Huber, a member of the government's own USDA National Plant Disease Recovery System, said the pathogen has evolved **because of GMO crops.**

Fortunately, some courageous members of Congress introduced a proposed law that would make Big-Agra companies — that are forcing their genetically modified food on you — label their products as "GMO" (genetically modified organism) or "GE" (genetically engineered).

I'm glad we have a few elected officials who will stand up to the giant Agribusiness companies that control our food supply. And I hope more will join them.

The House bill, called "The GE Food Right to Know Act," is a good first step.

In the meantime there are plenty of states that are looking to pass their own laws to force manufacturers to tell you when GMOs are in your food. Vermont, Connecticut, and California all have bills or ballot initiatives going.

There's even a coalition of about 450 groups, including health, agriculture, faith, parenting, and environmental organizations, that have a campaign and website called "Just Label It."

Because, as it stands right now, the crops and animals that are genetically tampered with are **not regulated.**

That's bad enough, but what troubles me even more is that if the food you're eating has been tampered with genetically, **no one has to tell you.**

Not only that, they don't have to release the studies on the effects of these foods, because the companies are private. Private companies don't have to release any information to you or anyone.

Let me give you an example.

Do you drink milk?

Monsanto, one of the worst GMO offenders in the world, genetically engineered a growth hormone to give to milking cows.

The FDA was shown *Monsanto's own study* on the hormone's safety. In other words, they saw exactly one study, and it was done by Monsanto itself. Monsanto tested this stuff, called rBGH, for only 90 days on only 30 rats.

The study was never published anywhere, nor was it peer reviewed like most scientific studies. Yet the FDA stated the results showed no significant problems and gave its okay for the hormone to be used on commercial milking cows.

But wait, it gets worse. In Canada, where Monsanto originally tried to strong arm the Canadian government into approving rBGH, scientists did their own rBGH study. They found some of the male rats developed cysts on their thyroids and abnormalities in their prostates.[2]

And rBGH can also cause mastitis in the cows. This is an infection brought on by inflammation that can cause pus and blood to be secreted into the milk.

Canadian government scientists testified that they were being pressured by higher-ups to approve rBGH against their better scientific judgment. And after eight years of study, Canada rejected Monsanto's application for approval of rBGH, joining the European Union, Japan, Australia, and New Zealand, which have all banned rBGH because of health concerns.

The U.S. government, on the other hand, continues to approve genetically modified milk. And crops, too. The government considers these crops safe and doesn't even regulate them.

What makes this an even bigger problem is that glyphosate, the weed killer Monsanto markets as Roundup and has modified the crops to resist, actually promotes these kinds of pathogens, or Frankenbugs.

Frankenbugs Transmitted to People

These new microscopic bugs that didn't exist until GMO crops were created can hurt plants, remove the plants' nutrients, and hurt the animals that eat the crops, too.[3]

Professor Huber says the new pathogen increases in soil treated with glyphosate, is then taken up by plants, and is transmitted to animals via their feed, and onward to people by the plants and meat we consume.

Monsanto has tried hard to discredit Prof. Huber.[4] But researchers have already proven that you can't trust what Monsanto says about what its weed killer does. Glyphosate has been found to kill human placental cells at concentrations below what's been approved by regulators. Roundup is lethal at even lower concentrations.[5]

And their GMO crops? Evidence of the dangers is leaking out from Europe, Russia, and many other countries around the world.

Here are just some of their findings:[6,7,8,9,10,11]

- Allergies increased. When GMO soy was introduced, allergies jumped by 50%. Allergen proteins were *seven times higher.* Some were unique *only* to GMO soy.

- It wreaked havoc on digestion and the absorption of nutrients. Digestive enzymes plummeted, and GMOs caused lesions in the digestive tract.

- Proteins that control stress response and energy creation in cells changed. This resulted in faster aging of cells.

- It caused reproductive problems. Sperm cells had trouble developing, and embryos showed altered genes. Offspring were smaller, and many more died.

So why do we need a Congressional act to force manufacturers to label their food as GMO when it should be the law that they do it?

The FDA ruled that GMO foods were not "materially" different from other foods, so they didn't need labels. You see, the Federal Food, Drug, and Cosmetic Act requires the FDA to stop misleading food labels that leave out "material" information.

But the FDA has limited that to what you or I can taste, smell, or otherwise sense.

Geneticall Engineered Food on the Market							
Product	Insecticide	Herbivore Tolerant	Hybridization	Disease Resistant	Altered Value	Altered Oil	Corporation
Canola	•						Bayer
Canola	•					•	Monsanto
Canola		•	•				Bayer
Chicory			•				Beyo Zaden

Crop							Company
Corn		•	•				Bayer
Corn		•					Bayer
Corn	•	•					Bayer
Corn		•					Dow/Mycogen
Corn	•	•					Dow/Mycogen/DuPont/Pioneer
Corn			•				DuPont/Pioneer
Corn	•						Monsanto/Dekalb
Corn		•					Monsanto/Dekalb
Corn	•						Monsanto
Corn	•	•					Monsanto
Corn		•					Monsanto
Corn	•						Synergia
Corn (pop)	•						Synergia
Corn (sweet)	•						Synergia
Cotton	•	•					Monsanto/Bayer
Cotton		•					Monsanto/Bayer
Cotton	•						Monsanto
Cotton		•					Monsanto
Flax		•					UnivSaskatchewan
Papaya				•			Cornell/Univ/Univ Hawaii
Potato	•						Monsanto
Soybean		•					Bayer
Soybean						•	DuPont
Soybean	•						Monsanto
Squash				•			Seminis Vegetable Seed
Sugarbeet	•						Bayer
Sugarbeet	•						Monsanto/Syngenta
Tomato					•		Agritope
Tomato					•		DNA Plant Technology
Tomato					•		Monsanto/Calgene
Tomato					•		Monsanto
Tomato					•		Zeneca/PetoSeed

Source: Union of Concerned Scientist; "Guides; Geneticall Engineered Foods Allowed on the Market"

And, because GMOs can't be detected by your senses, the food with GMOs is "substantially equivalent" to regular food according to the FDA. Companies, therefore, don't have to label foods as containing GMOs.

But until the "Right to Know" act is passed, I want to help you avoid foods with genetically modified organisms. Here's what I recommend:

For starters, beware of any food that has canola oil or corn in it. Seventy-five percent of canola and 73% of corn crops grown in the U.S. are GMO, according to the USDA. It's gotten so bad that even bees can't find nectar to make honey without getting it from GMO canola.

Even if the label says organic, most foods you buy with these in it will have been genetically changed. The good news is canola oil is not a healthy oil anyway, so you're not missing anything. Stick with healthier oils like olive, sunflower, or safflower.

Next, eliminate as much commercial beef and poultry from your food as you can. They are raised on GMO corn, soy, and grains. Instead, choose meat from another farm with pasture-raised animals.

As far as soy goes, most people would tell you to stay away from all soy because so much of it has been genetically modified. But I don't want you to deprive yourself. And the Japanese have enjoyed soy for hundreds of years. They simply use non-GMO soy, and instead of processing it, they ferment it naturally so you can eat it.

Natto, tempeh, and tofu are made from soy, but in Japan they use non-GMO organic soy. In fact, the soy that's grown here and sold to Japan by companies like Sow True Seed has to be GMO-free or the Japanese won't allow it into their country. The Non-GMO Sourcebook at *nongmosourcebook.com* tells you how and where to get non-GMO seeds and who sells non-GMO soy products.

Here is another good source — the Non-GMO Report site at *non-gmoreport.com*. Just click on "resources" on the left-hand menu. You'll see links to resources, companies, and even test kits.

And for news, there's the European Union's GM Watch at *gmwatch. eu.*

---

[1] Wetzel D. "Don Huber's Warning to Vilsack and his Cover Letter." *Green Pasture.* Mar. 30, 2011. Retrieved Dec. 14, 2011.

[2] Gilbert S. "More Bad News for Monsanto." *New York Times.* 1999. Retrieved Dec. 22, 2011.

[3] A.U. "Emergency! Pathogen New to Science Found in Roundup Ready GM Crops?" Institute of Science In Society. Retrieved February 27, 2012.

[4] Tukey P, "Monsanto begins smear campaign on Huber." *Safe Lawns Blog,* February, 2011. Retrieved Feb 27, 2012.

[5] Ho M, Cummins J. "Glyphosate toxic & Roundup worse." Institute of Science In Society. Dec 2005. Retrieved Feb 27, 2012.

[6] Smith, J. "Genetic Roulette: The Documented Health Risks of Genetically Engineered Foods." Yes! Books, Fairfield, IA USA 2007.

[7] Malatesta M, et al. "Ultrastructural analysis of pancreatic acinar cells from mice fed on genetically modified soybean." *J Anat.* 2002;201(5):409-415.

[8] Tudisco R, et al. "Genetically modified soya bean in rabbit feeding: detection of DNA fragments and evaluation of metabolic effects by enzymatic analysis." *Animal Science.* 2006;82:193-199.

[9] Vecchio, L, et al. "Ultrastructural analysis of testes from mice fed on genetically modified soybean." *European Journal of Histochemistry.* 2004;48(4):449-454.

[10] A.U. "Genetically modified soy affects posterity: results of Russian scientists' studies." *REGNUM.* 2005; regnum.ru. Retrieved February 27, 2012.

[11] Ermakova I. "Genetically modified soy leads to the decrease of weight and high mortality of rat pups of the first generation. Preliminary studies." *Ecosinform* 1. 2006;4-9.

Chapter 8

Chemical Warfare Camouflaged in Food

How to Win the Battle for Your Dinner Table

They're in every grocery store — brightly colored boxes of prepared foods loudly claiming how healthy they are.

But they're not what you think.

Unfortunately, nearly all of the prepackaged "low fat," "low carb," and "heart healthy" meals lining the shelves at the market are just shadows of real food, with literally no nutritional value.

Yet we're buying them in droves. In 2006 alone, the combined sales of *just the top four brands* of diet foods reached a whopping $1.925 billion. Talk about a health disaster in the making!

I'll uncover the hidden dangers of eating these chemically enhanced "health" foods, and how you can stay healthy by eating the way nature intended.

The Chemical 'Mind Control' of Packaged Food

Most people think of "flavor" as something that comes directly from the food it tastes like. For instance, most people assume that strawberry flavor comes from squeezing a bunch of strawberries and extracting the flavor from the concentrate.

But the truth is something else entirely.

The strawberry flavor found in many diet food snacks and desserts is made up of *50 different chemicals!* So your mind is tricked into believing that you're eating the flavor of fresh picked strawberries. It's kind of like mind control — your whole taste function is "hypnotized."

The science that goes into flavor making is quite advanced. And it's a closely guarded secret. An elite group of chemists create these mind tricks. Companies call them "flavorists," and they pay them a lot of money. After all, it is their art that really drives sales.

If something doesn't taste good, people won't buy it — plain and simple.

Corporate Fat Cats Know...
You Couldn't Stand Their Food *without* Tricks

Why do companies have to add "flavors"?

It's because the act of processing the food strips the flavor right out of it. Imagine what it takes to prepare a prepackaged "low-fat" roast beef dinner.

First, a factory processes the beef to remove the fat. While they're at it, they add chemicals to make sure it doesn't spoil. Then they add more chemicals, in the form of food colors, to make it look more appealing.

Next, they sterilize the food and cook it to excess to ensure there is no risk of bacterial contamination. Then it's tossed through handling and packaging machinery and sent to another machine where it's ultimately frozen.

With the extreme heat, machine handling and extended exposure to air, more vital nutrients are lost with each passing second.

It's a far cry from the roast beef dinner I used to eat on the farm when I was growing up. I'd ride with my dad to pick up a fresh roast from the butcher. Then my mom would cook it. The only processing it went through was a mouth-watering, slow roasting in the oven.

But a factory-prepared dinner — before added colors and flavors — would taste (and smell) bland, lifeless, and sterile. It definitely wouldn't make your mouth water!

That's where the flavorist comes to the rescue. You see, he's created a delicious new "roast beef" flavor. And it's *very* convincing.

If you were to close your eyes and smell their carefully crafted clear liquid potion, you'd swear someone had been slow cooking a perfectly seasoned pot roast all day in a Crock-Pot.

In other words, one micro-drop of this stuff and you'll think that mechanized, frozen roast beef dinner is as good as Mom used to make. But it's all a dangerous trick. These foods are chemical weapons in a box, plain and simple.

Could that Yummy 'Butter' Smell in Microwave Popcorn Give You Lung Disease?

The next time you open a bag of freshly popped microwave popcorn and take a big whiff of the buttery goodness inside, remember this. Hundreds of workers at popcorn plants that dealt with this butter flavoring have contracted a rare, irreversible, deadly lung disease called bronchiolitis obliterans. It's even known as "popcorn lung."

Popcorn lung is caused by inhaling butter flavoring made from diacetyl.[1] Diacetyl is that yellow liquid you may mistake for actual butter in your microwave popcorn. It smells like it, tastes like it, and it even looks like it.

And it's not just factory workers. There have been a couple of cases of popcorn lung in consumers as well.[2] Certainly, the cases were of people who consumed large quantities of microwave popcorn. However, since microwave popcorn has only been around since 1983, it's difficult to say what the long-term exposure to it will bring.

Plus, it's hard to tell if there are others. The disease is so rare it is often misdiagnosed — even in those who work in popcorn factories — as asthma, bronchitis, emphysema or pneumonia.[3] And the symptoms are innocuous — progressive, gradual shortness of breath, fatigue, wheezing, and coughing. You don't know that you have it until you need a lung transplant.

The government has been aware of this threat since at least 2000,[4] and is just now "fast tracking" the regulation of diacetyl handling for factory workers. Yet the FDA continues to give diacetyl its GRAS — generally recognized as safe — label, despite calls from the medical community for it to investigate the dangers further.[5]

This is just one example of the dangers lurking in these chemical concoctions.

The fact of the matter is that the FDA is asleep at the wheel when it comes to food safety. In its response to those calling for a ban on diacetyl, the FDA said it didn't reach a decision due to "limited availability of resources and other agency priorities."

In other words, the FDA fails to act even when it is handed evidence that a substance poses a threat.

Over the years, the FDA has banned 23 artificial flavors, colors, and preservatives in the U.S. Most were deemed unsafe only after years and years of human consumption. For example, it took 50 years for the FDA to ban the food dye Orange No.1 when it was shown to cause organ damage.

Plus, even when the FDA recommends banning a dangerous food additive, it can be overruled. Take Red Dye No.3, for example. The FDA proposed banning this common food dye back in 1983, but the Reagan administration chose otherwise. And it's still on the market today.

Likewise, the FDA wanted to ban saccharin in 1977. But the political forces at play at the time lobbied to keep it in use. And in 1997, the diet food industry pressured the government to remove saccharin from its list of cancer-causing chemicals altogether.

Still, several food additives are the target of independent food safety organizations today, including Red Dye No.3, saccharin, sodium nitrate/nitrite, potassium bromate, aspartame, and others.[6]

Take a look at the chart.

Ingredient	Used in	Caution
Blue 1	Beverages, candy, baked goods.	Suggestions of a small cancer risk.
Blue 2	Pet food, beverages, candy.	The largest study suggested, but did not prove, that this dye caused brain tumors in male mice.
Green 3	Candy, beverages.	A 1981 industry-sponsored study gave hints of bladder cancer.

Red 3	Cherries in fruit cocktail, candy, baked goods.	The evidence that this dye caused thyroid tumors in rats is "convincing," according to a 1983 review committee report requested by FDA.
Yellow 6	Beverages, sausage, baked goods, candy, gelatin.	Animal tests indicate causes tumors of the adrenal gland and kidney. In addition, small amounts of several carcinogens contaminate Yellow 6.
Sodium Nitrite, Sodium Nitrate	Bacon, ham, frankfurters, luncheon meats, smoked fish, corned beef.	Several studies have linked, but don't prove, consumption of cured meat and nitrite by children, pregnant women, and adults with various types of cancer.
Potassium Bromate	White flour, bread and rolls.	Causes cancer in animals. The tiny amounts of bromate that may remain in bread pose a small risk to consumers. Banned virtually worldwide except in Japan and the United States.
Saccharin	Diet, no-sugar-added products, soft drinks, sweetener packets.	Animal studies link to cancer of the bladder, uterus, ovaries, skin, blood vessels, and other organs. Increases the potency of other cancer-causing chemicals.
Aspartame	"Diet" foods, including soft drinks, drink mixes, gelatin desserts, low-calorie frozen desserts, packets.	Brain tumors in rats; lymphomas and leukemias, mammary (breast) cancer.
Acesulfame-K	Baked goods, chewing gum, gelatin desserts, diet soda.	Two rat studies suggest that the additive might cause cancer. In addition, large doses of acetoacetamide, a breakdown product, have been shown to affect the thyroid in rats, rabbits, and dogs.

Butylated Hydroxyanisole (BHA)	Cereals, chewing gum, potato chips, vegetable oil.	U.S. Department of Health and Human Services considers BHA to be "reasonably anticipated to be a human carcinogen."
Propyl Gallate	Vegetable oil, meat products, potato sticks, chicken soup base, chewing gum.	The best studies on rats and mice were peppered with suggestions (but not proof) that this preservative might cause cancer.
Olestra (Olean)	Lay's Light Chips, Pringles Light chips.	Diarrhea and loose stools, abdominal cramps, flatulence, and other adverse effects.
Trans Fats	Stick margarine, crackers, fried restaurant foods, baked goods, icing, microwave popcorn.	Promotes heart disease.

Source: Center for Science in the Public Interest

Bottom line: It's better to be safe than sorry. Avoid these packaged chemical weapons as much as possible, and concentrate on getting your nutrition from *real* foods.

Three Ways to Eat *Real* Food

Power up Your Metabolism with Protein — Your body stores fat when it doesn't get the fuel and nutrition it really needs. And your body relies on protein as the main source of fuel for every function in the body.

So when you don't get enough, your body thinks "Times are tough" and stores fat to use as fuel.

Eating more protein will tell your metabolism that it doesn't need fat. Besides, a thick, juicy steak is not only healthier for you than microwave "low-fat" lasagna — it is more satisfying.

But make sure you eat *grass-fed beef* only. Traditional beef is grain fed. This artificial diet makes the meat harmful because it changes the composition of fats in the animal.

Another great protein choice is eggs. They have every amino acid you need in perfect ratio. It's the most complete source of protein you can eat. And contrary to popular myth, they don't cause heart problems.

They help prevent them because they contain "good fats."

Choose Your Carbs Wisely — Most experts miss the point of "low carb." It's not about sugar or sweetness. It's about *starch*. Starch spikes the blood sugar and triggers insulin.

Insulin's job is to manage blood sugar and *build body fat*. So the higher the spike, the more insulin gets produced and the more fat is made.

You can find out how foods spike your blood sugar by using a *glycemic index*. You can find it in the back of this book. It gives the percentage on a scale of one to 100 of how a food will raise your blood sugar compared to pure glucose.

For maximum health, eat foods with 40 or less on the glycemic index.

Eat the Right Fats — Eating the right kind of fat is critical to feeling your best. Fats of all types play vital roles in nearly every function in the body.[7]

Here are the fats you need, and the ones you need to avoid:

- **Eat More Omega-3s** — Omega-3s protect you from cardiovascular disease. Eat plenty of fish, avocado, walnuts, and olives. Cod liver oil, Sacha Inchi oil, and nuts are also great sources.

- **Eat More Animal Fats** — Saturated fats are not only less dangerous than the media would have you believe, they're also vital to your health. They help your body absorb calcium[8] and boost your immune system[9] among many other things.

In fact, if you deprive yourself of animal fats, you're robbing yourself of what you need to absorb vitamins.

The best sources of saturated fats are pasture-grazed meats and other naturally produced animal products.

Choose Whole Foods — A whole food is a food that you can pick right out of the ground or off of the tree and eat it. It doesn't require any processing or packaging. Think apples rather than applesauce. Walnuts are a great whole food. Just be sure to look for organic fruits, vegetables, and nuts. Or, better yet, plant your own garden, and really take charge of the food you eat!

[1] FG van Rooy et al. "Bronchiolitis obliterans syndrome in chemical workers producing diacetyl for food flavorings," *American Journal of Respiratory and Critical Care Medicine*. 2007.

[2] Reuters UK. "FDA to probe popcorn link in man's lung disease," Sep. 5, 2007.

[3] US Dept. of Labor Occupational Safety and Health Administration. "Hazard Communication Guidance For Diacetyl And Food Flavorings Containing Diacetyl."

[4] Centers for Disease Control and Prevention. "Fixed obstructive lung disease in a microwave popcorn factory-Missouri," 2000-2002.

[5] Food and Drug Administration. "2006P-0379: To Urge the FDA's Prompt Action to Cancel the GRAS Designation for Diacetyl Until Testing is Complete and the Results are Independently Evaluated."

[6] Chemical Cuisine Learn about Food Additives." Center for Science in the Public Interest. 2014.

[7] Enig M, Fallon, S. "The Skinny On Fats." Weston A. Price Foundation. January 1, 2000.

[8] Watkins, B A, and M F Seifert, "Food Lipids and Bone Health," Food Lipids and Health, R E McDonald and D B Min, eds, p 101, Marcel Dekker, Inc, New York, NY, 1996.

[9] Kabara, J J, The Pharmacological Effects of Lipids, The American Oil Chemists Society, Champaign, IL, 1978, 1-14; Cohen, L A, et al,. *J Natl Cancer Inst*, 1986, 77:43.

Chapter 9

If You're Eating This Fish You Might as well Eat a Doughnut

Last weekend, my sister came into town out of the blue, and we went out to dinner to celebrate. She glanced at the menu and then put it down, saying, "I gotta eat healthy when I'm with you. I'll have the tilapia."

Most people are shocked when they hear the truth about tilapia. After all, it's fish. It's supposed to be good for you. The power of the omega-3s in fish is all over the news. Salmon is still the most popular, but tilapia is gaining on it because it has a mild taste and it's inexpensive.

But here's the thing: Eat tilapia and you get the same amount of "bad fats" as a typical doughnut!

The tilapia served as the "catch of the day" in restaurants across the country is usually farm raised. And researchers from Wake Forest University found that farm-raised tilapia has more omega-6s than bacon, doughnuts and hamburger.[1]

Instead of being good for your heart, it's flooding your body with inflammation — the main culprit behind heart disease! And on top of that, it's pumped full of gender-bending hormones!

The Real Dark Side of Fat

It's not that omega-6s are necessarily bad for you. They are essential fatty acids that your body needs. But we get so much of them that our bodies often have an unhealthy ratio of omega-6s to omega-3s.

In fact, the average American has an omega-6 to omega-3 ratio of 20:1. Your ideal ratio should be just 2:1. So, you need to eat foods that are high in omega-3s to balance out the omega-6s.

Unfortunately, farm-raised tilapia isn't a great source.

The omega-6 to omega-3 ratio in farm-raised tilapia is a whopping 11:1. Keep eating it, and it will do nothing to balance out the high levels of omega-6s in your body. It'll do just the opposite.

Those high levels of omega-6s can lead to obesity, diabetes, fatigue, and memory loss. They also cause dangerous inflammation in your body that leads to many health problems, including joint pain and heart disease.

You see, farm-raised tilapia has less than half a gram of omega-3s per 3.5 ounces of fish.[2] That's probably the lowest you'll find in any fish. Even farm-raised salmon has 12 times more omega-3s and farm-raised trout has four times more. In contrast, wild-caught salmon has 22 times more omega-3s than tilapia.

What makes tilapia so bad for you? It's the corn diet the fish are fed. Most wild-caught fish eat greens — or other fish that eat greens — which supplies them with omega-3s.

Corn, however, is loaded with omega-6s. When the fish eat the corn, they convert the omega-6s into arachidonic acid, the main cause of dangerous inflammation in the body.

Fish Undergoing Sex Changes

The fact that tilapia has too much omega-6 and not enough omega-3 fatty acids is reason enough not to waste your time eating it. But did you also know that young tilapia are pumped full of hormones that turn them all into males?

You see, farm-raised tilapia are kept in enclosed ponds and breed like crazy. It takes them just two to three months to mature and then they breed once a month. You might think this overabundance of fish would be good, but it causes overcrowding in the ponds and ends up stunting the growth of the fish.

So, the producers get an uneven harvest — some small, deformed fish and some larger fish (generally the male ones). In order to get a uniform "catch" of larger tilapia, fish farmers feed the stock the hormone 17 alpha-methyltestosterone, which turns all the fish into males.

This lets the fish farmers produce bigger fish in a shorter period for higher profits. No wonder this fish is becoming more popular every day. It's inexpensive. And its mild, white meat appeals to many consumers.

The hormone treatment is the chosen method used by tilapia farmers worldwide.[3] That means that just about all tilapia sold in supermarkets here in the U.S. are fed methyltestosterone.

There aren't any long-term studies to tell if this hormone is safe in humans eating tilapia. But the hormone itself is toxic to the liver and has been taken off the market in Germany.

This steady diet of corn and hormones just isn't the diet nature intended.

The Healthy Side of Omega-3s

Before the days of modern industry, your fish had abundant supplies of omega-3s. They dined on seaweed or algae and other fish below them in the food chain that ate these plants.

But these days, even some salmon has little to none of these essential fats. Farm-raised fish are fed corn, soy, those fish flakes that you feed the fish in your aquarium, and other unnatural foods.

Since your body can't make omega-3s on its own, it's critical that you find ways to get a steady supply through the proper food sources and supplements.

The benefits are practically endless when your body gets enough omega-3s. Many of my own patients have not only reversed disease but improved their mental and emotional lives as well. Omega-3s have been shown to:

- Prevent heart disease, cancer — even strokes;
- Lower blood pressure;
- Wipe out arthritis pain;
- Relieve depression;
- Lower triglycerides (blood fat);
- Raise HDL (good cholesterol);
- Boost memory and brain power;

- Lower your risk of macular degeneration;
- Protect blood vessels and nerves;
- Calm irregular heart rhythms, which can lead to sudden cardiac death.

Find the Best Fish for Your Omega-3s

Don't abandon fish altogether. They are still a great source of omega-3s.

I've put together a chart of the fish with the best ratios of omega-3s to omega-6s.

Omega-3 to Omega-6 Ratio of Wild-Caught and Farm-Raised Fish			
Wild Sockeye Salmon	19:1	Flounder	3:1
Wild Coho Salmon	10:1	Farmed Eel	3:1
Wild Trout	7:1	Farmed Salmon	2:1
Wild Eel	5:1	Black Bass	2:1
Cod	5:1	Farmed Catfish	2:1
Farmed Trout	4:1	Farmed Tilapia	1:11
Halibut	4:1	Swordfish	1:11

Source: *Journal of Diet Assoc* (July 2008); *American Journal of Clinical Nutrition* (1990)

As you can see, there are a number of fish varieties from which to choose that will give you the heart-healthy omega-3s you need.

Here are my general rules when shopping for fish:

Avoid Apex-Predator Fish. While tuna (albacore and bluefin) have good amounts of omega-3s, you should avoid them because they tend to contain high levels of toxins like mercury. Overall, stay away from top-of-the-food-chain fish like tuna, shark, swordfish, tilefish, and king mackerel because of their mercury levels.

Choose Smaller Fish. Try to stick to smaller fish that are lower down on the food chain. They don't typically eat other fish and fewer toxins get stored in their flesh. Good choices are herring, salmon, sardines, anchovies, trout, halibut, and haddock.

Always Buy Wild-Caught Fish. Farm-raised fish are simply fed an unnatural diet and become diseased and inflamed. The potential health risks could cost your body in the long run.

Because farm-raised fish don't have lots of room to swim and are prone to disease, they are often given antibiotics as well as preservatives and commercial dyes to give them a healthy color.[4]

For example, farm-raised salmon is not the nice pink color that you would see with wild salmon, so it is injected with dye. At your supermarket you will often see "color-enhanced" in small print under the farm-raised salmon sign.

Wild salmon, on the other hand, get their pink color from eating little sea creatures like krill. I prefer wild-caught salmon from the Pacific Ocean.

You can find good quality wild-caught fish at specialty markets such as Whole Foods or Fresh Market. I often order mine online from Grassland Beef (www.grasslandbeef.com) or Alaskan Harvest Seafood (www.alaskanharvest.com). It comes right to your door, fresh, packed in dry ice.

Make up for the Critical Nutrients You're Missing

Since your body doesn't make enough omega-3 fatty acids on its own, choosing species of fish that have the highest levels of omega-3s is one way to get your daily supply.

But this is not always possible, so supplementing with a good quality fish oil that is purified of contaminants is a sensible way to make sure you get enough to reap the health benefits.

There are two supplements I recommend.

Fish oil. I recommend taking an 1100 mg. fish oil supplement every day. I've developed a new fish oil capsule that comes from the pristine, non-industrial waters off the coast of Peru. It's safe, pure and provides a huge, healthy dose of omega-3s.

Cod liver oil. Cod liver oil is another great source of omega-3s. One teaspoon a day will give you the omega-3s you need. And I've developed an oil without the awful taste.

[1] Wake Forest Researchers Say Popular Fish Contains Potentially Dangerous Fatty Acid Combination." Wake Forest University Baptist Medical Center. July 8, 2008.

[2] "Farmed Fish & Omegas," Acres USA, September 2008.

[3] Barbara Minton. "Drug-Induced Fish: Hormone Causes Tilapia to Undergo Sex Change". *NaturalNews.com*. 4/6/09.

[4] "Wild vs. Farm or Ocean Raised Fish," *DeliciousOrganics.com*. viewed 5/27/09.

Chapter 10

Are You a Guinea Pig in the World's Largest Ongoing Experiment?

We are all in a kind of experiment. You never agreed to take part in it. But it's triggering infertility, tumors, kidney and liver disease and more.

The federal government not only allows it to happen, they're appointing people to key positions to make the experiment official policy. Case in point: President Obama's new "food safety czar" is a former vice president at Monsanto, one of the world's most powerful Big-Agra giants.

The political lobbying, the presidential appointments and their secretive policies are helping to put untested mutations on your dinner table in the form of GMOs — genetically modified organisms.

Genetically modified foods have never been proven safe. And the test results that reveal problems never see the light of day. When you eat them, you're taking part in a global Franken-foods experiment.

The facts — the few we're allowed to know — are scary. I'll show you how and why this horror show is unfolding and what you can do to avoid the crippling side effects.

President Appoints Fox to Guard Henhouse

Our president was elected on a platform of change. But when it comes to food safety it's business as usual.

Why would I say this? Look at President Obama's choices to head the USDA and the FDA: Tom Vilsack and Michael Taylor.

Mr. Vilsack is a long-time supporter of genetically modified foods. In fact, Vilsack recently pushed his GMO agenda at the Food Security Conference in Iowa.

But Michael Taylor, the new "food safety czar," is the proverbial fox guarding the henhouse.

Taylor has a long history of lobbying for — and being employed by — Big-Agra companies with a vested interest in GMOs. Not only was Taylor a vice president at Monsanto, he was one of the FDA officials who signed off on an FDA policy stating that GMOs don't need safety testing.

And who benefits? You guessed it: Monsanto.

Court Case Uncovers Monsanto Bribes of Government Officials

Back in 2000, Monsanto wanted to plant over 49,000 acres of genetically modified cotton in Indonesia. But hours before the agreement with Indonesia's government was to be signed, it was shot down by the Ministers of Economy and Environment. There had been no environmental assessment, as required by Indonesian law.

But just five months later, the Minister of Agriculture signed the agreement with Monsanto, *without the required environmental assessment.*

Why? As it turns out, it was a $50,000 bribe from a Monsanto employee that did the trick.

But that $50,000 was just the tip of the iceberg. As it turned out in U.S. court, Monsanto had paid some $700,000 in bribes to Indonesian officials, and wound up slapped with a $1.5 million fine.[1]

According to a report in the *Asia Times*, 140 Indonesian officials received bribes from Monsanto over the deal, including a former Minister of Agriculture, whose wife received a house worth $373,990.

Now, I realize that Indonesia was known at the time for official corruption. But if the genetically modified crop was really safe, wouldn't it be easier to simply prepare the required assessment?

Even more disturbing is an earlier U.S. government policy that cleared the way for us to become unwilling lab rats.

Mutant Killers Masquerading as Real Food

When giant agricultural corporations wanted to flood the market with genetically modified seeds, there was a problem. What about safety? What were the effects of eating an ear of corn laced with pesticide? What would happen if someone ate soybeans designed to survive the potent herbicide Roundup?

Not a problem, announced the federal government. As long as these "Frankenfoods" are "substantially equivalent" to the real thing, the GMO products would be deemed safe — and made available for sale.

So, if a GMO food — or other plant — is "substantially equivalent" in composition and nutritional characteristics, *it doesn't have to be tested for safety.*

Imagine for a moment if we applied this standard to children's toys.

Let's say you have the choice between two toy trucks that are nearly identical. One is painted with red, lead-free paint with plastic wheels. The other is identical, except that the paint contains lead. In other words, the two toys are "substantially equivalent," except for one tiny detail.

Which toy would you choose for your child? Obviously, you'd choose the one without the lead paint.

So what's the problem? The two toys are substantially equivalent. They're made of the exact same materials.

There's just that one tiny difference. But that difference can send you to an early grave.

This may be a simplified example of "substantial equivalence." But it certainly points out the problems we may face when new or modified foods are allowed on your store shelves without testing.

And responsible scientists weren't shy about pointing out the problems with the policy of substantial equivalence, either.

Geneva Sounds Alarm against Using the "Substantially Equivalent" Rule...

In 1998, Geneva's Center for Environmental Law argued against the World Trade Organization accepting "substantial equivalence" as a standard for GMO safety.

They pointed out that it was inadequate to prove safety… it would undermine meaningful standards in those countries that chose to enact them… and that substantial equivalence ignored scientific research that showed "substantially equivalent" GMO foods had significant negative health impacts.[2]

Unfortunately for all of us, commercial interests won out over science.

That's bad news. The American Academy of Environmental Medicine points out that GMO foods have been linked to:

- Infertility;
- Weakened immune system;
- Accelerated aging;
- Genetic problems with cholesterol, insulin control, cell signaling, and protein formation;
- Changes in the liver, kidney, spleen and gastrointestinal system.[3]

These Franken-foods may be "substantially equivalent," but the research shows they're substantially more dangerous, too.

But I'm not just quoting wild accusations. There's plenty of solid science at work here. Take a look at some of the studies I've found.

You're Playing Russian Roulette, American Style

In the rush to please the agribusiness giants, your government has sold you out. Today, as many as 85% of the processed foods on store shelves contain genetically modified ingredients.[4]

And that's not good, if the few studies on GM foods can be believed.

In 2008, Italian researchers found that GM foods had a negative impact on the immune systems of mice.[5] Turkish scientists found evidence of liver and kidney disease in rats fed genetically modified corn.[6] And Danish researchers found enough differences in rats fed genetically modified rice to question its safety.[7]

So where are the studies? A medical researcher in Spain found that there's an almost complete lack of proof that GM foods are safe.[8] And there's a good reason why.

Scientists Forbidden from Testing GMO Crops

So where is all the research on genetically modified crops? It simply doesn't exist.

Wouldn't you think that a new technology — one that holds both great promise and great questions — would be studied to the nth degree? I sure would. But here's why GMOs haven't been studied thoroughly…

The manufacturers won't allow it.

That's right. Monsanto — and the handful of other big producers of genetically modified crops — *don't allow scientific testing.*

If you want to get your hands on GMO seeds, you have to sign an "end-user agreement," just as if you were buying software. And these end-user agreements ban testing and comparisons to other products. The only testing that happens is testing that the manufacturers approve.

As *Scientific American* points out, the only tests approved are those that the manufacturers decide are "friendly."[9]

So, are genetically modified foods safe for you to eat? Sorry. That's on a need-to-know basis. And the manufacturers have decided that *you* don't need to know.

That leaves one important question. What can you do? Fortunately, you *can* do something to protect yourself and your family from Frankenfoods.

Four Simple Steps to Protect You and Your Family

1. Whenever possible, buy organic. The safest foods are certified-organic foods. If your grocer doesn't carry organic foods, let them know you'll shop elsewhere if they don't begin stocking them.

2. Find a farmer's market in your area: Eating locally is the best way to get the freshest organic food with no trace of GMOs. Try these websites: www.farmersmarket.com or www.localharvest.org

3. For dairy products and other packaged foods, look for a "non-GMO" label. This can be tricky, because the manufacturers of genetically modified foods are lobbying hard to get "non-GMO" labels banned. But for now, they're still legal. And, in my opinion, a good sign that these foods are safer.

4. When you can, "grow your own." Non-GMO seed companies have moved much of their seed production to Europe and Asia, where contamination is less likely. American agribusiness giants have less clout in these countries, and untainted seeds are still available.

5. Let your members of Congress and the Senate know you're concerned about this issue and demand that genetically modified crops be banned until proven safe.

---

[1] The seeds of bribery scandal in Indonesia." *Asia Times Online.* January 20, 2005.

[2] Stilwell M, Van Dyke B. "Codex, Substantial Equivalence and WTO Threats to National GMO Labeling Schemes." CIEL. 1998.

[3] ibid.

[4] Harlander S. Safety Assessments and Public Concern for Genetically Modified Food Products: The American View. Toxicologic Pathology, Vol. 30, No. 1, 132-134 (2002).

[5] Alberto Finamore, et al. Intestinal and Peripheral Immune Response to MON810 Maize Ingestion in Weaning and Old Mice. J. Agric. Food Chem., 2008, 56 (23), pp 11533–11539.

[6] Kiliç A and Akay MT. A three generation study with genetically modified Bt corn in rats: Biochemical and histopathological investigation. Food Chem Toxicol. 2008 Mar;46(3):1164-70. Epub 2007 Dec 5.

[7] Poulsen M, et al. A 90-day safety study in Wistar rats fed genetically modified rice expressing snowdrop lectin Galanthus nivalis (GNA). Food Chem Toxicol. 2007 Mar;45(3):350-63. Epub 2006 Sep 14.

[8] Domingo JL. Toxicity studies of genetically modified plants: a review of the published literature. Crit Rev Food Sci Nutr. 2007;47(8):721-33.

[9] "Do Seed Companies Control GM Crop Research?" **Scientific American.** July 20, 2009.

Chapter 11

This Modern "Health Food" May Be Poisoning Prisoners

Have you heard what has been known to happen in our prison system? If not, you're in for a shocker. In one case it even caused prisoners to sue their jailers. In the Illinois prison system, the diet of inmates was drastically changed to include large amounts of processed soy protein. Soy replaced cheese, meat and flour in the prisoners' diets.

When their diet changed, the inmates got seriously ill with chronic and painful constipation, alternating with debilitating diarrhea. Sharp digestive pains and vomiting occurred after soy-based meals. Fainting, heart palpitations, and panic attacks were common. Skin rashes, acne, thyroid problems, brain fog, fatigue, weight gain, frequent infections, and depression were also present.[1]

But the Illinois Department of Corrections ignored the prisoners' complaints. It also ignored the U.S. Food and Drug Administration (FDA) listing of close to 200 studies showing toxicity of soy in its Poisonous Plant Database.[2] Now the inmates are suing for a permanent injunction against the substitution of soy for meat in prison meals.

Isn't that the way guinea pigs are treated in science labs?

For Years You've Been Hearing About the "Miraculous" Benefits of Soy-Based Products

In 1999, the FDA endorsed soy protein as a way to lower saturated fats and cholesterol in the American diet, leading to an explosion in the food industry's use of soy-based products.

But beneath all the soy-health hoopla, I've found studies strongly suggesting that many of these products pose a number of serious health risks.

I'm going to tell you which soy-based products to avoid — and why. I'll also give you a few simple guidelines for eliminating them from your diet and replacing them with healthy alternatives.

The Dangerous Realities behind the "Soy Revolution"

In the January 2006 issue of the journal *Circulation*, the American Heart Association announced that soy has little effect on cholesterol and is unlikely to prevent heart disease.[3]

As I mentioned in Chapter 5, this doesn't mean that all types of soy are unhealthy. But it proves that soy isn't the "miracle food" the FDA and the food industry would have you believe.

Soy-based products are everywhere. And that's a problem. You may not realize it, but soy crops up in unexpected places. It's in your fridge and cupboard — from ice cream and yogurt to pasta and cereal. Not to mention the frying oil used in fast food.

How did this happen?

After FDA approval, the food industry jumped on the soy bandwagon in a big way. By 2004, 80% of all vegetable oils were derived from soy, and nearly all processed foods now contain some form of it.

Here are five facts about soy:

1. Soy and Indigestion:

The problems start with the soybean itself. In raw form, it's poisonous to the human body. In fact, eating raw soy can cause stomachaches, nausea, cramping, and gas.

Other soy ingredients prevent the body from absorbing essential minerals. Ironically, soy also makes it more difficult for the body to digest protein, the very thing soy was supposed to provide as an alternative to meat protein.

2. Soy and Hormonal Imbalance:

Even more serious, soybeans contain substances called "isoflavones" that mimic estrogen, the female hormone. Eating enough soy can disrupt a woman's menstrual cycle. One researcher calculated that, based on body weight, feeding your baby exclusively on soy formula is like giving it five birth control pills a day![4]

3. Soy, Gout, and Thyroid Problems:

As if that weren't enough, there's a chemical in soy that can cause gout and thyroid enlargement. Eating as little as 45 grams of soy products a day can cause thyroid malfunction within 3 months in healthy adult men and women.[5]

4. Soy, Cancer, and Harmful Fats:

Soy causes cancer in animal studies.[6] (By the way, soy makes its way into most industrial animal feed, which means it's also making its way to your table.) It's also high in omega-6 fatty acids — up to 18% of the whole bean. This is the kind of fat you're supposed to reduce in your diet.

5. Soy and Blood Clotting:

Another chemical in soy makes red blood cells cluster together. Among other dangers, this prevents the body from absorbing oxygen.

The Difference between Good Soy and Bad Soy

The Asian diet is famous for its soy-based products such as tofu and soy sauce. But why aren't the Japanese suffering from these ill effects? The answer lies in the way soy in Asian countries is traditionally processed.

For thousands of years, ancient farmers used soy as a fertilizer, not as food. They recognized that you would never want to eat raw soy.

The Chinese introduced soy into the human diet only after discovering that the natural fermentation processes rendered it edible. Fermented soy-derived foods such as tempeh, miso, and natto do NOT contain significant amounts of soy's toxins. In fact, they're very healthy.

Tofu, also a staple in traditional Asian cuisine, is not a fermented soy product. But the process of making tofu removes most of the harmful toxins in a different way.

And like some cheeses, tofu is made from the pressed "curds" of the bean. The "whey," or liquid left over after the pressing, is thrown out — and most of the toxins along with it.

Compare this with the modern industrial processing soy undergoes in the West to produce soy oil, flour, and other soy byproducts contained in most processed foods:

- Washing in alkaline;
- Boiling in petroleum-based solvents;
- Bleaching;
- Deodorizing;
- Adding chemicals;
- Heat-blasting;
- Crushing into flakes.

Does that sound appetizing to you?

What's more, soy in this country is genetically modified. The jury is out on how this may affect human health. What we do know is that some industrial processing techniques leave trace amounts of aluminum in soy products. Dietary aluminum leads to dementia according to some studies.

Four Simple Steps to Avoid Harmful Soy Byproducts

- **Avoid processed foods whenever possible.** This should go without saying, but I always recommend eating whole foods, grass-fed beef, and other minimally processed food products, across the board. These energize your body and result in vigor, strength, and long-term health.

- **Check the label.** Soy byproducts are everywhere, and they go by many (FDA-approved) names. Here are the ones to look out for:
    1. Vegetable protein;
    2. Soy protein isolate;
    3. Soy flour;
    4. Protein concentrate;
    5. Textured vegetable protein;
    6. Vegetable oil;
    7. Plant sterols.

I'm not saying small amounts of this stuff will kill you, but it's best to be mindful of how much you're consuming, given the potential health hazards. If you find these ingredients on the label, try to find substitutes without them.

- **Stick to traditional soy foods.** Tofu (in moderation), tempeh, miso, natto, and soy sauce are all fine. Other kinds of foods that substitute soy for meat, like soy-based hot dogs, are not healthy alternatives.

- **Limit your intake of traditional soy foods to no more than 25 grams per day.** It's worth watching how much soy and soy-based products are finding their way into your diet.

---

[1] Weston A. Price Foundation — Press Release — Washington, DC July 13, 2009.

[2] "FDA Poisonous Plant Database." FDA U.S. Food and Drug Administration.

[3] Sacks FM, Lichtenstein A, et al. Soy Protein, Isoflavones, and Cardiovascular Health. An American Heart Association Science Advisory for Professionals From the Nutrition Committee. *Circulation* 2006, 113:1034.

[4] Michael Fitzpatrick, MD as quoted in Lawrence, Felicity, "Should we worry about soya in our food?, *Guardian*, July 25, 2006.

[5] Kaayla Daniel as quoted in Nestor, James, "Too Much of a Good Thing? Controversy rages over the world's most regaled legume," *SFGate.com*, August 13, 2006.

[6] Rackis J, et al. The USDA trypsin inhibitor study, Background, objectives and procedural details. *Qualification of Plant Foods in Human Nutrition*. 1985, vol 35.

Chapter 12

Converted Diehard Vegetarian: "For 14 years I felt sick, nauseated, and bloated"

More and more diehard vegetarians are becoming meat eaters. Why the change of heart? It's simple: they're plumb tired of being sick and tired.

"For 14 years I felt sick, nauseated, and bloated," says Lierre Keith. She's the author of *The Vegetarian Myth*, one of the most important books on this subject. "Anything I ate became a bowling ball lodged in my stomach."

Her stomach was distended because her digestion was damaged from her vegetarian diet. To fix it, she had to return to eating meat.

Lierre understands all the "noble" reasons that made her a vegetarian for 14 years. Her book is a compelling insight into why she now eats meat.

Most vegetarians won't admit it, even to themselves, but they just can't stand the health consequences. They have no energy. They feel frail. They're getting sick. And they're getting old before their time.

They've also damaged their digestive systems. And they can't produce hormones like growth hormone, testosterone, and thyroid hormone.

Vegetarians often look down their noses at the rest of us, thinking they're morally and politically correct. It's elitist thinking. Vegetarians don't believe they owe a debt to the energy we all share in nature. They want to remove themselves from the real world so they don't have to participate.

But in the real world, you have to participate and play the game.

It's the same game we've played successfully for millions of years until *they* wanted to change it. You borrow energy by eating meat. Then one day you get eaten, and you give it back.

Of course, you can avoid being eaten by a predator in modern times. But in the end, you're going to be eaten by something. Eventually, your carbon, nitrogen, and your energy are returned back to the earth.

We're not really at the top of the food pyramid when we eat meat. Because it's not a pyramid at all. It's a circle. And you're a part of it.

Vegetarians like Lierre who convert back to meat eating have matured. They've stopped clinging to childlike arguments and wishful thinking. They act with what the ancients call "adult knowledge."

Adult knowledge is what our primitive ancestors knew instinctively. That we're indebted to nature from the moment we're born. We're *dependent* on other living creatures.

You can't opt out of this system. Even if you're willing to compromise your health and eat plants only, there is still a price to pay…

You Still Kill Animals by Eating Vegetables

Vegetarians talk about meat eaters like they're predators. But it's not a winning moral argument. Because when you eat grains, you're killing animals, too. And worse.

Agriculture and commercial farming is one of the most destructive things we've done to our own planet. We are destroying all the creatures that depend on it.

Grain destroys the environment. It's an annual grass that requires a huge amount of resources. It depletes the topsoil and is war on the ecosystem. You have to kill off every other plant to grow grain. When you do that, you kill off every animal in the ecosystem that depends on those plants. There's nothing moral about doing that.

Even if you only eat vegetables, you're still killing animals. Commercial farming practices have taken over and destroyed prairies, fields, and forests that animals have lived in for millions of years.

But when you eat animals that live in their native environment, there are no consequences *to* the environment. The environment continues

exactly as it was before. There is no energy expenditure. All that anni-
hilation of the environment goes away.

Vegetarians don't want to face it. But they are part of this cycle. There
is no getting out of it.

I'm not suggesting vegetarians run out to Outback Steakhouse. Or pick up
a sirloin at the market on their way home and throw it on the grill. Because
that is just as irresponsible as clinging to beliefs that make them sick.

The commercial farming industry is a travesty. But it's the ethics of the
system, not the meat, that's the enemy. *Eating meat is not ethically
wrong. But eating ethically wrong meat is wrong.*

Hidden Dangers of Grain

Feeding cows a grain diet is dangerous to the cow and to humans.

Cows are ruminants. They have four stomachs. The first is the rumen, designed to
digest plant matter. Cows "chew their cud" before it moves from one stomach to
another. The word "ruminate" comes from Latin and means "to chew over again."

When a cow's diet switches to grain, two things happen.

Rumination stops. The rumen can't digest grain properly. Instead, the grain
creates great amounts of gas called "feedlot bloat." It builds up inside the rumen
until it presses against the cow's lungs. Cows suffocate.

Cows develop acidosis from too much starch and sugar in the grain, just as we
develop acid indigestion. They stop feeding. They develop inflammation and disease.

When a cow's stomach is acidic, bacteria such as E. coli become resistant.
Grass-fed beef has 80% less E. coli. Switching from grain-fed beef decreases E.
coli by 10,000,000 times.[3]

Campylobacter is another bacteria passed on to humans. Fifty-eight percent of
grain-fed cows carry it compared to 2% of grass-fed cows.[4]

Grain-fed cows are injected with synthetic hormones. rBGH and rBST are
outlawed by the European Union, Japan, Australia, and Canada due to animal and
human risk. Both are used frequently in the U.S.[5]

This should be a rally cry for these converts. Former vegetarians who
now eat meat understand this concept. When you purchase grass-fed
beef from small, independent ranchers, it's *sustainable*. And much
healthier than hormone-stuffed burgers — or no burger at all.

Commercial farming practices create sick, diseased animals. But you buy them for dinner without a second thought.

You can't see the difference when you look at the meat in the butcher's case. You might not even taste the difference. But if you've never been to a commercial feedlot, let me give you an idea of what's going on.

First, bulls are castrated. Then they're injected with synthetic hormones to make them grow. They live out their lives standing in their own filth in cement sheds, never seeing the light of day. Their diet is so unnatural it makes them deathly sick. Then they're kept barely alive by antibiotics until they're slaughtered at an early age.

This is what you're served up at restaurants and in your own home, if you're like most people.

It might look good on the plate, but you're getting a dose of hormones with every bite. Commercial beef in the U.S. contains dangerous, synthetic hormones that are ending up in you and your children.

Why do you think young girls these days are going through puberty when they're still babies? Why are young boys developing breast tissue?

This is a worldwide health concern. Hormone-treated U.S. meat has been banned throughout the European nations since 1989.[1]

In the U.S., 70% of all antibiotics go to "healthy" livestock instead of people.[2] But commercial livestock isn't healthy. Commercial farmers use the antibiotics to keep dying animals alive just long enough to sell to you.

Why Grass-Fed Beef Is Better

1. Less overall fat and calories. A six-ounce grass-fed loin has 92 fewer calories than grain-fed. This saves an average American 16,642 calories each year.[3]

2. More Omega-3. Grass-fed beef has two to 10 times more omega-3s than grain-fed beef and a healthy ratio as little as 1:1. Grain-fed beef is as much as 14:1.[4]

3. More CLA. Grass-fed beef has two to five times more CLA than grain-fed.[5] CLA supports immune and cardiovascular function and lean muscle mass. Studies show women with highest levels of CLA have 60-74% lower risk of breast cancer.[6]

4. More Vitamin E. Grass-fed beef contains three to six times more vitamin E than grain-fed beef.[7]

5. More Carotenoids. Grass-fed beef has up to four times more beta-carotene than grain-fed beef.[8] Carotenoids promote eye and macular health.

6. More B Vitamins, CoQ10, and Zinc. Grass-fed beef has more B vitamins, CoQ10, and zinc than grain-fed beef.

Your Plan for Better Health

Step 1: Choose grass-fed, but don't stick to beef. Try buffalo, pork, venison, or other responsibly raised meat. Here is a comparison of basic nutrients you'll find in grass-fed meats:

Based on 3 1/2 ounces	Buffalo	Beef	Pork	Venison
Calories	141.89	281.8	246.08	156.47
Protein (g)	28.18	25.8	26.89	29.97
Fat (g)	2.38	19.05	14.59	3.18
Iron (mg.)	3.37	2.68	0.99	4.47
Sodium (mg.)	56.66	60.53	58.54	53.58
Potassium (mg.)	358.2	343.32	404.84	332.4
Saturated Fat (g)	0.9	7.58	5.33	1.24
Monounsaturated Fat (g)	0.94	8.29	6.46	0.87
Polyunsaturated Fat (g)	0.24	0.74	1.2	0.62
Cholesterol (mg.)	81.36	82.36	81.36	111.13

As you can see in the table above, buffalo has more protein than beef and almost no fat. If you haven't tried it, let me tell you, it really tastes great on the grill.

If you can't find a family owned farm or rancher in your area, go to the web. Many independent farmers advertise online and ship right to your doorstep.

If this is your first bite in years, go slow. It takes up to a week for enzymes in your body to adjust, but the benefits are well worth the effort.

Step 2: Try reintroducing organ meats. In the wild, predatory animals instinctively know that organ meat contains the most nutrients. Many cultures prize organ meat, but Americans still shy away. Try grass-fed organ meat such as liver, heart, or kidneys. Serve it for dinner or add small amounts to your favorite recipes for a nutritional boost.

To give you an idea what you're missing, here's a list of nutrients found in organ meat:

Vitamins	Minerals
A	Phosphorus
B1, B2, B3, B5, B6, B12	Iron
Biotin	Copper
C	Magnesium
D	Selenium
E	Zinc
Folate	Molybdenum
K	Iodine
EPA, DHA, and CLA	
Amino Acids	
Coenzyme Q10	

[1] "American Beef: Why is it Banned in Europe?" Cancer Prevention Coalition. 2003.

[2] "Judge Rules FDA Must Act to Protect Americans from Overuse of Antibiotics in Livestock," Union of Concerned Scientists. press release, March 23, 2012.

[3] Robinson, J. "Pasture Perfect: The Far Reaching Benefits of Choosing Meat, Eggs, and Dairy Products from Grass-Fed Animals." Vashon Island Press. 2004.

[4] Robinson, J. "Health Benefits of Grass-Fed Products." *Eat Wild*. Copyright 2002-2015.

[5] Robinson, J. "Grass-Fed Basics." Eatwild.com. 2010.

[6] Bougnoux, P., Lavillonniere, F., Riboli, E., "Inverse relation between CLA in adipose breast tissue and risk of breast cancer," *Inform* 10;5:S43, 1999.

[7] Smith, G.C. "Dietary Supplementation of Vitamin E to Cattle to Improve Shelf-Life and Case-Life for Domestic and International Markets." Colorado State University. Complete reference not known.

[8] Prache, S., A. Priolo, et al. (2003). "Persistence of carotenoid pigments in the blood of concentrate-finished grazing sheep: its significance for the traceability of grass-feeding." *J Anim Sci* 81(2): 360-7.

Chapter 13

Five Keys to Beating the Big Organic Hoax

I love shopping at the fruit and veggie stand near my house. It makes me feel good to know where my food is coming from.

I've gotten to know the farmer at my market personally. She's shown me the organic seeds she plants, and has let me see the type of soil she uses. We even talk about her natural methods of keeping nutrients in the soil and deterring bugs.

And now I don't need to go to a huge store any more to sort through all the produce stamped "organic." I'm feeding my family *better* than organic.

What's Wrong with Organic Fruit and Veggies at Your Grocery Store?

Ever wonder why the lettuce at your supermarket seems so lifeless? It has a lot to do with how it got there.

The food at major grocery stores travels an average of 1,500 miles to get there. A typical carrot is transported 1,838 miles.[1] And a lot of produce even comes from Mexico, Asia, Canada, South America and other countries.

By the time it lands at your supermarket, it just isn't the same as when it was fresh from the ground or picked off the tree. Produce loses nutrients during transport. And it loses more while it sits on the shelves at the store, and more nutrients are lost in your refrigerator.

This is true even for organic fruits and vegetables. Most don't come from anywhere near you. They are grown at large farms across the country. Then they get trucked hundreds of miles before they get to a store where you can buy them, losing potency the entire trip.

How do fruits and veggies lose their nutrients? By getting separated from their major nutrient source — the tree, the vine or the plant.

Generally, nutrient loss depends on how fruits and vegetables are processed and stored (especially the temperature and humidity levels of storage facilities and the processing machinery — or lack of machinery used). But some produce is especially sensitive to transport and storage.

Spinach is a great example. A Penn State University study published in the *Journal of Food Science* found that spinach stored at 39 degrees Fahrenheit for eight days loses most of its folate and carotenoids content.[2] But many trucks ship spinach across far distances at temperatures well above 39 degrees.

Folate is a form of vitamin B that helps to prevent birth defects. And carotenoids in fruits and veggies help to prevent blindness and some cancers.

But they aren't the only nutrients that crops lose during long transport. Vitamin C gets depleted, too. That's because vitamin C is sensitive to heat, light and oxygen. As a result, it tends to degrade very soon after harvest. University of California researchers found that fruits and veggies lose vitamin C the longer they're stored at higher temperatures.

This is true even in the case of citrus fruits, which tend to lose vitamin C at a slower rate due to their acidity. What's more, leafy greens, like spinach, need water to maintain vitamin C after harvest. Storing them at high temperatures in trucks can deplete their levels quickly.[3]

So the sooner you can eat fruits and vegetables after they've been pulled from their nutrient source, the more your body benefits. **And taking nutrients in through your food is the BEST way to get the nutrition you need.**

That's why...

Buying Your Fruit and Veggies from Local Farms You Trust is Better than Buying Organic — 100% of the Time

I buy fresh, local and organic food from small farms for many reasons.

First, the food is more nutritious because it's thousands of miles fresher (which also helps our planet). Many small farmers harvest their crops a couple of days or less before they sell them. So the produce still has plenty of vitamins and minerals.

That farm freshness makes the fruit and veggies taste good, too. Better than anything you'll find at a supermarket.

What's more, many small farmers use organic farming methods and seeds, even though their foods aren't certified organic. That's because they can't afford the government's expensive organic certification process.

At the produce stand, I also find varieties I can't get anywhere else. By "varieties" I mean slightly different types of the same fruits and vegetables. These selections have different genetic information that tells the plant how to grow. And this unique genetic makeup also influences flavor and appearance.

The Food and Agriculture Organization of the United Nations estimates that since 1900, about 75% of the genetic diversity of agricultural crops has been wiped out. And that's because large industrial farms only mass-produce crops that are resistant to disease, look uniform and can withstand long transport.[4]

But small farmers don't have any of these concerns. That's why they can raise several selections of crops — many which have been passed down through generations. The local fruit stand is one of the *only* places to find these rare selections.

But one of the best reasons I buy from local farms is that I want to support my community, especially in these tough times. There are less than one million farmers in the U.S. And they get paid as little as 18 cents per item at stores. When I buy directly from small farmers, they get all the profits. And those are profits that are invested in supplying natural food to my community.

So if you want to experience all these benefits, too…

Here Are Some EASY Tips for Buying *Fresh, Local and Organic*

1. Get the best food from the best sources.

- Farms stands and u-picks — Locations can range from a shed or truck to a warehouse, and you buy directly from the farmer. At u-pick farms, you can pick your fruit straight from the vine.

- Farmers' markets — These are outdoor markets where farmers sell their produce to the public. You can find unique varieties of fruits and veggies — as well as organic meat and cage-free poultry. Farmers are typically able to keep 80 to 90 cents of each dollar you spend there, too.[5] I use a great one here in my hometown of West Palm Beach. But I do find I have to talk to the vendors about their farming methods and sources.

- Community-supported agriculture (CSA) groups — These are partnerships between the community and a particular local farm. In a CSA, you can buy shares for weekly food allowances — then pick your food up right at the farm.

- Supermarkets — Some supermarkets offer a selection of locally grown produce. But remember they take a big cut of the profit. So if you want to support farmers, it's better to buy directly from them.

2. Check out these websites to get started buying locally today.

Alternative Farming Systems Information Center http://afsic.nal.usda.gov/	Your complete library of resources about local, fresh, organic food. It includes everything from articles to full reports and databases. So it will answer pretty much any question you have on the topic.
Community Involved in Sustaining Agriculture http://www.buylocalfood.org/	Includes an excellent list of general resources about buying locally.
Eat Well Guide http://www.eatwellguide.org/	Just type in your zip code to find fresh food sources in your community.

Food Routes http://foodroutes.org/	National nonprofit dedicated to rebuilding local food systems through outreach, events, local food guides, and educational materials. They have "Buy Fresh, Buy Local" chapters that'll connect you to your community's cleanest, freshest food.
Local Harvest http://www.localharvest.org/	Online community for buying local. It includes a national directory of small farms, farmers' markets, and other local food sources — that's constantly updated. Plus you'll chat online with others who share your interest in farm-fresh food here.

3. Don't assume all Mom-and-Pop farms use organic methods. Some could use chemical pesticides and fertilizers on their crops. So the only way to know for sure is to ask. If you're at a farmer's market, it's always good to find out where the produce was grown. Especially if they're selling out-of-season produce. It's also good to ask about the best ways to pack and store your food. And don't forget to ask when their fruits and veggies were picked — and whether they used organic seeds. Remember, *FRESH, local and organic* is the goal.

4. You can't get more local than planting your own crops. You can grow some herbs and keep them on your windowsill, or in a big backyard garden. There are countless books and online resources to get you started. With your own garden, you can make sure your family gets plenty of fruits and veggies. And you'll save money, too.

5. Plan meals in advance to make sure you use your fruits and veggies quickly. Also, keep your refrigerator set below 40 degrees to maintain freshness. Steaming veggies for a short time helps to preserve nutrients, too.

---

[1] Pirog, Rich and Benjamin, Andrew, "Checking the Food Odometer: Comparing Food Miles for Local Versus Conventional Produce Sales in Iowa Institutions," *Leopold Center for Sustainable Agriculture* July 2003

[2] Pandrangi, S., and LaBorde, L., "Retention of Folate, Carotenoids and Other

Quality Characteristics in Commercially Packaged Fresh Spinach," *Journal of Food Science* May 2006; 69: C702–C707

[3] Lee, Seung K. and Kader, Adel A., "Preharvest and Postharvest Factors Influencing Vitamin C Content of Horticultural Crops," *Postharvest Biology and Technology* 20; (2000) 207–220

[4] Food and Agriculture Organization of the United Nations, "Special: Biodiversity for Food and Agriculture: Farm Animal Genetic Resources," February 1998

[5] Pretty, J. "Some Benefits and Drawbacks of Local Food Systems," (PDF). *Briefing Note for TVU/Sustain AgriFood Network*. November 2, 2001.

Chapter 14

Beat the "National Eating Disorder"

Americans jump from one diet trend to the next — whether it vilifies a nutrient category like fat or deifies a single food as the savior. But just where has obsession with healthy eating gotten us? Obesity has continued to rise, now affecting one in five Americans.[1]

And incredibly, over 60% of American adults are now overweight.

Somehow, what I call our "national eating disorder" has turned us into the fattest people in the history of the world. We've also seen an explosion of other diet-related problems. And, so many of my new patients just can't figure out why they're so tired.

Americans want so badly to be healthy, but they're clearly missing out on something when it comes to what to eat.

How Did We Become Overfed Yet Undernourished?

Our tastes naturally guide us to food that's good for us. Unless our ancestors were starving, they didn't eat grains because grains just didn't taste good. Without processing, grains are hard, gritty, tasteless and difficult to digest. A natural balance ensued. The grains escaped mammalian predation and we stuck to foods we are adapted to eat.

With the advent of the milling of grains, cultures could feed more people. This allowed for both higher population densities and specialization. More people with trained, grain-fed soldiers out-competed hunters even though grain-fed peoples were smaller, weaker and more diseased than the numerically fewer hunters. Civilization made a huge leap forward. But we temporarily traded quantity for quality. Now, in the modern world, we have a choice.

Solve a Problem — Create a Problem

Fundamentally, the processing of grains created a problem. Many nutrients are different, and nutritional deficiencies appear in the archeological record at the time humanity switched to grains. But the biggest problem with grains had not yet fully developed.

Grains pack in starch. Not a huge problem for a sustenance farmer spending 10 hours a day in the field. But with the industrialization of farming, high-starch yields fuel another big problem. Starch triggers a rapid release of insulin in your blood. Insulin is your body's principal way of directing calories into building fat.

Grains are also inflammatory, wreaking all sorts of other damage, contributing to things like arthritis and Alzheimer's. Grain diets also cause a deficiency of fat. Studies of people eating low fat diets have found problems with calcium absorption, they've discovered low fat diets suppress the immune system, and they haven't found any evidence supporting the conventional advice that low-fat diets improve your weight, your blood pressure, or your overall health.[2]

Reversing What the Diet Trends Got Wrong

A study reported in *JAMA* specifically compared the effects of a diet low in fat to a diet low in glycemic load. A diet low in glycemic load doesn't cut carbs down to nothing. It limits foods that have densely

The people on the low glycemic load diet lowered their triglycerides, blood pressure, and levels of C-reactive protein compared to the low-fat group.[3] All of these are indicators of heart disease risk.

What's especially interesting to me about this is that eating low glycemic load foods is really simply your native diet. We evolved to eat like this. Whole, unprocessed foods. A good balance of meat, fish, vegetables, nuts, and fruits.

In the recent low-carb trend, Americans got a little closer to the mark, but they still didn't hit it. Not all carbohydrates are equal. Vegetables are a great source of carbs.

They're high in fiber, which slows the conversion of carbohydrates into glucose. That's important because it also slows your body's release of insulin. Fruits, nuts, and seeds are good as well. You can eat all these in their natural form and they are all good carbs.

Grains, potatoes, and corn can't be eaten without processing or cooking, and that turns out to be problematic. They're higher in starch and create huge amounts of blood sugar, eventually leading to insulin overproduction, which isn't good.

Lumping vegetables in with grains just because they're both carbohydrates ignores these critical differences and just doesn't make nutritional sense.

The Damage Done by Other Trends

We also narrow in on single foods, sometimes declaring the oddest things the path to true health. Take soy for example. Soy has been hailed as a preventer of heart disease and cancer, as a means to lower cholesterol, and as an all-around good thing to eat.

But it just ain't so.

Research links soy to decreased fertility, a higher risk of some cancers, and hormone imbalances. Still, Big Food grabbed hold of some promising study early on, some misleading tidbit of information, and created a booming market for soy. It's now in 70% of all processed foods.[4]

Overcoming the Marketing of Obsession

The sudden changes in our food beliefs give food marketers a way to create endless variations on processed foods. Whatever the trend is, they can easily exploit it, whether it is whole grain, low fat, or soy substitutes for real food. They can isolate one supposedly "healthy" element of a processed food and use that to market it to consumers.

It may be that Americans are so susceptible to food crazes because we don't have a stable culinary tradition to guide us. If you look at the French culture, they eat quite a number of high fat foods, but have lower heart disease rates than Americans. In a cross-cultural survey Americans were most likely to think about food in terms of health and least likely to think about it relating to pleasure.

Rebuilding Healthy Thinking about Food

Ask yourself, do you think more about good food to eat or more about what you are supposed to avoid? One perspective leads to fulfillment and satisfaction, making you likely to eat less. The other leads to guilt and regret and a propensity to eat more.

First, think about good food to eat:

- Eat more protein. Eggs from free range chickens are delicious.
- Grass-fed beef or bison are among my favorites.
- Eat more vegetables and fruits.
- Eat more nuts and seeds.
- Enjoy a bit of chocolate now and again.
- A glass of wine most days won't hurt either.

Next, how to eat:

- Don't skip breakfast.
- Make dinner an event. Plan the meal. Invite the family. Set the mood. And enjoy each other's company as much as you enjoy the meal.
- Chew. Slow down and savor the meal.
- Pause. Set your fork down between bites.
- Pay attention. When you feel comfortable and no longer hungry, stop eating.
- Think about your favorite foods. What are the things that make you really feel good when you're eating them? Don't deprive yourself of those foods. If they aren't healthy, just treat yourself occasionally.

Eating healthy is as simple as eating the foods you were built to eat. Having a healthy attitude toward food is as simple as enjoying the foods you eat, taking your time to taste them, and not worrying over the meal in front of you as you eat.

---

[1] Overweight and Obesity: At a Glance, The Department of Health and Human Services. 3/15/2005.

[2] Sears, Al MD. Eat for Life.

[3] Pereira, MA et al. Effects of a Low-Glycemic Load Diet on Resting Energy Expenditure and Heart Disease Risk Factors During Weight Loss, *JAMA* 2004; 292(20): 2482-90.

[4] The Truth About Soy, Dr Joseph Mercola's eHealthy News. December 4, 2004.

Chapter 15

It's Not Organic — but So What?

Have you heard what's been happening? Organic advocates, groups and media outlets are up in arms because breakfast cereal producers like Kashi and Mother's were caught switching from organic ingredients to "natural" ones.[1]

There are endless articles about how this or that cereal has almost no organic ingredients. There's even a giant report from the Cornucopia Institute called *Cereal Crimes*.[2] It describes how manufacturers are now deceiving you by lowering their organic content without telling you, but still charging high organic prices.

They're missing the point.

I'll tell you why in a minute, but first I'll let you in on a little secret that's not very well known: the entire reason cereal exists in the first place is because of the Kellogg brothers, who believed eating meat was wrong.

A hundred and fifty years ago, Americans ate pork, beef, or chicken for breakfast. In the nineteenth century, Americans ate breakfasts heavy on the meat and natural fiber, light on grains. Heart disease was extremely rare.

The Kelloggs ran a sanitarium and were vegetarians. They developed what we now call "granola" and eventually corn flakes to feed their patients instead of animal products. The patients started requesting it by mail after they left the sanitarium because they believed it was healthy. The Kelloggs started packaging it, and had a business on their hands.

To sell their products, the Kelloggs used shrewd advertising to convince you that cereal is good while meat and eggs are bad. Not because it's true, but because it was in their commercial interests. The Kelloggs had a commercial and vegetarian agenda that deceived people into thinking their product was "healthy" and traditional foods were not.

For decades now ads touting cereal as Mother Nature's wholesome solution for obesity and heart disease have been very effective. Kellogg's even has a "Mr. Breakfast" character to try and convince parents and children that cereal is the only breakfast food you need.

C.W. Post should know. He was a patient at the Kelloggs' sanitarium. His health didn't improve one bit while there, but he saw the business opportunity and started his own sanitarium. And his own Post Cereal Company. You might recognize his version of granola. It's the so-called health food called "grape nuts."

But what the Cornucopia Institute and others should be talking about isn't whether or not cereal is organic.

If they really wanted to be an advocate for you, they would admit that cereal is bad for you. It's not healthy. It will make you fat. It will spike your insulin and put you on the road to diabetes.

About the only thing good about cereal is that it won't lower your cholesterol — and you don't want to lower your cholesterol anyway.

The truth is, Mother Nature didn't intend for you to eat breakfast out of a box. In fact, it would harm your health less for you to eat the cardboard box than what's inside. At least you won't digest the box.

Your ancestors only ate grains in an emergency. They thrived on foods like eggs, meat, and fish. This is what gave them power, strength, and vitality.

I remember staying at my grandparents' place when I was a kid. I'd wake up mornings to the smell of steak and eggs and race down the stairs to get my place at the table.

Your grandparents ate this way, too. It's much better for you than what the media and food producers want you to believe.

Today, you're bombarded by commercials for low-fat granola, Cheerios, and Special K. You are encouraged to believe you're eating healthy products because they tell you it's "high-fiber, whole oat, and whole grain wheat."

And it has worked.

There is so much misinformation out there that most people believe cereals are "healthy" and natural. Few people think of cereal as being a threat to their health.

But no matter which one you choose, all those low-fat carbs throw your metabolism out of whack. And eventually, your health will suffer.

Among many other problems, breakfast cereals are high on the glycemic index (GI). A dose of high-glycemic carbs in the morning is the prescription for building excess body fat.

For instance, the GI rating of an average piece of chocolate cake is 38 — a Snickers bar is about 55. Still not bad.

Compare that to the GI of Kellogg's Corn Flakes, which registers a whopping 92.[3] That means corn flakes break down into sugar in your bloodstream almost as fast pure glucose, which has a GI of 100! Please see my GI in the back of the book.

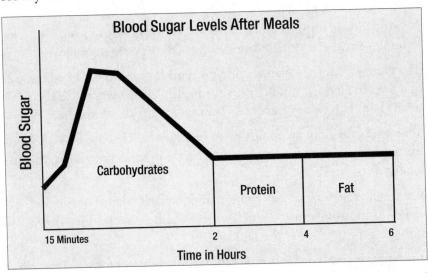

Remember, cereal grains spike your blood sugar after you eat them and high blood sugar triggers a wave of insulin. And insulin is the hormone that sends the message to build and store fat.

Even a "healthy" cereal like Grape-Nuts has a GI of 80. That's also very high.

Forget about the commercials you see on TV. Grains might be a fast fix when you're rushing to get your day started, but cereal in the morning will make you fat.

If you eat eggs and meat for breakfast regularly, and then grab a bowl of cereal and milk one morning you are in a hurry, you will be dizzy and weak by late morning. It's as if your body is telling you that cereal grains are no good for you.

If you want carbs, avoid the processed ones at all costs. Enjoy your carbs the way nature made them. Fresh and raw.

But please, don't skip breakfast. It's the most important meal of the day, and the one I enjoy the most. I try and change it up to keep it interesting, but meat or fish is always the centerpiece of my morning meal.

Here are three of my favorite breakfasts you might enjoy:

1. **Fried eggs with a side of steak:** Look for cage-free eggs at the grocery store. They come from antibiotic-free chickens raised in a natural, healthy environment. Fry them in organic butter.

   Make sure to buy grass-fed beef. Animal fat is good for you, as long as it's from disease-free livestock that haven't been injected with hormones or fed antibiotics. Stores like Whole Foods Market carry it, or see if your butcher can order it for you.

If you gravitate toward bacon, remember this is a highly processed food. So look for grass-fed and a brand that doesn't contain nitrates. They can cause cancer and changes to your DNA.

If you don't like frying, take a few extra moments and scramble some eggs. Before you throw the eggs in, sauté some sliced tomatoes and mushrooms. Maybe some onion, too.

2. **Cheese omelet with salmon:** Fish is a fantastic breakfast food. The Japanese eat fish and vegetables first thing every morning. They have for over 1,500 years, and have had virtually no heart disease or diabetes.

3. I like to add a leafy green vegetable to my omelets, usually spinach. For the cheese, look for 100% organic from grass-fed

cows, if you can. You get none of the hormones and antibiotics and far more nutrients. Buy wild salmon instead of farm-raised. It has no dyes, less toxins, and much higher levels of omega-3

4. Ackee with saltfish: This is Jamaica's national meal and the all-time best meal as far as I'm concerned. Ackee is a fruit, and it's a little bit tricky to prepare. The saltfish is a kind of cod. I also like to eat it with callaloo (amaranth).

Here's a recipe that serves four:

Ingredients:

1/2 lb saltfish (dried, salted codfish, also called bacalao)
1/2 lb fresh, shredded callaloo leaves
1 medium onion
1/2 tsp black pepper
3 tbsp of butter
1/2 Scotch Bonnet pepper
1 sweet pepper
1 chopped tomato
1 sprig fresh thyme or 1 tsp dried thyme

Optional ingredients:

2 cloves of garlic
4 scallion (or spring onions)
6 slices of bacon

Instructions:

- Cover the saltfish in cold water. Let soak overnight (minimum eight hours) changing the water several times (this removes most of the salt).

- Bring a pan of cold water to the boil and gently simmer the fish for 20 minutes (until the fish is tender).

- Chop the onion, sweet pepper, Scotch Bonnet pepper and tomato while waiting for the water to boil.

- Wash the callaloo in a pot of water and drain thoroughly.

- Remove the fish from water and allow to cool. Remove all bones and skin then flake the flesh of the fish.

- Melt the butter in a frying pan and add the onion, black pepper, sweet pepper, Scotch Bonnet and thyme. Fry for about five minutes.

- Add the callaloo and half a cup of water, cover and steam for 15 minutes.

- Add the tomatoes and flaked fish and steam for another 10 minutes.

When I leave the house, I'm full of energy. And I've never missed a day of work in my life.

If you really need a carb fix, save it for the occasional dessert. Don't make it a part of your breakfast. The addiction may be hard to break, but you'll be a lot happier — and more productive.

---

[1] Gomez, D. "Claim - "natural" cereals contain pesticides and GMOs." TG Daily. Oct 13, 2011. Retreive Oct. 28, 2011

[2] Valleys, C, et al. "Cereal Crimes: How 'Natural' Claims Deceive Consumers and Undermine the Organic Label—A Look Down the Cereal and Granola Aisle." *Cornucopia Inst.* October 11, 2011.

[3] "Breakfast Cereals and Related Products." Online Glycemic Index Database. Retrieve Oct 28, 2011.

PART 3

DITCH THE DIET ADVICE AND FEAST ON THE FATTY FOODS YOU LOVE

Chapter 1

After Atkins — Your Low-Carb Diet Update

It looks like the mainstream may finally be catching up with Dr. Robert Atkin's radical ideas, several years after his death. This may be direly needed relief. Americans have been wrapped up in a low-fat craze for the past half-century. Over that same period, heart disease has skyrocketed and environmental diabetes is up over 900%.

Yet Atkins didn't get the whole story correct. He was right about the problem, but not about the solution. I'll give you a few simple changes that will help you feel great, lose weight, and ensure heart health — the easiest and most natural way.

Exposing the Low-Fat Myth: Past and Present

Beginning in the '60s, Atkins argued that carbohydrates in the American diet — not fat, and not just calories — were responsible for soaring obesity rates. Implicit in this radical assertion: the *kind* of calories mattered when it came to weight loss.

This was — and remains — a difficult idea for nutritional experts to accept. Although his diet worked for millions of Americans, Atkins endured ridicule from the medical community throughout his life. Even after his death in April 2003, his critics kept attacking, going so far as to claim that he died of obesity and heart disease (he didn't).[1]

Scientific evidence from a recent Harvard study is now proving those critics wrong in other ways that are important to your health.

The study was one of the largest of its kind, with research involving 80,000 women over two decades. Published last month in the *New England Journal of Medicine,* it found that those who followed a low-carb, high-fat diet cut their risk of heart disease by 30%.[2] The Associated Press reported that these findings are "easing fears that the popular Atkins diet and similar regimens might set people up for eventual heart attacks."[3]

I can personally attest to the low-fat diet myth's persistence. For my Barry University (Florida) nutrition course, I looked through 26 nutrition textbooks. Every one listed a low-fat diet as the ideal. Did you ever try eating low-fat without increasing carbs?

Real science tells us that your body responds differently to carbohydrate, protein and fat. Starchy, high-carb foods spike your blood sugar and trigger an insulin response. The more insulin, the more fat your body stores. So over time, you turn to fat.

This does not mean you have to avoid carbs entirely. You can use a system to grade just how much any particular carb will contribute to the overproduction of insulin.

Carbs and the Glycemic Index

The Glycemic Index (GI) ranks foods in terms of how rapidly they spike your blood sugar as a percentage of that caused by eating straight sugar. For example, a food with a glycemic index of 50% will cause half of the rapid rise in blood sugar that glucose (pure natural sugar) would. Here's a table listing common foods and their glycemic index.

Glycemic Index of Common Foods		
Low (0 to 55)	Medium (56 to 69)	High (70 or More)
Eggs	Whole Wheat Pita	Rice Cakes
Oranges	Ellueherrs Muffin	Kellogg's Corn Flakes
Milk	Cantaloupe	Pretzels
Carrots	Raisins	Bagels
Meat	Whole Grain Snack Bars	Pasta
Poultry	Snickers Bar	White Bread
Broccoli	Ice Cream	Corn Chips

A few surprising observations emerge from looking at the above chart. For instance:

- Rice cakes raise blood sugar levels more than candy.

- Corn flakes raise blood sugar twice as much as orange juice.

- You get more blood sugar from spaghetti than from ice cream.

Most people think sweets are the problem. You can now see that starches are the main culprits. They cause a much more prolonged elevation of sugar and insulin than simple sugars do. This does not mean, however, that any fat automatically makes sense. While fat doesn't trigger an insulin response, as with carbs, there's more than one kind of fat.

Some Fats Are Better

For example, the Atkins diet regarded bacon, cheese, and heavy cream as acceptable because they are low-carb. The problem is that these foods have too much of the wrong fat: omega-6 fatty acids. We need this fat in moderate amounts. However, excess omega-6s are inflammatory and can lead to arthritis, diabetes, and heart disease.

Atkins recommended far too much of it and not enough of its beneficial cousin, omega-3 fatty acids. These are in fish, nuts, eggs, avocados, walnuts, and grass-fed meats.

Here are just a few of the benefits of these "healthy" fats:

- Low triglycerides and better heart health.

- Sharper memory, mental focus and brainpower.

- Better eyesight and a lower risk for age-related macular degeneration.

- Better skin health and hair luster.

- Anti-inflammatory protection from arthritis.

The Adulterated Diet of the Modern World

Sadly, much of the fat we eat today contains the toxic byproducts of our industrialized society. Hormones, antibiotics, pesticides and other chemicals generally wind up in the fat of animals exposed to them. When you eat this fat, you're also absorbing its stored toxins.

Modern farming techniques worsen the problem. Animals aren't fed their natural diet and don't get exercise. Today's livestock feed violates their natural dietary needs. Cows, for instance, eat grain feed despite their natural diet of grass. The result is obese animals unnaturally high in omega-6 fats.

By contrast, grass-fed beef contains a higher ratio of omega-3 fats to omega-6 than fish. This gives you some idea of how distorted our food supply has become, and how negatively it affects our health.

And modern food processing yield fats not seen in nature. The "trans" fatty acids fall into this category, and they are extremely harmful to your health.

Hydrogenated vegetable oils are the chief culprit. Because it isn't a naturally occurring fat, your body doesn't know what to do with it. As a result, it binds to your arteries and puts you on the fast track to heart disease.

Back to the Future — the Optimal Diet

Early humans ate low-carb foods naturally. Before the days of farming (and grain-based agriculture) our ancestors lived on meat, wild vegetables, nuts and berries that gave them the strength, stamina and muscle growth they needed to survive under harsh conditions. It also afforded them the right mix of the essential fats for optimal health.

By returning to a diet that is natural to the human condition, you can easily — and naturally — lose those extra pounds and prevent heart disease. Here are a few simple guidelines to help you sidestep the worst of the "low-fat" mistakes and the flaws of Atkins while enjoying real foods for native health.

- Know what kind of fat you are eating. Eat foods high in omega-3s: fresh oily fish (like salmon and mackerel), seeds, nuts, eggs, avocados, and walnuts. Look for grass-fed beef, free-range chicken, and other forms of naturally raised animal fat.

- If you have difficulty incorporating omega-3 rich foods, consider supplementing your diet. Cod liver oil is one of the very best forms.

- Avoid processed foods and anything containing hydrogenated vegetable oils.

- Avoid starchy carbohydrates like potatoes and bread. Consult the Glycemic Index to determine which carbs are best. Reduce (drastically if you can) the amount of foods that score high, and substitute lower-scoring foods.

---

[1] McLaughlin, K. "Report Details Dr. Atkins's Health Problems." *Wall Street Journal*. February 10, 2004.

[2] "Low-Carbohydrate-Diet Score and the Risk of Coronary Heart Disease in Women," *New England Journal of Medicine* 2006; 355(1.9):1991-2002.

[3] Associated Press. "Carbs may be worse for heart than fatty foods: Long-term study eases concerns about risk of Atkins, other low-carb diets." MSNBC. November 8, 2006.

[4] Goodman, Jonathan. *The Omega Solution: Unleash the Amazing, Scientifically Based Healing Power of Omega-3 & -6 Fatty Acids.* New York: Prima Lifestyles, 2001.

Chapter 2

Turn Your Body into a Fat-Burning Furnace — by Eating MORE Fat

Have you seen this ad for one of those fake butter spreads?

It features a 1950s family called the "Buttertons." The mother serves the family entire sticks of butter shoved into baked potatoes. The voiceover says something like, "Back then we didn't know much about cholesterol and saturated fats. Today, we know better."

That means they're telling you that you shouldn't eat fat. It's remarkable that this message is still dominant in the mainstream media.

The truth is we don't eat a high-fat diet. We eat less fat than our ancestors did. And yet we're the ones with obesity, heart disease, high cholesterol, clogged arteries and high blood pressure.

In direct contradiction of what you commonly hear in the media — like in that ad — real butter is good for you. Saturated fats are a natural part of your diet and are essential to life. Fat makes up the basic building blocks of compounds that help your body perform everyday functions. This includes things like regulating blood pressure, blood clotting and bolstering your immune system.

Saturated fats have been on the media hit list for over 50 years. Butter is just one example. Red meat is another. But one of the worst victims of this low-fat propaganda is coconut oil. Like butter, it's been vilified for decades.

But a new study shows that coconut oil can lower your total cholesterol, boost your HDL "good" cholesterol, lower your LDL "bad" cholesterol, and shrink your waist size. Compare that to soybean oil, which did the opposite — lowered HDL, raised LDL and total cholesterol, and did nothing for your belly size.

And it's not the only study to reach that conclusion. Several other studies back up those findings and find even more benefits of coconut oil.

Coconut oil can protect your heart, boost your immune system, and help you lose fat faster and easier than ever before. And I'm going to show you how to use it.

Make the Switch from Corn Oil and Watch Your Waistline Shrink

Coconut oil is rich in medium-chain fatty acids, medium-chain triglycerides (MCTs).

Unlike longer-chain fatty acids, the medium-chain fatty acids in coconut oil are tiny enough to enter your cells' mitochondria directly.

This means your cells use the fat from coconut oil for energy instantly, instead of storing it for later use.

A Boston University study gave one group corn oil (longer-chain fatty acids) and the other medium-chain fatty acids.

After 90 days, those that got the medium-chain fatty acids lost weight, increased their insulin receptivity and even lowered their overall cholesterol.[1]

Another study published in the journal *Lipids* compared coconut oil with soybean oil. The women taking coconut oil saw their waist lines shrink and their HDL "good" cholesterol levels increase. Meanwhile, the women taking soybean oil didn't see any change in their waist size. Plus, LDL, or "bad," cholesterol levels rose and HDL levels dropped.[2]

Another study found that coconut oil can help reduce the symptoms of type-2 diabetes and that "people who incorporate medium-chain fatty acids, such as those found in coconut oil, into their diets can lose body fat."[3]

Coconut oil can help turn your body into a fat-burning furnace.

Plus, it can help you eat less. It controls your hunger by leaving you feeling satisfied, longer.[4]

Boost Your HDL Levels

Contrary to what mainstream medicine tells you, eating high amounts of fat does not automatically equal higher cholesterol. And that's certainly the case with coconut oil.

The War Against Saturated Fat

The war against saturated fats started way back in the late 1950s.

A researcher by the name of Ancel Keys was investigating cardiovascular disease. His goal was to prove eating high amounts of saturated fat was linked to heart disease.

He published the "7 Countries Study," successfully showing fat as the major cause of heart problems.

His research was praised and soon became gospel. He even became known as the "father" of the Lipid Hypothesis. That's the theory that high cholesterol causes heart disease... and in turn, eating a lot of fat causes high cholesterol.

But there was a slight problem with Keys's research. Something he deliberately ignored. Keys only chose to use data from seven countries that matched exactly what he wanted to prove.

The truth is there were at least a half dozen other countries with examples that proved the exact opposite. Countries where people routinely ate tons of fat — yet rarely experienced heart disease. When it didn't fit his hypothesis, he ignored the data.

Unfortunately, Keys's research caught on over the years. One group in particular — the Center for Science in the Public Interest (CSPI) — ran with Keys's ideas. They launched what began an all-out war against all saturated fats. In fact, CSPI coined the term "artery-clogging" fat.

Sadly, coconut oil got caught up in it all.

Decades ago, food manufacturers used tropical oils like coconut oil in their baked goods. Movie theatres used it for their popcorn.

CSPI argued that coconut oil was terrible for your health. It was laden with saturated fat.

Instead, they demanded that these companies use vegetable oils instead (this of course benefited the American Soybean Association, who in the past has made generous donations to CSPI).

The food industry gave in. Coconut oil became taboo. Even the government joined in.

The National Cholesterol Education Program even issued a statement, encouraging margarine and partially hydrogenated fats, stating that "… coconut oil… should be avoided."

Today, we know better.

The truth is it does the exact opposite. It helps improve your HDL to LDL ratio ("good" vs. "bad" cholesterol), lower overall blood levels of serum cholesterol, and reduce the amount of fat your body stores.

In fact, in Sri Lanka, about 50% of calories from the typical diet come from coconut oil. Yet heart disease there is virtually nonexistent.[5]

Researchers, perplexed by this, decided to see what would happen if they took a group of young men and had them substitute their coconut oil with corn and soybean oil.

The results weren't pretty.

Their HDL level plunged 42% — which put them far below what's considered healthy. Their LDL/HDL ratio increased 30%.[6]

That's a recipe for heart disaster.

These results simply confirm what countless studies are finding. Coconut oil is good for your heart and helps increase your good HDL cholesterol.

For example, a study published in the *Journal of Nutrition* studied 25 women. They were given three different diets. A diet high in coconut oil, a low-fat diet with small amounts of coconut oil, and a diet high in polyunsaturated fats. Each diet lasted three weeks.

As you might guess, the highest increase in HDL was when the women ate the high fat, coconut oil diet.[7]

Bulletproof Your Immune System

Coconut oil contains lauric acid, a powerful immune system booster.

Lauric acid has antiviral, antifungal, antibacterial and antiprotozoal properties that help bulletproof your immune system against everything from free radicals to a latent virus that's waiting to wreak havoc.

It's so powerful, in fact, that preliminary research suggests it's effective against lipid-coated viruses, such as HIV.

A recent study took a group of 15 men with HIV. They had not received any prior treatment. After three months of supplementing with coconut oil, half of the patients showed a decrease in viral load.[8]

Good Health Can Taste Great

It's pretty easy to get all the coconut oil you need in your diet.

Just follow any one of these simple tips:

Fry with it. Coconut oil has a high smoke point. That means that it won't degrade at high temperatures — leaving all the fatty acids intact. It's especially great for pan searing. If you do cook with it, consider getting it with no flavor. This is known as "expeller-pressed" coconut oil.

A favorite of mine is to grab one banana. Dip it in plain yogurt. Then roll it in finely chopped coconut. Afterwards I put it in the freezer and eat it whenever I want a quick snack.

Make a smoothie. Scoop a healthy serving of coconut oil (it'll probably be solid, but that's okay) into the blender. Mix in your favorite fresh fruits. Maybe even add some protein powder. Add organic milk and a little ice. Blend it all and enjoy a tasty, heart-healthy smoothie.

Bake with it. It's okay to have your favorite foods from time to time. And if you like to bake cookies, brownies, or anything else, go for it. Just substitute expeller pressed coconut oil for vegetable oil. Not only will everything taste better, but most of the fat you'll be eating will get burned off right away.

---

[1] Han JR, et al. "Effects of dietary medium-chain triglyceride on weight loss and insulin sensitivity in a group of moderately overweight free-living type 2 diabetic Chinese subjects." *Metabolism.* 2007 Jul;56(7):985-91.

[2] Assunção M, et al. "Effects of Dietary Coconut Oil on the Biochemical and Anthropometric Profiles of Women Presenting Abdominal Obesity." *Lipids.* Volume 44, Number 7 / July 2009

[3] News and Events. "How Coconut Oil Could Help Reduce The Symptoms Of Type 2 Diabetes." Garvan Institute. September 8, 2009.

[4] Van Wymelbeke V, Himaya A, Louis-Sylvestre J, Fantino M. "Influence of medium-chain and long-chain triacylglycerols on the control of food intake in men." *Am J Clin Nutr.* 1998 Aug;68(2):226-34.

[5] Kaunitz, H. "Medium chain triglycerides (MCT) in aging and arteriosclerosis." *J*

Environ Pathol Toxicol Oncol. 1986 6(3-4):115.

[6] Fallon Morell, S. "Know Your Fats Introduction." Weston A. Price. February 24, 2009.

[7] Müller H, et al. "The Serum LDL/HDL Cholesterol Ratio Is Influenced More Favorably by Exchanging Saturated with Unsaturated Fat Than by Reducing Saturated Fat in the Diet of Women." *J. Nutr.* 133:78-83, Jan 2003.

[8] Tayag E, Dayrit CS, Santiago BC, Manalo MA, Alban PN, Agdamag DM, Adel AS, Lazo S, Espallardo N. "Monolaurin and Coconut Oil as Monotherapy for HIV-AIDS."

Chapter 3

Get a Clearer Picture

He was nearly blind.

The pain in his eyes was so intense he thought he would go insane.

But he kept hiking, stumbling along over a small plateau high in the Rocky Mountains.

His sight was so far gone that he almost stumbled into two grizzly bear cubs and their enormous mother bear.

He was lucky he wasn't attacked… and he knew he couldn't walk much farther in the mountains and stay alive.

The prospector came to the mouth of a rocky pass, sat down and started sobbing. He was sure he was never going to see his family again.

As he sat there holding his throbbing head, he suddenly heard a voice behind him…

It was an old Indian who had been tracking that same bear. The two of them couldn't speak with each other, but the Indian understood that the prospector's eyes were hurting him.

The elder Indian led the stranger down to a nearby stream, and set a trap made of stones in the running water. The Indian then waded upstream and drove a few trout into his trap.

He caught one of the fish and threw it onto the stream bank. He had the prospector eat the flesh of the head, and especially the eyes and the tissue at the back of the fish's eyes.

Within a few hours, his pain was nearly gone. Within two days, the prospector's sight had almost returned to normal.[1]

How did the Indian cure the prospector so quickly? He gave him one of the very best sources of vitamin A you can find in nature.

Ancient cultures knew the value of the whole, fresh foods they ate, and what to do with them. Unfortunately, this way of looking at things with an eye on nature has been discarded and forgotten.

The prospector was a doctor of engineering and science. Yet he almost went blind and died looking for gold and silver in the Rocky Mountains in the 1930s. He was a scientist, but he had no idea what to eat, where to find it, how to eat it, or why. All because modern science ignores ancient wisdom passed on through thousands of years of trial and error.

Today, we have all of these individualized categories of study being looked at by very smart people. But we're not as smart as we think. The people who interpret the information they're getting don't have the wisdom to apply it.

They keep trying to break nature down into component parts, and then give it back to you one by one. But these attempts to outsmart nature run into predictable problems.

Vitamin A was the first vitamin isolated and studied by modern science. And until a few years ago, we told people just to take vitamin A for their eyes. That turned out not to work. It solved one problem but caused others down the road. And too much vitamin A at once can be toxic to your liver.

Then we discovered a natural vitamin A precursor called beta-carotene. Pick up any multi-vitamin formula today and you'll see beta-carotene.

But that turned out not to be a complete solution either. Beta-carotene is a carotenoid, and in a carrot it does what all carotenoids do. It gives the plant its color, and helps protect the plant's delicate and very sensitive photosystems.

Your body can use beta-carotene the same way. It can protect your own photosystem — your eyes — by turning into vitamin A. The problem is that if your body has enough vitamin A, it won't convert beta-carotene.

A Diet Rich in Beneficial Carotenoids		
Vegetable	Lutein/Zeaxanthin, pg	Beta-carotene, pg
Kale	21,900	4,700
Raw spinach	10,200	4,100
Broccoli	1,900	700
Leaf Lettuce	1,800	1,200
Green peas	1,700	350
Brussel sprouts	1,300	480
Corn	780	50
Green beans	740	44
Raw carrots	260	7,900

Note: A half cup serving is recommended at two to four servings per week. Source: Bergin CL

Today, we are finding other carotenoids that are not only better than vitamin A but better than beta-carotene. In fact, they're up to 100 times more powerful.

So it's a good thing we're so smart now, and we don't just recommend pure vitamin A or pure beta-carotene as the total solution. Because what you really need are these other carotenoids… right?

Not so fast. My instinct is that we're still only catching a very thin slice of that pie. The truth is they're going to find a whole bunch more things next year or in 10 years.

We should learn from this that you can't break Mother Nature into tiny little pieces and build it back. We have to presume that you need things as natively as possible, rather than get them in a refined or processed form. Because we're always going to miss something for the foreseeable future.

That's why you're always better off eating whole fresh vegetables and wild-caught fish to take care of your eyesight. Because your eyes depend on good, balanced nutrition, just like the rest of your body does.

If you give your eyes the building blocks and maintenance materials they need most, you can reverse many of the common symptoms of vision loss. And you may also prevent the major causes of blindness — glaucoma, cataracts and macular degeneration, or AMD.

Telling Fish Tales

Do you know how many fish get their color? They eat plants that have carotenoids and use those plant colors as their own. Even rainbow trout do this. It could be one of the reasons eating fish is so beneficial for your eyesight.

The Association for Research in Vision and Ophthalmology published two important studies that prove other ways in which eating fish protects your vision.

Age-related macular degeneration (AMD) is a common eye problem related to age. Macular degeneration is a disruption of nerves in the retina. This disruption causes loss of sight. AMD is one the leading causes of blindness in older people.

Researchers from the National Eye Institute found that DHA, one of the omega-3 fats found in fish, supports the nerves in the retina. They looked at over 4,500 people ages 60-80 and found that people who ate two servings of fish a week were 50% less likely to develop AMD that those who ate no fish.

100 grams (3.5 ounces) fesh filet of:	Total Omega-3 Fats	Ratio of Omega-3 to Omega-6 Fats*
Wild Coho Salmon	.92 grams	15.3
Wild Rainbow Trout	.77 grams	2.3
Wild Channel Catfish	.29	1.2

*The higher the ratio of omega-3 to omega-6 fats, the more able the body is to use the omega-3 fats.

Another study performed by Harvard's Schepens Eye Research Institute found that fish protects you from dry eye syndrome. When a person's eyes do not make enough moisture, the dryness can damage the cornea.

The study followed over 32,000 people. Those who ate more fish had up to 66% less chance of developing dry eye syndrome.

Eat good quality fish like wild-caught salmon a couple times a week to keep your eyes in top condition.

My favorite fish dish is the national dish of Jamaica, Ackee with salt-fish. Ackee is a fruit, and it's a little bit tricky to prepare because it's toxic if it's not quite ripe.

You can get a little sick from it. They call it "Jamaican morning sickness" and it's not fun. I experienced it myself before I really knew what I was doing trying to choose the ripe ackee.

The saltfish is a kind of cod, and I also like to eat it with callaloo (amaranth). It's no coincidence that the local Jamaicans have been eating callaloo with fish for centuries… it's loaded with lutein and zeaxanthin, the two most powerful carotenoids for your eyes.

Your Eyes May Know Best

Fruits and vegetables are the most potent sources of eye-healthy carotenoids. Fruits and vegetables are natural multivitamins, multiminerals and multiantioxidants. In choosing them, you can use your vision to protect your vision. Choose combinations that are pleasing to the eye.

Benefits of Colorful Fruits and Vegetables		
Color	Foods	Benefits to the Eye
Orange and Yellow	Pumpkin, squash, yellow peppes, carrots, mango, peaches, apricots	Lutein, zeaxanthin & other cartenoids protect eye from sun & age damage
Red and Pink	Tomatoes, red peppers, guava, watermelon, grapefruit	Range of cartenoids protect eye from free radicals
Green	Broccoli, zucchini, green peppers, spinach, kale, asparagus, other "greens"	Potent antioxidants prevent age-related damage to the eye
Blue and Purple	Purple cabbage, eggplant, plums, cherries, blueberries, grapes	Anthocyanin, which protects the eye from cancer

Eat a variety of different colored fruits and veggies every day. Eat as many colors as you can because the type of carotenoid determines the pigment and the health benefits.

For example, plants with zeaxanthin tend to be yellow, and those with lycopene tend to be red. The more colorful your plate is, the more nutrients you are getting.

It's best to get at least 6 mg. per day of the important eye-healthy carotenoids from a mix of fruits and vegetables.

I always recommend food as the most natural way to get your nutrients. But the most recent Continuing Survey of Food Intakes by Individuals (CSFII) found that 85% of Americans don't eat even the USDA's minimum recommended amount of fruits and vegetables. Even if you did, that's only the bare minimum you need, not the amount you should get for optimal eye health.

This makes a good case for complementing your food with a mixed carotenoid supplement. I recommend doubling the dose on the bottle if you are already suffering any vision problems. For best results, store them in your fridge and take them with food.

But a supplement should never replace real, whole, fresh foods. Real food comes intact with all the micronutrients, minerals and co-factors that nature designed them to have, and that make them so healthy in the first place. Natural whole foods are almost always your first best choice.

Beef liver is still your best food source of vitamin A, but other good sources include dark green leafy vegetables, egg yolk, apricots, pumpkin, and sweet potatoes.

---

[1] Weston A. Price, *Nutrition and Physical Degeneration* (Lemon Grove, CA: Price-Pottinger Nutrition Foundation, 2008).

Chapter 4

Cook with Fire for a Better Brain and Healthier Heart

Summer is grilling season. And that's good news.

Grilling is the oldest and most natural, original form of food preparation. Grilling appeals to our sense of natural order — that is, as long as you keep it natural.

Keeping it natural also means there's no need to cook your meat into shoe leather. For healthy grilling, it also matters how you prepare your meat for grilling. And these days, you don't have to hunt your evening meal but you do want quality meat and fish for your grill.

I will show you:

- How to choose meat with more vitamin E, omega-3 and conjugated linoleic acid (CLA).
- Why rarer is better.
- Recipes to keep the pre-processed junk off your grill.

Real Cows Don't Eat Grain

No amount of sauce, rub or marinade is going to compensate for nutritionally inferior food. Choose animals that eat their "original" diet. "Grass-fed" animals and wild fish are the way to go. Here's why...

Grass-fed animals roam the pasture freely, dining on a variety of grasses as they choose. Some people think we raise all animals we eat that way. Unfortunately, it's far from the standard practice. The truth is most animals live in confined and dirty spaces. They eat a diet of grains. This is not natural to them and it makes them abnormally fat and unhealthy. To combat these diseases they get regular doses of antibiotics. Livestock account for the largest percentage of antibiotic use — and they're passing it all on to us, even when we don't need it.

Free range is an improvement but it's not the same as grass-fed. Grass-fed means free-range, but free-range does not necessarily mean grass-fed. "Free-range" suggests that animals have access to the outdoors. But with no standards or certification, conditions may still be cramped and unhealthy and you'd never know. Also, the animal's diet may still be unnatural, and they may be injected with antibiotics and hormones.

Then there's the term "organic." Since 1999, farmers can certify their meat and poultry as organic as long as they don't use hormones or antibiotics and they use 100% certified organic feed. But it doesn't mean the animals get their original diet, and it doesn't tell you anything about their living conditions.

Grilled Salmon with Habanero-Lime Butter

Submitted by Mike Smith to www.allrecipes.com

Serves 4

¼ cup vegetable oil
½ cup orange juice
4 tbsp. lime juice
1 tbsp. tequila
1 tbsp. grated lime zest
1 tbsp. minced habanero pepper
1 clove garlic, minced
4 (5 ounce) salmon steaks
¼ cup butter, softened
¼ tsp. garlic salt
2 tsp. minced habanero pepper
2 tsp. grated lime zest

In a bowl, stir together vegetable oil, orange juice, 3 tablespoons lime juice, 1 tablespoon lime zest, 1 tablespoon habanero pepper and garlic. Reserve a small amount to use as a basting sauce, and pour the remainder into a shallow baking dish. Place the salmon in the shallow dish, and turn to coat. Cover, and refrigerate for 2-4 hours, turning frequently.

In a small bowl, mix together softened butter, garlic salt, 1 tablespoon lime juice, 2 teaspoons habanero pepper, and 2 teaspoons lime zest. Cover and refrigerate.

Preheat grill for medium heat. Lightly oil the grill grate, and place salmon on the grill. Cook salmon for 5-8 minutes per side or until the fish can be easily flaked with a fork. Transfer to a serving dish, top with habanero butter, and serve.

Another Fishy Farming Industry

Fish is a good addition to the American diet in recent years — with indisputable health benefits. But just like their four-legged friends, how fish grow and eat determine if they belong on your grill.

Let's look at salmon, currently the most consumed fish in America. Farmed salmon live in extremely crowded conditions and eat food tainted with PCB's. No, you're not having a flashback. We banned PCBs in the 1970s — but they are persistent chemicals that are still found in high levels in farm fish feed. A recent study found that farmed Atlantic salmon contains 10 times more dioxins, PCBs, and other cancer-causing contaminants than wild Pacific salmon.[1]

Wild fish is the ocean's version of grass-fed meat.

Get 350% More Vitamin E the Natural Way

Natural meats and fish taste better and contain greater quantities beneficial nutrients. They are lower in harmful omega-6 fatty acids and higher in omega-3 fatty acids and conjugated linoleic acid (CLA).

A steak from a grass-fed steer has more omega-3 fatty acids than even wild fish do.[2] These "good fats" form in the cells of the leaves of green plants and algae. Animals and fish whose diets are high in these plants naturally have higher levels of omega-3. Studies have shown a steady decline in the levels of stored omega-3s in commercially raised or farmed animals and fish.

People with high levels of omega-3s have lower rates of high blood pressure and are 50% less apt to suffer a heart attack.[3] Omega-3s are also essential to building and maintaining your brain and nerves. They reduce depression, attention deficit disorder and Alzheimer's disease. Finally, they reduce your risk of cancer.[4] Research has shown that CLA fights cancer as well.[5] It also is effective against arteriosclerosis, reduces body fat and can prevent diabetes.

Grass-fed meat is higher in vitamin E, an essential nutrient for heart health and cancer protection as well as for its anti-aging properties. One study showed that cattle from the pasture have almost four times more vitamin E than grain-fed cattle do.

Choosing grass-fed meat and wild fish for your summertime grilling sessions will make for a much tastier — and healthier — season. Try hunting them down at your grocery store, but if they don't carry them, here are a couple of websites you can order from: **www.alaskaseafood. org** and **www.grassfedbeef.2ya.com**.

Sizzling Hot and Healthy

Now that you have the right meat, it's time to get it ready for your grill. Be careful picking a pre-made sauce. They're usually full of the worst kind of sugar. It's easy to make your own marinade or spice rub. Here are some simple tips:

- Marinade is a seasoned liquid composed of three parts: an acidic liquid for tenderness such as soy sauce, vinegar, lemon or lime juice, wine; an oil to keep it moist; and seasonings for flavor. Follow these guidelines for marinating times.

Protein	Marinate Time
Seafood	30 minutes for most
Poultry	1 hour
Beef, Lamb, Pork	At least 4 hours, 24 hours better

Here's an easy and delicious marinade recipe for you to try.

Garlic Mustard Easy Marinade

1/3 cup white wine vinegar
1/3 cup Dijon mustard
2 tsp. chopped fresh thyme
2 cloves garlic, chopped
2 tsp. olive oil
¼ tsp. salt
¼ tsp. pepper

- Spice rubs cut down on prep time — you just rub on and cook. My favorite spice combo is garlic, fresh thyme, dried cumin, salt, and cayenne pepper.

- Plain and simple — you went through the trouble of selecting the best natural, flavorful meat; why cover it up? A little salt and pepper can be plenty. Just don't salt the meat too far in advance or you'll dry it out.

How Would You Like That Done, Sir?

An equally important consideration when grilling is to cook the meat without charring. When the proteins in meat are burned by high heat, they can produce a harmful reaction, causing the creation of carcinogens called HCAs (heterocyclic amines) and PAHs (polycyclic aromatic hydrocarbons). The more rare the meat, the less of this reaction and the tastier the meat.[6]

I also use natural charcoal, sometimes called charwood. And for that great smoky, old-fashioned flavor, you can add some water-soaked hardwood chips (like oak or hickory). Just soak them for an hour and toss them right onto your coals.

Tips for Safe and Healthy Grilling

Here are some tips for healthy grilling.

- Wash your grill with hot water before grilling or turn it on high and scrape off any residue.

- If you use wooden skewers, soak them in water for an hour before use so that they don't burn on the grill.

- Use tongs instead of a fork to turn meat so it doesn't pierce the meat and let the juices out.

- Don't let the meat char or turn black — this part of the meat can contain carcinogens. If your meat does char, trim that portion off.

- If you marinade raw meat, don't reuse the sauce. It can pick up bacteria from the meat. (This will be killed in the mat over the heat on the grill but can replicate in the sauce.)

- Touch your meat for doneness. Your forehead has the consistency of well-done meat. The tip of your nose feels like medium doneness. For the feel of rare meat, touch the tip of your chin.

Meat will continue to cook for a few minutes after you remove it from the fire, so take it off the grill a few moments before the desired doneness.

---

[1] Sucher, L, Moore L. "First-Ever U.S. Tests of Farmed Salmon Show High Levels of Cancer-Causing PCBs." Environmental Working Group, Washington, DC. 2003, July 30 press release.

[2] Duckett, S, Wagner D. et al. (1993) "Effects of time on feed on beef nutrient composition." *J Anim. Sci.* 71 (8): 2079-88.

[3] Siscovick, D, Raghinathan T. et al. "Dietary Intake and Cell Membrane Levels of Long-chain n-3 Polyunsaturated Fatty Acids and the Risk of Primary Cardiac Arrest." *JAMA* 274(17): 1363-1367.

[4] Simopolous, A.P. and Robinson J. *The Omega Diet.* 1999. New York, HarperCollins.

[5] Rose D, Connolly J, et al. "Influence of Diets Containing Eicosapentaenoic or Docosahexaenoic Acid on Growth and Metastasis of Breast Cancer in Nude Mice." *Journal of the National Cancer Institute.*1995; 87(8):587-92.

[6] Smith, G. "Dietary supplementation of Vitamin E to cattle to improve shelf life and case life for domestic and international markets." Colorado State University, Fort Collins, Colorado. Knize M, Salmon C, Pais P, Felton J. "Food heating and the formation of heterocyclic aromatic amine and polycyclic aromatic hydrocarbon mutagens/carcinogens." *Advances in Experimental Medicine & Biology.* 1999;459:179-93.

Chapter 5

Throw a Steak on the Grill and Forget about Heart Disease

Did you fire up some steaks this 4th of July but then felt guilty? Or did you stay away from red meat altogether because your doctor told you to?

If you think juicy animal fat is bad for you, I have good news. Not only does your body need animal fat — *it thrives on it.*

Your heart uses animal fat for fuel. In fact, your heart is covered with a layer of "animal fat" that it uses as an energy booster during times of stress.[1]

All native cultures put animal fats at the center of their diet and show no trace of heart attacks or heart disease. The Inuits of Alaska, better known as the Eskimos, eat a diet that is over 80% animal fat. And before they were exposed to the typical Western diet they had no history of heart disease.

Now I'll expose the myths about animal fat (which you probably know as saturated fat). This "forbidden pleasure" is good for you, and your body needs it to stay vibrant and healthy — especially your heart.

Meet One of Nature's Most Important Nutrients

Saturated fat is one of your body's basic building blocks. It makes up at least 50% of all cell membranes. Many key hormones and hormone-like substances are made up of this kind of fat.

Every time you eat fat, it slows down your body's absorption of food and keeps you from feeling hungry. And of course it's a source of concentrated energy. This is why people who don't worry so much about fat are often slimmer and more vigorous than those who do.

More good news about 40% saturated fat: it's the carrier for a variety of key nutrients, including the "fat-soluble" vitamins A, D, E, and K (butter's packed with these, by the way), and the heart's most critical fuel, CoQ10. Without fat, your body couldn't absorb and use them.

It also needs saturated fat to convert some vital compounds into usable form. For instance, it uses saturated fat to turn carotene into vitamin A. These are nutrients your body must have to maintain optimum health across the board, from eyesight, bone and muscle strength to proper insulin levels, a sense of well-being — and a reduced risk of heart disease.

Here are a few more benefits you won't hear much about:

- Saturated fat is an immune booster.
- It lowers Lp(a), a substance in the blood that indicates how likely you are to develop to heart disease.
- It protects the liver from alcohol and other toxins and chemicals (including Tylenol, which can cause liver damage).
- It helps keep your bones healthy and strong. In fact, my research suggests that at least 50% of your dietary fat intake should be saturated to insure optimal calcium absorption.
- You need saturated fat to make use of omega-3 fatty acids. Omega-3 remains in your bodily tissues longer with a diet rich in saturated fats.
- Saturated fat possesses important antimicrobial properties. It protects you against harmful microorganisms in the digestive tract.

When Americans Jumped on the Low-Fat Bandwagon, Heart Attacks Skyrocketed

You'd think that ever since the 1950s, when the government began making "low-fat" dieting official policy — and people started eating less animal fat — heart disease rates would drop off a cliff. But the opposite has happened.

The proportion of traditional animal fat in the average American diet fell from 83% to 62% between 1910 and 1970. During the same period, the percentage of fat from vegetable sources — including shortening, margarine, and refined oils, shot up by about 400%.

Since then, more people have been getting fatter and dying of heart disease than ever before — forty percent of all deaths each year in the U.S. alone. It's become our nation's number one killer.

So what's changed to cause such a drastic rise in heart-related deaths?

One thing that hasn't — our fundamental physiology, which evolved over millions of years to rely on saturated fat as a major energy source. There's a reason you have a taste for this kind of fat. It's good for you, and your genetic make-up adapted to make use of it.

Consider this: if you look at the wild game our prehistoric ancestors most commonly hunted and ate, including the nutrient-packed organ meat as well as the flesh of the animal, their body fat was *heavily* saturated.[2]

Animal Food Source	% Saturated Fat
Camel	63
Wild Boar	41
Buffalo	56
Buffalo Kidney	58
Antelope	56
Antelope Kidney	65
Elk Kidney	62
Mountain Goat (Kidney)	66
Mountain Sheep	50

The nuts and seeds they foraged were also rich in fat. To take one example, pecans — a staple of the Native American diet in the Southeast — are 85% fat.

Mainstream medicine continues to blame animal fat for the rise in heart-related deaths. But modern science shows the opposite is true.

In one of the largest studies of its kind, researchers looked at the diets of 6,000 people from the town of Framingham, Massachusetts. They compared two groups in five-year intervals for four decades: those who ate diets low in cholesterol and saturated fats, and those who consumed relatively high amounts of saturated fat and cholesterol.

The creators of the Framingham Study expected to find much higher rates of heart disease in the high-fat, high-cholesterol group. But after 40 years, the facts spoke for themselves.

The director of the project had to make a reluctant confession:

> In Framingham, Mass., the more saturated fat one ate, the more cholesterol one ate, the more calories one ate, the lower the person's serum cholesterol ... We found that the people who ate the most cholesterol, ate the most saturated fat, ate the most calories, weighed the least and were the most physically active.[3]

A British study involving several thousand men found the same thing. Half quit smoking, switched over to a restricted diet with lowered saturated fat and cholesterol, and ramped up their consumption of "healthy" fats like vegetable oils and margarine. The other half ate what they pleased and even kept on smoking. After only one year, the group who stuck to the "good" diet experienced 100% more deaths from heart-related illness than those on the "bad" diet.[4]

Finally, a team of researchers at the Northwest Lipid Research Clinic in Seattle found that a diet rich in saturated fats actually *slowed* the progression of heart disease in patients already showing signs of poor heart health.[5]

And if you compare rates of heart disease and fat consumption around the world, you find the same thing: more dietary fat means fewer heart attacks. To take just three examples:

- Scientists in India discovered that people in the northern part of the country ate 17 times more animal fat than people in the south, but their overall incidence of heart disease was *seven times lower.*[6]

- The French eat more saturated fats in the form of meat, liver, pâté, butter, cream, and cheese than people in almost any other Western nation. Yet the heart-related death rate among middle-aged men there is 145 per 100,000, compared to 315 per 100,000 in the U.S. And heart-related deaths in France are actually *lowest* in Gascony, the region in France where people eat the most fat.[7]

- Most people think the Japanese eat a low-fat diet. But this is a myth. The truth is that they get plenty of fat from eggs, chicken, beef, pork, organ meats, and shellfish. The amount of animal fat in their diet has gone up steadily since World War II. Yet rates of heart disease there are among the lowest in the world — and their average life span has actually increased.[8]

Bottom line: your body needs saturated fat and is optimally designed to make use of it.

Enjoy These "Fat Foods" — Guilt-Free

While it's true that your body literally thrives on saturated fat, there's an obvious but overlooked fact about it: in order for it to be truly nutritious, it has to come from natural sources.

Fats from animals raised on their natural diets, with as little processing as possible, are automatically suited to your body's nutritional needs. Wild game, for example, survive entirely on the food sources their instincts tell them to eat.

Societies that eat a lot of saturated fat with low rates of heart disease generally maintain higher standards of purity than American commercial food makers do. They also raise more of their domestic livestock on grasses, not grains.

The result is that the fat in their meat is in exactly the right proportion for optimum health. Grass-fed cattle, for instance, yield meat that's packed with omega-3, which we normally think of as coming from fish.

Saturated fat from commercially raised animals today, on the other hand, *is* bad for you. Cattle, pigs, chickens, and other livestock from modern feedlots are forced to eat grains instead of the grasses they evolved to digest and get pumped full of hormones, antibiotics.

The result is a diseased animal with the fat content in its meat thrown out of healthy balance. Even worse, many pesticides and other toxins get stored in the fat of the animal.

This is where the Atkins diet went wrong. Dr. Atkins was right about the nutritional importance of fat, but he failed to take into account the consequences of an adulterated food supply.

You also can't really eat fat to your heart's content, as many people who followed Atkins believed. But you can get up to 35% of your total daily calories from fat without worry.

Look for meat and animal-derived products that come from organic, grass-fed, and free-range animals. Remember, enjoying meat doesn't have to mean always cooking a New York Strip on the grill. Here are some other options.

- Buy a brisket and drop it in the slow cooker and let it sit for eight hours. Throw in some veggies and you can get two or three good meals out of it.

- Cook up some flank steaks and slice them up for a low carb wrap.

- Try using ground sirloin for better burgers. Skip the bun.

And don't forget about cream and butter. They get a bad rap, but they are not the artery clogging villains everyone makes them out to be. Your nineteenth-century ancestors used lots of cream and butter in their recipes back in the days when heart disease was almost unheard of. So, don't be afraid to enjoy them.

---

[1] Fallon S, Enig M. "The Cave Man Diet." *Price-Pottenger Nutrition Foundation Health Journal.* 21(2).

[2] Castelli W. Archives of Internal Medicine. 1992. 152(7):1371-1372.

[3] Rose, et al. "The United Kingdom Heart Disease Prevention Project. Incidence and Mortality Rates." *Lancet.* 1983. 1:1062-1065.

[4] Knopp, et al. "Saturated fats prevent coronary artery disease? An American Paradox." *American Journal of Clinical Nutrition.* 2004. 80(5):1102-1103.

[5] Malhotra, S. *Indian Journal of Industrial Medicine.* 1968. 14:219.

[6] O'Neill, M. "Can Foie Gras Aid the Heart? A French Scientist Says Yes." *New York Times.* Nov 17, 1991.

[7,8] Koga Y, et al. "Recent Trends in Cardiovascular Disease and Risk Factors in the Seven Countries Study: Japan." Lessons for Science from the Seven Countries Study, Toshima, et al.Springer : New York, NY. 1994, 63-74.

Chapter 6

Will Anyone Stand Up for Salt?

A recent eight-year study of people with high blood pressure found that people on low-salt diets had more than *four times as many heart attacks* as those on normal salt diets.[1]

Salt maintains the electrolyte balance inside and outside your cells and *natural* salt contains vital minerals your body needs.

Here are just a few more of the many benefits of salt. Salt:

- Stimulates salivation and helps to balance and replenishes all of the body's electrolytes.
- Provides renewed energy.
- Gives you a high resistance to infections and bacterial diseases.
- Supplies all 82 vital trace minerals to promote optimum biological function and cellular maintenance.
- Balances alkaline/acid levels in the blood.
- Restores good digestion.
- The natural iodine in salt protects against radiation and many other pollutants.
- Aids in relieving allergies and skin diseases.
- Eliminates toxins in the body to help prevent infection.

Plus it brings out the flavors in your food when you cook.

With all the negative press on salt, how could this be?

Ignore the Government and Stick with Your Gut

When I was in med school we were taught that salt causes high blood pressure, and you read about the "evils" of salt everywhere you turned. The reason doesn't appear to be science but that there's just not much money in naturally occurring salt compared to proprietary foods and drugs.

There's a lot of money to be made in altering your food. But here's the catch — first they have to convince you that the natural food we've been eating for eons will kill you — now you have to buy their new-fangled package of modern substitute food.

Even so, when I looked at the results used to justify the "salt is bad" campaign I was shocked. The studies I discovered showed exactly the opposite of what you'd heard.

Here's a summary:

- A health outcomes study in Finland, reported to the American Heart Association, revealed that no health benefits could be identified and concluded "our results do not support the recommendations for entire populations to reduce dietary sodium intake to prevent coronary heart disease."[2]

- A ten-year follow-up study to a massive Scottish Heart Health Study found no improved health outcomes for those on low-salt diets.[3]

- An October 2007 analysis of a large Dutch database published in the *European Journal of Epidemiology* documented no benefit of low-salt diets in reducing stroke or heart attack incidence nor lowering death rates.[4]

Get the *Real* "Salt of the Earth"

Standard table salt is not only highly refined — it's chemically cleansed and unfriendly to the human body. Unrefined sea salt, on the other hand, is a naturally occurring complex of sodium chloride and a complement of essential trace minerals.

This is the form of salt your body is designed to digest — the kind of salt that's been around since humans first walked the earth. Refined table salt, on the other hand, is a modern invention, artificially designed to look white and pour easily. Your body was never meant to absorb it.

Natural salt is a source of 21 essential and 30 accessory minerals that are essential to our health. That's why I use sea salt. It's unrefined and packed with all the trace elements the ancients prized for maintaining health and vigor.

Here are just a few of the key minerals and elements you'll find in most sea salts:

Mineral	Function
Chloride	Chloride, along with sodium, regulates the acid/alkali balance in the body. It is also necessary for the production of gastric acid which is a component of hydrochloric acid (HCl).
Iron	Necessary for cell function and blood utilization. It's used to make hemoglobin, which carried oxygen in the blood. Blood loss is the most common cause of iron deficiency.
Sulfur	Found in all cells, especially in skin, connective tissues, and hair. Inadequate dietary sulfur has been associated with skin and nail diseases. Increased intake of dietary sulfur sometimes helps psoriasis and rheumatic conditions.
Calcium	Necessary for the formation and maintenance of bones, blood coagulation, and heart, nerve and muscle function. Calcium depletion can result in a number of symptoms, most notably osteoporosis which results in decreased bone mass and increased chances of bone breakage.
Copper	Copper facilitates in the absorption of iron and supports vitamin C absorption. Copper is also involved in protein synthesis and an important factor in the production of RNA.
Potassium	Stimulates nerve impulses and muscle contractions. It regulates the body's acid/alkali balance, stimulates kidney and adrenal functioning, and assists in converting glucose to glycogen. It's also important for biosynthesis of protein.
Zinc	Required for growth, immune system function, sexual development and the synthesis of insulin. Proper zinc metabolism is needed for wound healing, and carbohydrate and protein metabolism. It is considered an antibacterial factor in the prostatic fluid, and may contribute to the prevention of chronic bacterial prostatitis and urinary tract infections.

Silicon	Silicon is necessary for normal growth and bone formation. With calcium, silicon is a contributing factor in good skeletal integrity. Silicon is a main component of osteoblasts, the bone forming cells. Silicon may help to maintain youthful skin, hair and nails.
Sodium	Sodium regulates the pH of intracellular fluids and with potassium, regulates the acid/alkali balance in the body. Sodium and chloride are necessary for maintaining osmosis and electrolyte balance.
Magnesium	An important mineral because it aids in the activation of adenosine triphosphate (ATP), the main energy source for cell functioning. It also activates several enzyme systems and is important for the synthesis of RNA and DNA. Magnesium is necessary for normal muscle contraction and important for the synthesis of several amino acids.
Cobalt	Cobalt is essential to the formation of vitamin B12.

Switching to sea salt is easy to do. You can find it in most supermarkets, health food stores — even online.

Worried about Sodium?
Bring it into Balance Naturally

More important than the amount of sodium in your diet is the ratio of sodium to potassium. Recent research suggests this ratio is critical. While many studies have focused on high sodium content in the diet, it appears that problems with hypertension may be related more to an inappropriate ratio of sodium to potassium.

Sodium has a special relationship to potassium. Sodium is the major electrolyte outside the cells, and potassium is the major electrolyte *inside* the cells. These two elements work together to maintain fluid balance, transmit nerve messages and control muscle contractions.

The body monitors the amount of salt and potassium in the bloodstream, as the body has no mechanism for storing electrolytes. When a shortage of either exists, the body secretes hormones that drastically reduce excretion of electrolytes and fluids.

If you're worried about your sodium levels you can bring them into balance by making sure you get enough potassium in your diet. Potassium helps neutralize the effect of sodium on your blood pressure, lowers your risk for stroke and heart attack, and even prevents the bone loss that can lead to osteoporosis. (Notice that sea salt is rich in potassium.)

You can eat many potassium-rich foods but it will do you little good unless you are consuming adequate sodium as well. Your body cannot properly digest raw vegetables without salt. People used to eat a salty soup before a meal to enhance digestion.

Salt re-enriches your saliva so your body can manufacture the proper digestive juices to break down the complex carbohydrates, celluloids and chlorophyll from the vegetables which contain potassium. *Without salt no digestion is possible.*

Unfortunately, you probably aren't getting enough potassium through your diet alone. On an average day, the typical man gets about 3,000 mg. — women closer to 2,300 mg. For optimum health, I recommend getting around 5,000 mg. of potassium per day.

It's easier than you think. Most people think bananas are the best source, but you might be surprised. Cantaloupes, raisins and avocados are all rich in potassium.

The following page shows a table of potassium-rich foods. Try adding a few of them to your diet.

Fruits			
Avacados (One whole)	1.483	Figs (dried, 5 pieces)	675
Raisins (1/2 cup)	644	Apricots (1/2 cup)	611
Cantaloupes (1/2 melon)	853	Orange Juice (1 cup)	496
Watermelon (2 cups)	320	Grapes (1 cup)	310
Bananas (1 whole)	490	Grapefruit juice (1 cup)	400
Seafood, Beef & Poultry			
Clams (10 steamed)	597	Halibut (3 oz. cooked)	490
Snapper (4 oz. baked)	590	Carb Meat (1 cup)	481
Pork (3 oz. cooked)	310	Tuna canned (2 oz.)	130
Salmon (3 oz. cooked)	390	Flounder (3 oz. cooked)	290
Chicken (3 oz. cooked)	200	Beef (3 oz. cooked)	270

Vegetables (1/2 cup cooked)			
Swiss Chard	480	Acorn squash	450
Brussels sprouts	250	Zucchini	230
Artichokes	220	Collard greens	210
Nuts (1/2 cup)			
Almonds	520	Pistachios	620
Brazil Nuts	420	Cashews	387
Chestnuts	424	Peanuts	491
Other			
Milk (1 cup)	370	Lima beans (1/2 cup)	490
Lentils (1/2 cup)	370	Pinto beans (1/2 cup)	290
Pumpkin seeds (1/2 cup)	915	Wheat germ (2 Tbs)	270

[1] Alderman, et al. "Low urinary sodium associated with greater risk of myocardial infarction among treated hypertensive men." *Hypertension.* 1995. 25(6):1144-1152.

[2] Valkonen, V-P. "Sodium and potassium excretion and the risk of acute myocardial infarction." Presented October 15, 1998 to the American Heart Association Scientific Sessions, Dallas, TX (unpublished).

[3] Tunstall-Pedoe, H. "Comparison of the prediction by 27 different factors of coronary heart disease and death in men and women of the Scottish heart Health Study: cohort study." *British Medical Journal.* September 20, 1997. 315(7110):722-9.

[4] Geleijnse, J, et al. "Sodium and potassium intake and risk of cardiovascular events and all-cause mortality: the Rotterdam Study." *European Journal of Epidemiology.* November 2007;22(11):763-770.

Chapter 7

Ditch the Modern-Day Diet Deception

I recently read through a reproduction of a very old cookbook. The contrast between then and now was remarkable to see: the American diet before 1900 was rich in animal fat — at least 35% to 40% of calories coming from fats, mostly dairy fats in the form of butter, cream, whole milk and eggs.

Folks back then relied on lard or tallow served for frying. Dishes like headcheese and scrapple — packed with saturated fats — were popular. Heart disease, on the other hand, was rare.

The cookbook dated from 1895. It's called *The Baptist Ladies' Cook Book.*[1]

Just about every single recipe for *any kind of food you could think of* called for plenty of fat.

Their first fish recipe? "Fish a la Crème." It included a sauce made from whole milk, butter, salt and pepper. This delicious dish uses "one half-cup butter and two-thirds pint or more of cream."

Here's a great recipe for chicken croquettes, from one of the Ladies named Jessie Weir:

One pint chopped chicken, fine, one-half cup of cream, one-half cup stock, one tablespoon flour, three tablespoonfuls butter, four eggs, yellow only. Cream the butter and flour, and add to the cream stock when boiling, then the eggs, well beaten, and lemon juice. Work five minutes. Pour over the chicken. Salt and pepper to taste, mix thoroughly. When cold, shape into small balls, dip into egg, roll in cracker crumbs and fry in hot lard.

Another typical example, for scrapple, submitted by Mrs. Flora Hyde:

Take a hog's head, heart, tongue and part of the liver. Cleanse thoroughly and soak in salt water twenty-four hours. Put on the boil in cold water. Cook until all the bones can be easily removed. Then take out in a chopping bowl and chop fine. Season highly with sage, salt and pepper. Return it to the liquor on the stove, which you must strain. Then thicken with cornmeal and a teacup of buckwheat flour until the consistency of mush. Then dip out in deep dishes, and when cool, slice and fry a rich brown, as you would mush. It is very nice for a cold morning breakfast. If you make more than you can use at once, run hot lard over the rest and you can keep it all through the winter.

I couldn't turn the pages fast enough to see what else the cookbook contained. Just about every single recipe for *any kind of food you could think of* called for plenty of fat.

Here's just a sample of what those Baptist Ladies and their families were getting out of their truly "rich" diet. They're all vital to lifelong vigor and perform many essential biological functions:

Nutrient	Function	Source
Thiamin (Vitamin B1)	Releases energy from carbohydrates; promotes normal growth and keeps your appetite up.	Pork, organ meats
Riboflavin (Vitamin B2)	Maintains healthy skin and eyes; maintains a normal nervous system; releases energy to your body's cells during metabolism.	Organ meats, milk, cream, butter, cheese
Niacin (Vitamin B3)	Helps growth and development; maintains your nervous system and gastrointestinal tract health.	Organ meats, milk, cream, butter, cheese, eggs, poultry, fish, beef
Folic Acid (Vitamin B9)	Cell division and reproduction, red blood cell production.	Organ meats, eggs
Cobalamin (Vitamin B12)	Metabolism and health of every cell in your body.	Organ meats, beef, pork, fish, shell fish, milk, cream, butter, cheese, eggs
Pyridoxine (Vitamin B6)	Helps you digest fat, supports your nervous system; DNA integrity and gene expression.	Organ meats, beef, ham, egg yolk, fish

Vitamin A	Helps bone and tooth development; promotes good night vision; maintains healthy skin and membranes.	Organ meats, egg yolk, milk, butter, cream, cheese
Selenium	Prevents breakdown of fats and other body chemicals; promotes virility.	Seafood, meat, egg yolk, chicken, milk, cream, butter, cheese
Zinc	Required for growth, immune system function, sexual development and the synthesis of insulin.	Shellfish, meat, fish, poultry, nuts, eggs
Magnesium	Synthesis of RNA and DNA; necessary for normal muscle contraction and important for the synthesis of several basic biological building blocks.	Shellfish, liver, beef
Iodine	Critical to healthy thyroid function, hormone production, metabolism.	Shrimp, oysters, lobster, shellfish

This "Old Fashioned" Diet Would Be Condemned by Modern Science… but There's Clinical Proof That Proves the Power of Good Fat

The chart above shows a partial list of vitamins and nutrients found in the Victorian-era diet. It gives you some idea of just how "unhealthy" the pre-industrial diet really was.

Folks back then were getting a broad range of vital nutrients from their animal-based diet, all of which went out the window once they started listening to the mainstream medical establishment's misguided advice on diet.

The science refutes the claim that fat's bad for you, too. In fact, it proves the opposite: a low-fat, high-carb diet can be deadly.

To take one example, a British study involving several thousand men found that fat wasn't the culprit behind heart disease. Half the people in the study quit smoking, switched over to a restricted diet with lowered saturated fat and cholesterol, and ramped up their consumption of so-called "healthy" fats like vegetable oils and margarine.

The other half ate what they pleased and even kept on smoking. After only one year, the group who stuck to the "good" diet experienced **100% more deaths** from heart-related illness than those on the "bad" diet.[2]

A team of researchers at the Northwest Lipid Research Clinic in Seattle found that a diet rich in saturated fats actually *slowed* the progression of heart disease in patients already showing signs of poor heart health.[3]

Probably the most notorious — and underreported — proof came from one of the largest studies of its kind, the Framingham Study, involving over 30,000 men and women for decades.

The creators of the Framingham Study expected to find much higher rates of heart disease in the high-fat, high-cholesterol group. But after 40 years, the facts spoke for themselves.

As I've noted in the past, the director of the project had to make a reluctant confession:

In Framingham, Mass., the more saturated fat one ate, the more cholesterol one ate, the more calories one ate, the lower the person's serum cholesterol... We found that the people who ate the most cholesterol, ate the most saturated fat, ate the most calories, weighed the least and were the most physically active.[4]

So how could people back then eat so richly and stay free of chronic disease?

The answer's simple: the fats they ate were natural, and the foods they cooked with were literally *packed* with nutrients.

The foods we eat today don't contain the same amount of nutrients as they did at the turn of the century.

A study by Kushi Institute studied nutrient changes from 1975 through 1997. It found vitamin and mineral content declined by as much as 25-50% in both fruits and vegetables.[5]

Combine this with earlier (pre-ripened) picking, longer storage, and more processing of crops, and it's not surprising that we may be getting fewer nutrients in our food than we were 100 years ago.

One *must* take supplements to get the same amount of nutrients and minerals our grandparents were getting naturally from food.

Before you go out and start loading up on these rich, delicious foods, there are a few things to bear in mind, some of them obvious, some not so much.

Eat real foods, the kind the Baptist Ladies did.[6] I recommend sticking exclusively to natural, organic, grass-fed or wild-caught animal meats and other animal products. This is what our forebears ate, and the sad fact is that today's animal fat is exactly where most toxins are stored. That includes pesticides, chemicals, and unnatural additives.

Don't be afraid to eat cream, butter, milk, lard, and other animal-derived foods, so long as they come from grass-fed, organic sources. (In moderation, of course.) The Baptist Ladies sure didn't, and they got all the nutritional benefit these nutrient-packed foods supply.

These should be supplemented with organic fruits, nuts, seeds, and wild-caught fish. Keep carbs to a minimum. This is the way our prehistoric ancestors ate (not to mention folks in the 1800s). Your body will stay lean and optimally healthy without the calorie-counting and carb-heavy dietary regime the USDA's brainwashed everyone into thinking of as healthy.

- Steer clear of processed or prepared foods. There's a bounty of carbohydrates and sugars hidden in most commercial food products, including high levels of high fructose corn syrup (HFCS). This stuff is an artificial, high-carb sugar that overloads your liver and packs on the pounds. It puts you on the fast track to heart disease.

- Bear in mind that not all fats are the same. "Good fats" include those from healthy animals raised as Nature intended, on foods their bodies were designed to digest (grasses for cattle and other ruminants, fruits, root vegetables, and flowers for pigs). The fat in the meat from these animals actually contain omega-6 and omega-3 in the right ratio (about 2:1).

- Forget about cholesterol. This is the great red herring of modern medicine. The fact is that, as the authors of the Framingham study discovered, there's no real link between heart attack and cholesterol intake. The key is to get the right balance of LDL and HDL. As long as your HDL levels are high — 85 or so — it doesn't matter if your total cholesterol's 150 or 350.

- Don't go "hog-wild" on fats. The old way of eating meant you got about 30-40% of your calories from fat.[6] The same should be true today. The rest of your diet should be low-carb, with (organic) fruits, vegetables, seeds, and nuts playing the major roles.

- Skip the cheap meats. Sure, you might save money by going for that 99 cents per pound ground beef. But it's not worth the risk. Cheap commercial meat's packed with hormones, antibiotics, pesticides, and chemicals from fertilizers used to grow their grain-based feed. This stuff is poison, wreaks havoc on your health over time, and leads to a host of lethal diseases, including cancer.

- Get your omega-3s. You already know about the importance of these essential fatty acids, and you'll want to make sure you get the right balance of fats. Integrating them into your diet ensures you're getting the right amount of fat in the right ratio (the animal products of our forebears actually contained plenty of omega-3s). I recommend cod liver oil as a good nutritional supplement — about a tablespoon per day.

- Exercise. Plain and simple. The fact is that back in the nineteenth century, nearly every sector of the economy — food production and distribution, construction, transportation, communication, consumer goods, resource extraction, land management—all of these were largely the direct or indirect result of hard manual labor. People spent *a lot* more time outdoors engaged in physical activity. I suggest you do the same.

[1]. *The Baptist Ladies' Cook Book: Choice and Tested Recipes.* Monmouth, IL: January 1, 1895.

[2] Rose, et al. "The United Kingdom Heart Disease Prevention Project. Incidence and Mortality Rates." *Lancet.* 1983. 1:1062-1065.

[3] Knopp, et al. "Saturated fats prevent coronary artery disease? An American Paradox." *American Journal of Clinical Nutrition.* 2004. 80(5):1102-1103.

[4] Castelli, W. "Concerning the Possibility of a Nut...." 1992. 152(7):1371-1372.

[5] Jack, A. Nutrition under siege. *One Peaceful World Journal.* 1998;34(1):7–9.

[6] Fallon,Enig. "Americans Now and Then." *Price-Pottenger Nutrition Foundation Health Journal.* 1999;20(4):574-7763.

Chapter 8

Three Big Reasons Why You Don't Want to Be a Vegetarian

Meat Is Your ONLY Source of These Must-Have Nutrients

When I ask my university students if they're vegetarians or meat eaters at least two-thirds of the class claims to be vegetarians. But most of them admit to eating fish, poultry and dairy products.

This wishful thinking is common to vegetarians. Even nutrition students are misinformed. Avoiding red meat doesn't make you a vegetarian — and it doesn't make you any healthier.

Here's the bottom line: if you follow a true "vegetarian" no-meat diet, you may be robbing yourself of three critical nutrients you need to stay healthy.

I'll show you how this happens and how you can avoid it. I'll also give you easy-to-follow guidelines for safely enjoying the kind of red meat your ancestors thrived on.

On a Vegetarian Diet There's a 93% Chance You're Not Getting Enough Zinc

By avoiding beef, you are over seven times more likely to suffer a zinc deficiency.[1] Check out this graph:

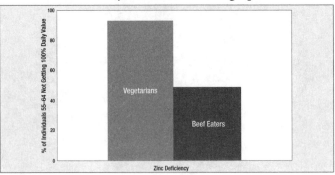

And that's bad news. As a mineral, zinc is second only to iron in concentrations in the body. It helps in the production of hundreds of enzymes that are responsible for regulating your bodily functions.

The prostate has the highest concentration of zinc in the body. And a deficiency has been linked to inflammation of the prostate known as *prostatitis*.

Zinc also has many anti-aging benefits. It is essential for making super-oxide dismutase (SOD), the most *potent* antioxidant that your body has. It also gives your skin a more youthful look. Zinc is essential for your body to use collagen which makes your skin more resilient and elastic — to fight off wrinkles and saggy skin.

Zinc also keeps your vision sharp by transporting vitamin A to the retina, improving night vision. And it protects retinal cells from free-radical damage while helping to slow down the progression of age-related macular degeneration (AMD).

The list of zinc's crucial role in your health is long, including:

- Promote a healthy immune system.
- Growth of reproductive organs.
- Fertility and conception.
- Prevent acne and regulate the activity of oil glands.
- Aid in protein synthesis and collagen formation.
- Cell reproduction and wound healing.
- Perception of taste and smell.
- Protect the liver from chemical damage.
- Bone formation.
- Maintain both vitamin E and vitamin A in the blood.
- Decrease the amount of copper absorbed.

Zinc deficiency is just the start of "veggie-only" dangers. There are two other critical nutrients you only get from red meat.

Avoiding Beef Robs You of Energy...

You've heard me talk about it before: CoQ10 is vital to your heart's survival.

Every cell in your body uses CoQ10 for high-octane energy. And your heart needs *massive* amounts of energy to pump blood... around the clock... every day.

I hope you're paying attention, vegetarians, because red meat is the ONLY dietary source of *heart-critical* CoQ10.

In my own practice I see it all the time — vegetarians with critically low levels of this vital nutrient.

CoQ10 is not only vital to your heart's ability to pump blood, it's essential to *life itself.* That's because *every single organ in your body* uses CoQ10 to get the energy they need to function. And if you don't eat red meat, you're not getting enough from your food. Period.

...and Weakens Your Mind

Here's the third critical nutrient missing from vegetarian diets: vitamin B12.

The body uses B12 to create red blood cells. It also helps maintain the nervous system, and is critical for brain health. B12 forms a protective layer around the nerve cells in your brain. Without that protective layer your brain can't function properly.

Deficiency can cause memory loss, "brain fog" or worse — not to mention anemia and neuropathy where the degeneration of nerve fibers causes irreversible neurological damage.

And even vegetarians admit you can't get reliable dietary sources of B12 from anything but animal sources like liver, fish, eggs, and meat.

Urban Legend versus Real Science

Vegetarian ideas are not backed by real science. Many are simply myths or urban legends. And some of them are *dangerous.*

Here are a few examples:

Animal fats cause heart disease — Studies have shown that the plaque in arteries that causes heart disease is mostly made of *unsaturated fats,* especially polyunsaturated ones (in *vegetable* oil), not the saturated fat of animals like vegetarians believe.[2]

In fact, *the body needs saturated fats* to be able to use other key nutrients, like fatty-acids and fat-soluble vitamins.

Here's another vegetarian slip-up:

Vegetarians live longer and have more energy — This one is misleading. The reports of vegetarians living longer are likely due to the fact that most of them also choose to exercise, eat less junk food, and not smoke.

One massive study on heart disease by Russell Smith, PhD, showed that when the consumption of animal products increased, mortality rates decreased![3]

Moreover, a study by Burr and Sweetnam in 1982, revealed that, although vegetarians did have a slightly lower (0.11%) rate of heart disease than meat eaters (again, probably due to other healthy choices), the *overall death rate was much higher for vegetarians!*[4]

In spite of the evidence, religious and politically correct groups co ntinue to perpetuate the myth that meat-eating peoples have shorter life spans.

Here's another baseless myth:

Humans evolved as vegetarians — Think so? Here's a fact: <u>There are NO native vegetarians</u>. Every native culture known to man — both past and present — has prized meat above all else.

You can start by looking at the modern equivalents to our ancestors. There are many native people today who live in a fashion similar to our caveman ancestors, and they have much lower rates of heart disease and other degenerative conditions *than we do*. What are they eating? *Lots of animal fats.*

- Take the Aborigines of Australia. They eat a diet rich in animal products, and are renowned for their longevity (at least before Western diets entered the picture).[5]

- Explorers report remarkably old ages among the Eskimos or Inuit (again, before western influence) who eat large quantities of whale and seal fat.[6]

- How about the Russians of the Caucasus Mountains? They live to great ages eating fatty pork and whole raw milk products.

- Then there are the Hunzas, mountain people of northern India, who are legendary for their robust health and longevity. They eat large portions of goat's milk which has higher saturated fat content than cow's milk.[7]

Yet, the mostly vegetarian Hindus of southern India have the shortest life spans in the world! That's partly because of a lack of food, but also because of a distinct lack of animal protein in their diets.[8]

The bottom line: vegetarians say that a diet of meat and animal fat leads to a premature death. Anthropological data from primitive societies do not support that claim.[9]

Here's a common vegetarian misconception I would find *laughable* if it weren't for how tragic the results can be:

You can get what you need by substituting meat and dairy with soy — Hello? Has anyone preaching the "vegetarian gospel" even *read* the facts?

The *fermented* soy foods like miso, tamari, tempeh and natto are definitely healthful in certain amounts, but the super-processed soy products that most vegetarians consume are not. This is because unfermented soy is high in phytic acid.[10] That's an *anti-nutrient* that actually binds to minerals and *carries them out of your body!*

Vegetarians are known for their tendency to be mineral deficient. And the high grain and legume-based diet, which are full of phytates, is to blame.[11, 12]

Just look at the nutrition of soy. Like all legumes it's low in cysteine, methionine, and tryptophan, all vital amino acids. Worse, soybeans contain *no vitamin A or D*, both of which are needed by the body to absorb the beans' proteins![13]

Check this out. Here are three key nutrients the body needs for optimal health. This chart shows beef versus vegetarian sources. You be the judge.

Vegetarian Foods Contain ZERO B12 and CoQ10			
	Vitamin B12	**CoQ10**	**Zinc**
Daily Value	6 mcg.	N/A	15 mg.
%Daily Value			
Beef (3oz)	37	2.6 mg.	39
Tofu (1/2cup)	0	0	8
Pinto Beans (1/2 cup)	0	0	6
Black Beans (1/2 cup)	0	0	6
Chickpeas (1/2 cup)	0	0	8
Peanut Butter (2T)	0	0	6
Almonds (1oz)	0	0	6

Source: U.S. Department of Agriculture; Iowa State University

As you can see by the table above, there are no vegetarian sources of vitamin B12 or CoQ10, and only limited sources of zinc. That makes a balanced diet difficult.

Soy is no substitute for meat. Not only does soy rob you of essential nutrients, it can actually damage your health. Soy has high levels of phytoestrogens. Phytoestrogens feed tumors and can destroy your cognitive function. And they can severely affect development in children. Parents who feed their infants soy-based formula are feeding them the *hormonal equivalent of five birth-control pills a day!*[14]

Vegetarians Don't Like to Admit It, but We Were All Born to Eat Meat

Simple fact is our ancestors thrived on meat. It's part of the metabolism that is in your DNA. It's perfectly natural to crave it, and to want to sink your teeth into a juicy steak. Don't let myths or political correctness make you feel guilty about that.

Your body is telling you what you need. But you need to get *real* meat, not the poor excuse for meat that big corporations are shrink-wrapping for your local grocers.

Grass-fed beef is a much better option. It has a potent nutritional value, and is packed with CoQ10, zinc and vitamin B12 — and it has the proper ratio of omega fatty-acids. Commercial grain-fed cattle is poisonous by comparison.

Follow These Five Simple Guidelines for Finding High-Quality Beef

- Grass-fed beef is growing in popularity so you may find it at one of your local grocery stores. Places like Whole Foods Market usually have a wide selection of grass-fed meats, and they are often locally raised.

- The best option I've found is at www.uswellnessmeats.com. I've been buying from them for years and I know the owner personally. Their quality is exceptional and they have a number of other raw and grass-fed products on hand. Their butters and cheeses are out-of-this-world delicious. By the way, when you order online, your order is shipped to you by overnight mail — and your food is never compromised.

- If you can't get grass-fed, your best bet is beef raised without hormones or antibiotics. This meat will most likely be grain-fed but it's widely available and clearly marked on the package. Usually grocery stores will separate this meat from the rest. If you're unsure, just ask someone behind the meat counter and they'll point it out if they have it. And don't be shy about striking up a conversation. Even if your grocery store doesn't sell grass-fed or hormone-free beef they can often tell you where to find it.

- If you're not sure about the quality, here's a simple rule of thumb: the cheaper the meat, the more contaminated it's likely to be. When you see those super-saver sales, like the kind advertised on TV or stuffed into your mailbox at home, you can assume that it's grain-fed and pumped full of every chemical and hormone known to man. It doesn't pay to eat cheap meat.

- Same rule applies when you're going out to eat — meat from fast food restaurants is the worst. Especially those places offering you an entire burger or sandwich for 79 cents or whatever their offer of the moment happens to be. It's poison.

If you're still not convinced that a vegetarian diet is a disaster waiting to happen, and wish to remain a vegetarian, then you need to be vigilant about your supplements. You need a full range of B vitamins, minerals and a powerful CoQ10 source — get the reduced ubiquinol — not the ubiquinone. This is critical — *no* exceptions.

I recommend a homocysteine-reducing formula for your B vitamins, as they usually have a powerful blend of the ones you need most. They're easy to find at your local vitamin store. For minerals — aside from zinc — I recommend you take chromium, selenium and boron. You can find them at vitamin or health food stores. Just follow the directions on the label.

For boron I recommend taking three to six mg. a day. Selenium you should get at least 55 micrograms a day, and for chromium, 100 to 200 micrograms a day.

Diehard vegetarians should have regular blood tests to protect against deficiency — especially for CoQ10. Many of my vegetarian patients have low CoQ10 levels, (1 mcg/ml or below). Try and at least double that. And for therapeutic levels, shoot for three to four mcg/ml.

If your doctor won't order a test for CoQ10, you can go to Quest labs. You can find a location near you by searching their website: www. questdiagnostics.com.

---

[1] Waylett, D.K, et.al. "The Role of Beef as a Source of Vital Nutrients in Healthy Diets."*ENVIRON*. Prepared for National Cattlemen's Beef Association. Arlington, VA. July 1999.

[2] Felton CV, et al. "Dietary polyunsaturated fatty acids and composition of human aortic plaques." *Lancet*. 1994; 344:1195.

[3] Smith R, Pinckney E. "Diet, Blood Cholesterol, and Coronary Heart Disease: A Critical Review of the Literature--vol. 2." Vector Enterprises, CA. 1991.

[4] Burr M., et al. "Mortality in vegetarians and nonvegetarians: detailed findings from a collaborative analysis of 5 prospective studies." American Society for Clinical Nutrition. 1999.

[5] Price W. *Nutrition and Physical Degeneration*. 163-187.

[6] Stefansson V. *The Fat of the Land*.Macmillan; NY. 1956.

[7] Pitskhelauri. G. "The Long Living of Soviet Georgia." Human Sciences Press, NY.1982. ; Moore T. *Lifespan: What Really Affects Human Longevity*. Simon & Schuster, NY. 1990.

[8] Abrams, H. "The relevance of paleolithic diet in determining contemporary nutritional needs." *J Appl Nutr* 1979l; (31)1,2:43-59.

[9] Abrams H. "Vegetarianism: An anthropological/nutritional evaluation." *J Appl Nutr* 1980, 32:2:53-87.

[10] JN Freeland-Graves and others. "Zinc status in vegetarians." *J Am Diet Assoc* 1980 Dec 77:655-6

[11] BF Harland and others. "Nutritional status and phytate: zinc and phytate x calcium:zinc dietary molar ratios of lacto-ovo vegetarian Trappist monks: 10 years later." *J Am Diet Assoc* 1988; 88: 1562-6

[12] Sandberg AS., "The effect of food processing on phytate hydrolysis and availability or iron and zinc." *Adv Exp Med Biol.* 1991;289:499-508.

[13] L. Dunne. The Nutrition Almanac, 3rd edition, 306.

[14] Fitzpatrick M. "Soy Isoflavones: Panacea or Poison?" *Jnl of PPNF.* Fall 1998.

Chapter 9

Don't Discard Centuries of Nutrition Wisdom

My dad was health conscious in an old-fashioned way. He practiced holistic health care before it had a name. He knew how to keep himself lean and muscular without much effort.

He would beat all the neighbors at parties in push-up contests. Women would steal glances at his biceps and men would marvel at his feats of strength. Many people probably assumed it was good genes. Yet I believe it was about life choices.

Our culture has been critical of the health choices of our fathers. They have become politically incorrect — even taboo. Yet before you throw away these centuries of wisdom, let's reexamine them in light of today's science.

Dad never lifted a weight in his life. He did rounds of push-ups, pull-ups and crunches. He said his diet of raw eggs, wild game and spicy food would "make a man out of you." Most tips he got from his father and older brothers. They were their own men's club. He passed these health tips down to me, and now I want to share them with you.

Eat Wild Game, Grass-Fed Meat

My dad was a hunter. We always had rabbit, squirrel and quail — and occasionally deer or wild boar. He claimed that eating meat could make you strong and "put hair on your chest."

I never took this literally until decades later, when I found research that red meat is the best source of muscle building creatine, provides the highest concentration of heart-fueling CoQ10 and increases testosterone levels.

As testosterone drops, men lose body hair. As testosterone rises, men experience increases in body hair in a masculine distribution. You were right, Dad; meat really does put hair on your chest.

The meat we ate was either wild game or from nearby farms. The majority of the meat we eat today comes from commercial farms. Farmers feed the cattle grain, animal by-products, and synthetic hormones and antibiotics.[1]

Feedlot cattle do not eat what nature intended them to eat. As a result, the cattle often have a difficult time digesting the starch and get sick or die. To combat the disorders caused by a starchy diet, farmers inject the animals with antibiotics.

The percentage of livestock that is salmonella resistant to five different antibiotics has increased from less than 1% in 1980 to 34% in 1996.[2] The numbers continue to rise. A growing body of evidence incriminates feedlot growth hormones as a risk factor for gastrointestinal cancers.[3]

How can you follow this tradition? Eat wild game and grass-fed beef. You can find these products at the grocery store if you ask and you can order them online. The prices are a bit higher, but the health benefits are substantial. Grass-fed beef and wild game is higher in omega-3, CoQ10, beta-carotene and vitamin E.

This reduces your risk of heart disease, certain cancers, depression, high blood pressure, and diabetes. What's more, grass-fed beef is five times higher in CLA than feedlot beef. CLA helps convert fat to lean muscle.[4]

Spicy Foods Protect Your Heart

Dad was fond of the spicy foods that nutritionists have been telling us to avoid. He grew a variety of his own peppers and dosed much of the food he ate with hot pepper sauces. He said they were good for your heart. He also enjoyed daring me to eat them.

It turns out that many spicy foods contain powerful antioxidants that protect against heart disease. Plants in the pepper family contain capsaicin, which has been shown to speed up your metabolism and your ability to burn calories.[5]

Dad's love of hot sauce may have helped him stay lean. If you like spices and peppers, don't be afraid to throw some in your next meal.

Drink a Raw Egg Daily

Right after his nightly set of push-ups, Dad drank a raw egg. He said his father would take one directly from the chicken coop, punch a hole in it with his pocketknife, put it to his lips and suck it down. He thought it was important for me to learn this technique but usually we would break it into a glass. The eggs we bought in those days came right from the farm.

Dad always said that eggs were the perfect food, but they were better if eaten raw. I don't know how he knew this, but after devoting my life to natural nutrition and health, I couldn't agree more.

Eggs are the only food known to man to have a protein quality rating of 100. They have every amino acid you need in exactly the ratios you need them. The white has every B vitamin and the yolk has every fat-soluble vitamin. They are an excellent source of essential fatty acids and the hard-to-get brain and heart nutrients DHA and CoQ10.

Eating eggs raw maintains their chemical makeup. When you cook eggs, the protein is denatured, the B vitamins decrease, and it may destroy the DHA. Raw eggs are additionally much easier for your body to absorb. A raw egg is absorbed in 30 minutes while it takes about four hours to digest cooked eggs. In addition, eating eggs raw saves time. You don't have to clean pots or pans.

The risk of salmonella poisoning is very unlikely from consuming raw eggs. The U.S. Department of Agriculture estimates that 0.00003% of eggs in the U.S. have salmonella.[6] I have eaten raw eggs for 40 years and have never suffered. However, you lessen your chances even more by purchasing organic eggs.

My dad's diet of meat, raw eggs and spicy food helped him stay strong and masculine, burn fat, feel great and still enjoy his life.

He taught me a reverence for health and diligence to my own body that I will never forget. I share his story as an example that I hope helps you take action to promote wellness in your own life.

---

[1] Cordain L., et al. "Origins and evolution of the Western diet: health implications

for the 21st century." *The American Journal of Clinical Nutrition.* 2005.

[2] Robinson, Jo (2000). *Why Grassfed is Best! The Surprising Benefits of Grassfed Meat, Eggs, and Dairy Products.* Washington: Vashon Island Press.

[3] Epstein, SS (1996). "Unlabeled milk from cows treated with biosynthetic growth hormones: A case of regulatory abdication." *International Journal of Health Services,* 26: 173-185.

[4] Rule D.C. (2002). "Comparison of muscle fatty acid profiles and cholesterol concentrations of bison, beef cattle, elk, and chicken." *Journal of Animal Science,* 80: 1202-1211.

[5] Hot peppers help control weight. Yoshioka M., et al. *Br J Nutr* 1999 Aug;82(2): 115-23.

[6] Hope BK, Baker R, Edel ED, Hogue AT, Schlosser WD, Whiting R, McDowell RM, Morales RA. (2002) An overview of the Salmonella enteritidis risk assessment for shell eggs and egg products. *PubMed Risk Anal:203-18.*

Chapter 10

You Should Avoid Fast Food. Right?

Not So Fast. I'll Show You How to Feast on *REAL* Fast Food

Picture this: A patient walks into my office. When I look up from her chart, I advise her to eat *more fast food*. She flashes me a look of horror — as if I had just told her to jump off a bridge.

Let me explain. I'm not talking about a bucket of fried chicken from the Colonel or a cheeseburger combo meal from your local drive-thru window.

I'm talking about *real* fast food… what I call **whole food**. Whole foods are healthy and unprocessed. It can be as fast as picking up an apple and taking a bite — or as simple as a fistful of walnuts and a bag of dried cranberries.

Whole foods are foods that come to you as nature intended — without corporate or chemical interference. But you don't have to sacrifice on taste, flavor or satisfaction. How about a grass-fed New York Strip or a marinated chicken breast with mango salsa? These whole foods are fast and easy to prepare. And they represent real value. Whole foods keep you happier, healthier and alive longer.

It's easy to be tempted by dollar menus and drive-thru windows — especially when the economy is bad. But these foods are not really fast. (They take months to prepare.) Even worse, the chemical additives and fake fats put you on the fast track to chronic disease.

Exposing the Big Lie in Your Drive-Thru Bag

When you pull away from the drive-thru window, visions of a fresh, hot hamburger dance in your head. But what's really inside that wrapper is far from what you're imagining.

Imagine growing up on a farm as I did. You'd savor the smell of a fresh hamburger cooking and couldn't wait to sink your teeth into it. From start to finish, that burger was the result of a very simple process:

- A cow was born.

- It grew up eating grass in the pasture.

- At full maturity (roughly three to four years), you took the cow to the butcher.

- You brought the fresh hamburger meat home and cooked it.

That's it. That was the complete lifecycle of a hamburger. It was a whole food — complete in nutrition, with nothing altered or stripped from what nature intended.

Now let's take a look at the lifecycle of a modern drive-thru "junk food" burger:

- A cow is born.
- Ranchers rip the un-weaned calf from its mother and send it off to a commercial feedlot.
- The calf lives with tens of thousands of other cows among giant mounds of manure. It gorges daily on a concoction of corn (a completely unnatural food for cows), antibiotics (to fight the bacteria of its living conditions) and hormones (to make it grow fatter faster).
- The cow begins to get sick from the unnatural diet and living conditions (13% of all cows at slaughter have abscessed livers[1]). It's given more antibiotics and a hormone implant.
- At only 14 to 16 months old, the sick and obese cow is sent to slaughter.
- An industrial slaughterhouse processes as many as 400 cows per hour. The speed of the lines in the name of profit makes it difficult to keep manure out of the meat. This is why, out of all foods, ground beef is the leading source of E. coli infections in the U.S.[2]
- The slaughterhouse sends the meat to a food processing plant, where they mix the ground beef with chemical flavorings,

preservatives, and other ingredients.

- They cook the meat, freeze it, package it, and ship it to your local junk food restaurant.

- Your junk food vendor reheats your burger from frozen to done in around 40 seconds.

- They top your burger with chemically enhanced condiments. McDonald's mayo has 19 ingredients including preservatives and coloring. There's also the pickles and ketchup — equally as chemically laden.

- They wrap your burger and put it under a heat lamp where it sits for an undetermined amount of time until you pull up to the window.

Hardly a natural process, is it? Now you know why it's called *junk food*.

"Okay," you think. "You're right. I should limit my drive-thru stops to breakfast on my way to work." Sorry, but it's no better.

Even breakfast is an overprocessed chemical nightmare at the mega-chain drive-thrus. For example, if you ordered eggs you'd expect… well, eggs. But here's the official McDonald's ingredient list — word for word — of two plain scrambled eggs from their menu:

"*Pasteurized whole eggs with sodium acid pyrophosphate, citric acid and monosodium phosphate (all added to preserve color), nisin (preservative). Prepared with liquid margarine: Liquid soybean oil, water, partially hydrogenated cottonseed and soybean oils, salt, hydrogenated cottonseed oil, soy lecithin, mono- and diglycerides, sodium benzoate and potassium sorbate (preservative), artificial flavor, citric acid, vitamin A palmitate, beta carotene (color).*"[3]

As you can see, the commercial junk sold by mega-corporations isn't really "fast food."

If you want to save your health, it's time you learn about *real* — and healthy — fast, whole foods.

Discover the Holy Grail of Lifesaving Nutrition

The "processing" of whole food is simple. Mother Nature grows it; the farmer harvests it; you eat it. What could be simpler — or faster? It is food the way nature intended you to eat it — the "holy grail" of food.

With whole food, there is no giant "processing plant" between the field and your stomach… no factory making chemical preservatives to inject into your food… and no laboratories inventing ways to enhance the flavor or color.

It's clear: Big corporations focus on profit — not nutrition. Massive food processing plants smash, grind, boil, nuke and chemically alter your food in the name of convenience and flavor. When they do that, they destroy vital nutrients in the food — nutrients your body needs.

Think about this for a moment. Which one is a whole food: an apple, or applesauce? Here's the "process" of eating an apple: You (or a farmer) pick an apple from a tree, and you eat it — *that's it*. It's perfect… whole… and nutritious.

But to sell you a jar of applesauce, "mega-food" corporations grow nutrient-poor apples (due to over-farming and using chemical fertilizers and pesticides). Then they wash the apples in a chemical bath, peel them, cook them, and finally add chemical preservatives, colors and flavors.

Which one do you think has more nutrients intact?

In fact, check out this table. It shows you just how much of the nutrition is lost from common processing methods.

Typical Maximum Nutrient Losses (as compared to raw food)					
Vitamins	**Freeze**	**Dry**	**Cook**	**Cook+ Drain**	**Re- heat**
Vitamin A	5%	50%	25%	35%	10%
Retinol Activity Equivalent	5%	50%	25%	35%	10%
Alpha Carotene	5%	50%	25%	35%	10%
Beta-Carotene	5%	50%	25%	35%	10%
Beta Cryptoxanthin	5%	50%	25%	35%	10%
Lycopene	5%	50%	25%	35%	10%
Lutein+Zeaxanthin	5%	50%	25%	35%	10%
Vitamin C	30%	80%	50%	75%	50%
Thiamin	5%	30%	55%	70%	40%
Riboflavin	0%	10%	25%	45%	5%

				Cook+	Re-
Niacin	0%	10%	40%	55%	5%
Vitamin B6	0%	10%	50%	65%	45%
Folate	5%	50%	70%	75%	30%
Food Folate	5%	50%	70%	75%	30%
Folic Acid	5%	50%	70%	75%	30%
Vitamin B12	0%	0%	45%	50%	45%
Minerals	**Freeze**	**Dry**	**Cook**	**Cook+ Drain**	**Re- heat**
Calcium	5%	0%	20%	25%	0%
Iron	0%	0%	35%	40%	0%
Magnesium	0%	0%	25%	40%	0%
Phosphorus	0%	0%	25%	35%	0%
Potassium	10%	0%	30%	70%	0%
Sodium	0%	0%	25%	55%	0%
Zinc	0%	0%	25%	25%	0%
Copper	10%	0%	40%	45%	0%

Source: USDA Table of Nutrient Retention Factors (2003)

As you can see, you lose a lot of nutrition when you process foods using even traditional methods. But here's the thing: the giant food processing plants that make your modern food are processing to the *extreme*.

They're not just cooking — they're blasting. They don't just chop — they mutilate. It's what happens when machines replace humans.

Then there's the additional processing like the addition of chemicals and irradiation. What do you think irradiation does to your food?

The only way to avoid this insanity — and stop it from stealing your health — is to eat whole food. Whole food gives you all of the nutrition, and none of the junk.

My Top Five Whole Food Favorites for Supercharged Health

You'll not only find whole foods to be healthier when you calculate cost per serving. Of course, you have to make an accurate comparison — just how many processed burgers would it take to get the same nutrition as one natural burger?

Here are my top four favorite whole foods:

1. Grass-Fed Beef — Your body relies on protein for nearly every function it performs. And beef is one of the best sources of whole food nutrition there is. The emphasis here is on *grass-fed* beef.

Most commercial beef is grain fed, which causes an imbalance in the fatty acids of the cow. You get an unhealthy ratio of omega-6 to omega-3 fatty acids when you eat grain-fed animals. It's that imbalance, not animal fats in general, that contribute to heart disease.

You can find grass-fed beef at health food stores, or online. I prefer U.S. Wellness Meats. Find them at http://www.grasslandbeef.com/.

2. Eggs — Eggs offer the most complete protein of any food. They contain all the amino acids (the building blocks of cells) used by the human body.

It's important to eat only eggs that come from free range, natural farming methods. Commercial farming practices have hurt the healthy nutritional makeup of eggs too.

3. Dark Green Veggies — Dark green vegetables are a great source of antioxidants, vitamins and minerals. A few of my favorites are kale, spinach, celery, eggplant, and especially… broccoli. In addition to many other nutrients, broccoli is rich in magnesium and calcium.

And yes, commercial farming has even managed to mess that up too. For example, today's broccoli has less than 50% of the calcium it did just 10 years ago.[4]

So, just like other foods, be sure to get organically grown produce. Local is even better.

4. Nuts — In addition to being a good source of protein, nuts also contain omega-3 fatty acids that help ease inflammation. I like Brazil nuts, almonds, pistachios, hazelnuts, and my personal favorite: walnuts.

I grew up eating walnuts. In addition to being the highest source of omega-3 of any nut, they are full of heart healthy flavonoids and arginine, which helps dilate the blood vessels.

You should know that peanuts aren't really a nut. They're a tuber, and they promote inflammation. Stay away from them.

So avoid nuts that have been processed and/or cooked with peanut oil. And don't eat them with other processed ingredients like sugar-coatings, colors, and preservatives.

In the end, if you feel you must eat what the mainstream call "fast food," be conscientious about it. Choose the healthiest option you can.

For example, Boston Market offers decent nutrition in a hurry. Their selections have little trans fats or processed carbs, and there are several high-protein choices.

But if you just can't shake that addiction to your favorite mega-chain burger joint, at least keep these things in mind:

- **Choose the Leanest Red Meats** — The saturated fats of *quality beef* are actually healthy for you. But that's a *far cry* from what you're getting from fast food chains. Fast food chains are all about profit, and that means buying the cheapest beef possible from commercial sources. The fats in this beef are out of balance, and are quite harmful.

- **Pitch the Bun** — The processed carbs in white bread are high in glycemic load, and cause a host of problems such as blood sugar problems and arterial damage. Eat your burgers "naked."

- **Skip the Dressing** — Even the dressings for the "healthier" salads offered by fast food chains are a toxic nightmare. Full of artificial and chemical flavors, they are also full of trans fats, a big culprit in hardening of the arteries.

- **Drink Water** — It's an automatic reflex for most people to order a soda with that meal deal. But look before you leap. The amount of sugar in a typical soda is shocking. You're drinking around 12 teaspoons in a 16-ounce soft drink. Now, do the math on how much you're getting once you've been "supersized" to that 64-ounce cup!

---

1. Pollan M. "Unhappy Meals." *The New York Times*. January 28, 2007.
2. Centers for Disease Control and Prevention, "Disease Listing, Escherichia coli O157:H7." CDC, 2006

3. McDonald's. "It's all about delicious choices: Nutrition Choices. Changing. Together." 2010-2015.
4. Farnham M. "Calcium and Magnesium Concentration of Inbred and Hybrid Broccoli Heads." *Journal of the American Society for Horticultural Science.* Feb 15, 2000.

Chapter 11

Why I "Prescribe" Meat to My Patients

Have you seen any of these headlines?

- "Too much red meat will kill you" (*The National Business Review*)

- "Want to live longer? Cut back on red meat" (CNN)

- "Meat-heavy diet linked to early death" (*USA Today*)

So why in the world would I "prescribe" eating red meat to my patients — when the mainstream media are screaming to the masses that it will kill you?

Because, in my opinion, there's a huge difference between factory-farm GRAIN-FED beef and pasture-raised GRASS-FED beef.

Here's why.

Get the Truth about Grain-Fed Beef

Cattle aren't supposed to eat grain. They're natural-born grass eaters. But factory farmers feed cattle high-calorie, high-octane grain to fatten them up faster... bring them to market faster... and reap higher profits.

Unfortunately, you wind up paying for it. Grain-fed beef has up to three times more fat than grass-fed beef.[1]

And grain isn't the only "unnatural" food these farmers serve cattle, either.

You know the saying, "You are what you eat?"

Well, think about this:

Factory farmers have also been known to feed cattle:

1. Recycled human food, such as stale candy, pizza, potato chips, brewery wastes, and hamburger buns.

2. Parts of our fruits and vegetables that we don't eat, such as orange rinds, beet pulp, and carrot tops.

3. STUFF YOU DON'T WANT TO KNOW ABOUT, including chicken manure, chicken feathers, newsprint, cardboard, and "aerobically digested" municipal garbage.

And here's something even more disturbing.

In the mid-1990s, a team of animal researchers conducted a study to see what would happen if they fed cattle stale chewing gum — still in its wrappers."[2]

The conclusion? Here's a direct quote from the researchers. (I'm not making this up.)

"… gum and its packaging material can safely replace at least 30% of growing and finishing diets without impairing feedlot performance or carcass merit."

Fatten cattle up on stale bubblegum and aluminum wrappers and pass on the end product to you and your family.

Would you eat something that was raised on stale candy, garbage, bubblegum, aluminum wrappers, cardboard and chicken crap? Or feed it to your family?

I'll tell you something — the fact that the USDA lets this fly is absolutely insane.

And then there are all the synthetic hormones, low-level antibiotics, and chemicals they pump into factory-farm cattle…

… or how the cattle may "accidentally" get fed cow parts — which leads to the deadly "mad cow" disease…

… or how the massive, corporate-owned feedlots cram huge numbers of cattle into inhumanely small spaces (which places huge amounts of stress on the animals — and makes them highly susceptible to disease).

The list of negatives goes on and on and on.

With all this in mind, in my opinion, it's no wonder that red meat has been linked to certain chronic health concerns. How could any cow that's raised in such a way remain healthy and produce healthy beef?

It's next to impossible.

The bottom line is factory-farm red meat is simply horrible stuff. And you have every right to be scared to death of it.

However, pasture-raised, grass-fed beef could not be any more different. You have nothing to fear when you make it a part of your diet. In fact, pasture-raised, grass-fed beef is so loaded with health benefits, I'd even go as far as to call it a "super food."

Seven Health Benefits of Pasture-Raised, Grass-Fed Beef

For starters, here are seven reasons why making grass-fed beef a regular part of your diet is such a wise health decision.

Health Reason No. 1. Less Overall Fat and Calories than Grain-Fed Beef: A six-ounce loin from a grass-fed cow has, on average, 92 fewer calories than a six-ounce loin from a grain-fed cow. Now, the average American eats 67 pounds of beef per year.[3] This adds up to, on average, a 16,642 calorie difference. So if you switched to grass-fed beef and did nothing else, you'd lose 9½ pounds in two years just by switching to grass-fed!

Health Reason No. 2. More Omega-3s: You need omega-3s to survive. That's why they're called "essential fatty acids." Omega-3s:

- Help promote a healthy heart, brain, and immune system.
- Encourage strong bones, teeth, and nails.
- Support a positive, happy mood.
- Help maintain sharp vision for decades — and more.

And where do omega-3s originate from? Green plants (including grass, the food of choice of grass-fed cows.) As a result, grass-fed beef has two to ten times more omega-3s than grain-fed beef.[4]

Health Reason No. 3. A Healthier Ratio of Omega-6s to Omega-3s: Omega-6s and omega-3s are both essential fatty acids. You need them to survive. The problem is when you have too many omega-6s. Omega-6s have a pro-oxidation effect if your diet is too heavy in it, which the typical American diet tends to be. This can impact your overall health and well-being, including heart and brain health.

Many health experts believe the ratio of omega-6s to omega-3s should be no more than 4:1.[5] Grain-fed beef has an omega-6 to omega-3 ratio of 5:1 to 14:1. Way too high. Grass-fed, on the other hand, has a much healthier ratio of less than 1:1 to 3:1.[6]

Health Reason No. 4. More CLA: Grass-fed beef contains two to five times more CLA than the grain-fed variety.[7,8] CLA is a newly discovered "good fat" that research suggests helps support immune and cardiovascular growth. It also appears to help promote lean muscle mass.[9]

Health Reason No. 5. More Vitamin E: Vitamin E is an extremely powerful antioxidant. It helps protect you from free radicals, which are considered the leading cause of premature aging. Vitamin E also boosts your immunity and helps promote a healthy heart.

Grass-fed beef contains three to six times more vitamin E than grain-fed beef.[10]

Health Reason No. 6. More Carotenoids: A diet rich in carotenoids has multiple health benefits, including promoting eye and macular health. Grass-fed beef has up to four times more beta-carotene than grain-fed beef.[11]

Health Reason No. 7. More B Vitamins, CoQ10, and Zinc (and SAFE!): When you eat grass-fed beef, you are getting more B vitamins, CoQ10, and zinc than you would with grain-fed beef.

Aside from grass-fed beef's amazing health benefits, there's one other thing I haven't mentioned yet.

And I think you'll like this as much as I do.

It's the Best Beef I've Ever Tasted

One of the biggest misconceptions about grass-fed beef is that it tastes dry or gamey — that because it has no fat, it has no flavor.

This couldn't be further from the truth.

When it's raised and finished properly, it's actually far superior, in my opinion, to grain-fed beef. And I'm not alone in thinking this, either.

Here's what gourmet critics in several mainstream publications had to say about the flavor of grass-fed beef:

"... superior to the meat harvested from grain-fed animals."

— New York Times

"Grass-fed beef tastes better than corn-fed beef."

— Atlantic Monthly

"... delicious, rich and full-flavored, but without the excessive fattiness on the finish of some prime beef."

—Wine Spectator

I'm telling you — it's delicious!

There is one caveat about grass-fed beef, however. And it's something you should know about as well.

Because it takes so much more TLC to raise grass-fed cattle, it costs a little more than the cheap grain-fed stuff.

And it hasn't been that easy to find, either. It requires more effort to get it onto your plate. But I sure think it's worth it, especially when you consider:

- The welfare of the animals (grass-fed cattle are raised in a natural environment).
- The well-being of the local farmers that raise grass-fed cattle (supporting local farming benefits the community — instead of massive corporate-owned farms).
- Your health. (Now that you know the facts, what would you rather eat?)

So in the end, it's definitely worth it to "go grass-fed."

And here's some good news.

I've just made it easier than ever for you to give grass-fed beef a try.

Sample Some Delicious Grass-Fed Beef in Your Own Home

Not long ago, a friend put me in contact with a man who owns a cattle ranch in the foothills of Virginia's Appalachia country.

He's got about 700 cattle. What's more:

- The cattle are pasture-raised and grass-fed.
- The beef is "Certified Humane."
- The feed is free of animal proteins.
- They don't EVER use hormones or steroids on the cattle.
- They don't give the cattle unnecessary antibiotics.
- The beef is dry-aged for 14-21 days (to ensure maximum flavor).

If you would like to order some grass-fed beef for yourself and your family, try visiting this website: www.grassfedbeef.2ya.com

---

[1] Robinson, J. *Pasture Perfect: The Far Reaching Benefits of Choosing Meat, Eggs, and Dairy Products from Grass-Fed Animals*. Vashon Island Press. 2004.

[2] ibid.

[3] ibid.

[4] Robinson, J. "Health Benefits of Grass-Fed Products." *Eat Wild - Getting Wild Nutrition from Modern Food*. 2002-2015.

[5] Simopoulos, A.P. "The Importance of the Ratio of Omega-6/Omega-3 Essential Fatty Acids," (2002). *Biomed Pharmacother* 56 (8): 365-79.

[6] Robinson, J. "Health Benefits of Grass-Fed Products." *Eat Wild - Getting Wild Nutrition from Modern Food*. 2002-2015.

[7] Dhiman, T.R., G.R. Anand, L.D. Satter, and M.W. Pariza. (1999). "Conjugated Linolenic Acid Content of Milk from Cows Fed Different Diets." *J Dairy Sci 82*, (10): 2146-56.

[8] French, P., C. Stanton, F. Lawless, E.G. O'Riordan, F.J. Monahan, P.J. Caffrey, and A.P. Moloney. (2003) "Fatty Acid Composition, Including Conjugated Linolenic Acid, of Intramuscular Fat from Steers Offered Grazed Grass, Grass Silage, or Concentrate-Based Diets." *J Anim Sci 78*, (11): 2849-55.

[9] Platzman, A., MS, RD, CDN. "Crank Up Your Body's Furnace with these Fat-Burning Foods." *Meals on Fire*. 2007.

[10] Smith, G.C. "Dietary Supplementation of Vitamin E to Cattle to Improve Shelf-Life and Case-Life for Domestic and International Markets." Colorado State University. Complete reference not known.

[11] Prache, S., A. Priolo, et al. (2003). "Persistence of carotenoid pigments in the blood of concentrate-finished grazing sheep: its significance for the traceability of grass-feeding." *J Anim Sci* 81(2): 360-7.

Chapter 12

Enjoy Fun, Food, and Cold Ones at Your Next Super Bowl Party

The Super Bowl is a truly American tradition that brings families and friends together for a day of good fun and good food.

And good beer.

Many of the low-carb diets claim that beer has a high-glycemic index and will make you fat. But that's not necessarily true.

I'll show you why this claim is bogus and how it misses a more import-ant point — the *glycemic load.*

And I'll show you the best beers for your Super Bowl party. You can still enjoy the fuller flavor of "real" beers without having to suffer the watered-down, low-calorie beers that taste like dust, or worse.

You'll also discover:

- What can cause a "beer belly."
- How to tell the difference between carbs that matter and those that don't.
- How you can pick up a beer with confidence instead of guilt.

Good News for Beer Lovers — It's Good for Your Heart

A study from Israel adds evidence that a beer a day may help keep heart attacks away. Men with heart disease drinking one beer a day for a month decreased cholesterol levels, increased antioxidants, and reduced levels of fibrinogen, a clot-producing protein in the blood.[1]

Lower fibrinogen levels are associated with lower rates of heart attacks and strokes. Several population studies have linked moderate beer con-sumption to a reduced risk of coronary heart disease and heart attack.

But as you've been hearing in recent years, excess carbs will give you excess belly fat. With a beer weighing in with an average of 11 grams of carbs per bottle, it's leaving carb-counting beer drinkers a little parched.

Yet there is more to the story of carbs and beer. To understand this point, let's take a quick look at how beer is made.

Let the Yeast Take Care of the Carbs

Beer makers start with malted barley. When they brew barley malt, the liquid contains a lot of the sugar, *maltose*, and other starches from the grains. Does this equal high carbs? Yes. But wait...

During the next step — the fermentation process — they add yeast. Yeast cells eat carbohydrate. They convert it into alcohol and natural carbonation: the beverage you know as beer. The longer this fermentation process goes on, the higher the alcohol content and the less unfermented carbohydrates remain.

But what about the supposed high-glycemic index of carbs in beer?

In the Real World, Glycemic *Load* Matters

The glycemic index measures how fast and high a specific food or beverage increases your blood sugar. A lower glycemic index indicates a food will stimulate less blood sugar and is a "good" carb. A higher one means it's a "bad" carb. This system is useful but fallible because it doesn't account for your carbohydrate serving size. A better measure is your *glycemic load*.[2]

Glycemic load measures the effect of the total amount of a food on your blood sugar. To find the glycemic load of any food or beverage, simply multiply the glycemic index by the number of carbs per serving and then divide by 100.[3] What's a healthy number? Shoot for 10 or less.[4]

This distinction happens to be critically important when it comes to beer...

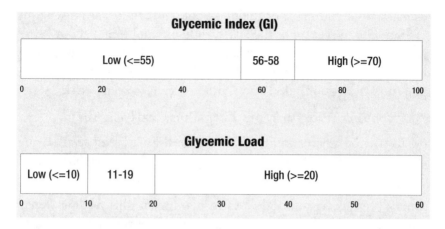

It's best to eat foods that have a lower glycemic index (GI) — less than 50. An even more useful measurement is the glycemic load (GL). This tells you the effect on your blood sugar depending on how much you actually eat. Try to eat foods that have a GL of less than 10.[5]

Beer Is Bad? The Diet Books Get It Wrong

Now back to the low-carb diet books telling you that beer has a high-glycemic index that will make you fat. You'll wonder how they came to this conclusion after you look at the tests to determine glycemic index.

We measure the glycemic index by having a test subject consume 100 grams of a carbohydrate test food or beverage all at once. It has to be consumed within 15 minutes.

We then measure blood sugar every half hour over the next two hours. Then we compare these blood sugars with the blood sugars produced in response to 100 grams of sugar water.

To test beer's glycemic index, a test subject would consume 100 grams of carbohydrate. With an average of 11 grams per beer, you would have to drink nine beers all at once. To test a light beer, you have to drink more.

If someone tells you that a low-carb beer with 2.6 grams of carbs will make you fat because it has a high-glycemic index, ask them, *"Who drank 24 beers within 15 minutes?"* **Even if you use only 50 grams of carbs, beer can't be tested without causing test subjects excessive drunkenness!**[6]

So what should you make of the diet books' glycemic warnings about beer? Ignore that section of the low-carb books and forget about beer's glycemic index. If you limit yourself to a couple of beers, there's simply not enough carbs to conduct a meaningful test — or to have a meaningful impact on your blood sugar. But you can do even better.

Drink a Six-Pack, but Keep Those Six-Pack Abs

Now for the best news about carbs and beer. Since yeast feed on the carbs in beer, to lower the carbs all a brewer has to do is let the fermentation proceed for longer.

Recently brewers have found ways to manipulate this feeding frenzy to allow the yeast to remove naturally nearly all of the carbs. This also has the advantage of avoiding the watering down of low-cal light beers.

Anheuser-Busch produced the first low-carb beer. For about a year, Michelob Ultra was the only low-carb on the block. Busch reports it had the fastest growth of any new brew they have ever introduced. In less than a year, it shot to number 7 in sales for premium beers, eclipsing the acceptance of light beers a couple of decades back.

Now other brewers are looking for their share of this fast-growing market. In recent years, beers like Labatt and Coors have joined Michelob Ultra. These beers boast less than three grams of carbs per bottle. They have less than half of the carbs but twice the flavor of some light brands.

Here are the lowest carb beers you can buy:[7]

Beer	Carbs
Greens Trailblazer	0.53
Budweiser Select 55	1.9
DAB Low Carb	2
Rock Green Light	2.4
Miller Genuine Draft Light 64 (MGD 64)	2.4
Molson Ultra	2.5
Labatt Sterling	2.5
Sleeman Clear	2.5
Aspen Edge	2.6

Michelob Ultra	2.6
Bootie U95	2.6
Schmidts Light	2.8
Iron City Light	2.8
SeyBrew Lager	2.8

Here's how the popular brews stack up when it comes to carbs:

Popular Brew	Carbs
Miller Lite	3.2 g
Amstel Light	5.0 g
Coors Light	5.0 g
Bud Light	6.6 g
Heineken	9.8 g
Budweiser	10.6 g
Coors	11.3 g
Michelob Light	11.7 g
Rolling Rock	13.0 g
Miller Genuine Draft	13.1 g
Guinness	17.6 g

Note that you get fewer carbs in four Michelob Ultras (10.4 g) than in one Michelob Light (11.7 g). You could drink five Rock Green Lights (my pick) and have fewer carbs at 12.0 than if you drank one regular Rolling Rock, which has 13.0. What's more, each of these new low-carb brews seems to outperform the last, in terms of flavor and fullness.

They all have full-bodied taste but have the lowest carbs, as these are the specially formulated low-carb brews. You can find some European imports that will top off at 30 grams of carbs.

You'll want to partake in these in moderation, if at all. Also, the "beer alternatives" such as wine coolers and hard ciders are in no way healthier and much worse when it comes to carbs. They *start* at around 26 grams and go up from there. If you're cutting carbs, give those a wide berth.

Try a taste test of the lowest on the list and see which you prefer. If you like a beer now and then, you may be able to kick back and enjoy a cold one this Super Bowl with a little less guilt.

---

[1] Gorinstein S, et al. "Structural Changes in Plasma Circulating Fibrinogen after Moderate Beer Consumption as Determined by Electrophoresis and Spectroscopy." *J. Agric. Food Chem.* 2003.

[2] "Glycemic index, glycemic load, and risk of type 2 diabetes," Walter Willett, JoAnn Manson, and Simin Liu, *American Journal of Clinical Nutrition* 2002; 76 (suppl): 274S-80S.

[3] "Glycemic index: overview of implications in health and disease," David JA Jenkins, et al., *American Journal of Clinical Nutrition* 2002; 76 (suppl): 266S-73S.

[4] "Glycemic index and heart disease," Anthony R. Leeds, *American J. of Clinical Nutrition*, 2002; 76 (suppl): 286S-9S.

[5] Foster-Powell K, Holt SH, Brand-Miller JC, "International table of glycemic index and glycemic load values: 2002." *American Journal of Clinical Nutrition*, 2002; 76:5-56.

[6] U. of Sydney Glycemic Index Research. 2011.

[7] "Lowest Carb Beers." Beet Tutor. 2005-2015.

Chapter 13

Atkins without Beef — What's Next?

Have you heard about this "Eco-Atkins Diet" that a bunch of researchers dreamed up to please vegetarians?

Dr. Atkins must be spinning in his grave.

These veggie-wackos want a diet that offers "Atkins without animal fat." They call it, "Eco-Atkins."

Holy cow!

The Atkins Diet is *all about* eating animal protein. So how do you eat a high-protein diet without animal fat? Turns out we're supposed to bulk up on soy burgers and wake up to the smell of vegetarian bacon — whatever that is!

Beef Is the Best Source of These Essential Nutrients:

Protein: Meat is a complete protein. Vegetables are not. Vegetarians have to combine foods to make a complete protein. They're also lower in protein content than meat sources. For instance, three ounces of beef contain 50 grams of protein compared to two tablespoons of peanut butter, which contains 16 grams.

B12: Animal products are the primary source of B12. This is a serious problem for vegetarians, especially vegans. Lack of B12 causes anemia and can cause nerve damage leading to irreversible conditions like blindness.[5,6]

Iron: Vegetarians not only get less iron, but the type of iron from a vegetarian diet is different. The type of iron from a vegetarian diet is absorbed 70% less than from a meat diet.[7] This is especially dangerous to children and pregnant women. Children develop behavior problems and delays in their development. Pregnant women deliver pre-term.[8,9]

Zinc: Beef is the number one source for zinc, and all animal products are good sources. Vegetarians not only get less zinc to begin with, they absorb up to 35% less of it.[10] A zinc deficiency affects your immunity, and can stunt your growth and the way your brain functions.

CLA: Almost 98% acid (CLA) comes from meat. CLA has been shown to reduce the risk of cancer.[11] It also helps with fat loss.

CoQ10: Beef is the best source of Coenzyme Q10. There is next to none in fruits and vegetables. CoQ10 is in every cell of our body. It creates energy. CoQ10 improves heart function and diabetes, and helps prevent autoimmune disease.[12]

Don't be deceived. This crazy veggie-plan is in no way eco-friendly, sustainable, or healthy. The diet is based on multiple allergens such as soy, gluten, and dairy. They use processed foods like veggie bacon, deli slices, and breakfast links.

What's worse:

- Up to 30 times the maximum level allowed for a toxic chemical called melamine has been found in soy products. Melamine is a hazardous air pollutant that affects the brain. It's banned from organic food, yet it's finding its way into soy.[1]
- Commercial soy farmers in South America are taking over and driving peasant farmers off their land.[2]
- Soy is grown on stripped and deforested lands in the Amazon rainforest.[3]
- Inferior and contaminated soy is quietly being imported from China.[4]

This concept is disconnected from our past, and it screams of ignorance.

For millions of years, our ancestors were part of an ecological system that had a perfect balance in nature. They relied on fresh-caught meat and food gathered from the ground, bushes, and trees. Their diet was high-protein, high-fat, and low-carbohydrate. Diseases of modern day were nonexistent.

Vegetarians want to replace this with processed, low-fat starch products that can ruin your health.

Where's the Beef?

The study they've based their conclusions on has nothing to do with Atkin's diet plan. Atkin's diet is based on beef. In the study, one group ate a vegetarian diet, and the other a vegan diet. The diets are hard to follow for most people, and the products aren't readily available. But what's more important, vital nutrients are missing.

Meat eaters are more likely than vegetarians to get 100% of the protein, iron, zinc, and B vitamins they need.

This veggie Atkins imitator is a far cry from the natural and healthy diet handed down through millions of years of evolution. Eco-Atkins goes against our own biology and history.

Ancient Is Eco-Friendly

Step back in time with me for a moment.

A Stone Age diet is similar to the original Atkins plan. Primitive man hunted animals that fed on wild grasses. Meat was pure, fresh, and full of nutrients. They supplemented with fruits, vegetables, nuts, and seeds. They drank fresh water. Very little was based on grains, gluten, or soy. Their diet certainly was not based on processed, prepackaged veggie links.

Our bodies were designed to digest meat, yet vegetarians still think it's bad for you. They don't understand that eating grass-fed beef is healthy and low in fat, and contains essential nutrients they're missing from their diet. Our ancestors' diet allowed prehistoric man to have a stored energy source for times of famine. Today, it gives us a great backup fuel system for our bodies.

By eating like our ancestors, we naturally lower our intake of carbohydrates. With fewer carbohydrates, our bodies switch to using fat as fuel. We are fully satisfied *and* lose body fat. Our blood sugar levels out. Our LDL and HDL cholesterol levels improve, along with triglycerides.

There's more...

Natural sources of animal protein:

- Have higher nutritional value. Grass-fed beef is low-fat with fewer calories than grain-fed. It also has more omega-3s, B vitamins, CoQ10, zinc, vitamin E, and beta-carotene.

- Avoid common allergic triggers such as milk, soy, egg, and wheat.

- Offer important nutrients that fuel the brain and stabilize mood.

- Satisfy the appetite. They keep hunger away longer, making dieting easier.

Benefits of Grass-Fed Beef

1. **Less Overall Fat and Calories:** A six-ounce grass-fed loin has 92 fewer calories than grain-fed. This saves an average American 16,642 calories each year.[13]

2. **More Omega-3:** Grass-fed beef has two to ten times more omega-3s than grain-fed beef and a healthy ratio as little as 1:1.14 Grain-fed beef is as much as 14:1.[15]

3. **More CLA:** Grass-fed beef has two to five times more CLA than grain-fed. CLA supports immune and cardiovascular growth and lean muscle mass.[16]

4. **More Vitamin E:** Grass-fed beef contains three to six times more vitamin E than grain-fed beef.[17]

5. **More Carotenoids:** Grass-fed beef has up to four times more beta-carotene than grain-fed beef.[18] Carotenoids promote eye and macular health.

6. **More B Vitamins, CoQ10, and Zinc:** Grass-fed beef has more B vitamins, CoQ10, and zinc than grain-fed beef.

Dr. Atkins was a visionary. He taught people to eat like our primitive ancestors. But there is one area where he went wrong.

You've got to watch out for trans fat and eliminate it from your diet. Trans fat comes from partially hydrogenated oils. You find it in processed and fast foods. Trans fat raises bad cholesterol (LDL) while lowering good cholesterol (HDL).

You also need to watch the ratio of omega-3 to omega-6. We get too few 3s and too many 6s. When you cut down on processed and fast foods, you decrease 6s. Another way is by switching to grass-fed beef. A high-protein, low-carb diet is good for you, as long as you're getting the right fats.

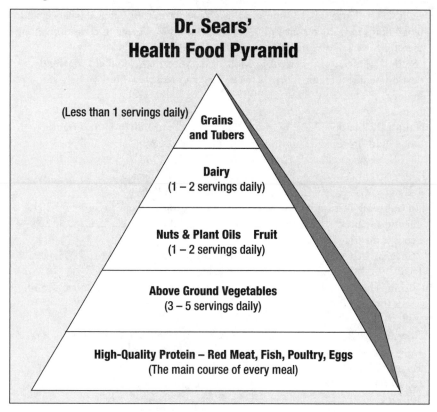

Here's how to get back to the basics:

- Make protein the main course of every meal. Base your diet on grass-fed beef, buffalo, wild game, and free-range eggs. For variety, add an occasional wild-caught, cold-water fish.
- Eat quality, low-glycemic complex carbohydrates. Stick to above-ground vegetables, fruits, and berries.
- Eat quality fat and increase your omega-3s. Throw in a handful of nuts, avocados, and some healthful oils.
- Avoid packaged and processed foods.

[1] Institute of Medicine, Food and Nutrition Board. Standing Committee on the Scientific Evaluation of Dietary Reference Intakes. Dietary Reference Intakes for Thiamin, Riboflavin, Niacin, Vitamin B6, Folate, Vitamin B12, Pantothenic Acid, Biotin, and Choline. Washington, DC: National Academy Press, 1998.

[2] Milea, D. "Blindness in a strict vegan." *N. Engl. J. Med.* 342: 897- 898; 2000.

[3] Hunt, J.R.; Matthys, L.A.; Johnson, L.K. "Zinc absorption, mineral balance, and blood lipids in women consuming controlled lactoovovegetarian and omnivorous diets for 8 weeks." *Am. J. Clin. Nutr.* 67: 421- 430; 1998.

[4] Lozoff, B.; Jimenez, E.; Hagen, J.; Mollen, E.; Wolf, A.W. "Poorer behavioral and developmental outcome more than 10 years after treatment for iron deficiency in infancy." *Pediatrics* 105: e51; 2000.

[5] ibid.

[6] Hunt, J.R.; Matthys, L.A.; Johnson, L.K. "Zinc absorption, mineral balance, and blood lipids in women consuming controlled lactoovovegetarian and omnivorous diets for 8 weeks." *Am. J. Clin. Nutr.* 67: 421- 430; 1998.

[7] Kelley NS, Hubbard NE, Erickson KL. (2007). "Conjugated linoleic acid isomers and cancer." *J Nutr* (UC Davis, Ca, USA) 137 (12):2599-607.

[8] Linus Pauling Institute. "Micronutrient Information Center." Accessed 02 2010.

[9] "Behind the Bean: The Heroes and Charlatans of the Natural and Organic Soy Foods Industry." 2009.

[10] "Paraguay may limit soy farming in land reform," Interview 12 Sep 2008 16:59:39 GMT: Reuters. By Mariel Cristaldo.

[11] "Behind the Bean: The Heroes and Charlatans of the Natural and Organic Soy Foods Industry." 2009.

[12] ibid.

[13] Robinson, J. *Pasture Perfect: The Far Reaching Benefits of Choosing Meat, Eggs, and Dairy Products From Grass-Fed Animals.* Vashon Island Press. 2004.

[14] Rule D.C. (2002). "Comparison of muscle fatty acid profiles and cholesterol concentrations of bison, beef cattle, elk, and chicken." *Journal of Animal Science,* 80: 1202-1211.

[15] Paul, R. "Health Benefits of Grass-Fed Products-Eat Wild! Local Harvest. Jan 23, 2011.

[16] Dhiman, T.R., G.R. Anand, L.D. Satter, and M.W. Pariza. (1999). "Conjugated Linolenic Acid Content of Milk from Cows Fed Different Diets." *J Dairy Sci.* 82, (10): 2146-56.

[17] Smith, G.C. "Dietary Supplementation of Vitamin E to Cattle to Improve Shelf-Life and Case-Life for Domestic and International Markets." Colorado State University Department of Animal Sciences.

[18] Prache, S., A. Priolo, et al. (2003). "Persistence of carotenoid pigments in the blood of concentrate-finished grazing sheep: its significance for the traceability of grass-feeding." *J Anim Sci* 81(2): 360-7.

Chapter 14

New York City Takes on Salt

The Real Issue ... and Why You Need to Know About It

New York City's former mayor Michael Bloomberg once named salt his "Public Enemy #1."[1]

His health department had already banned trans fats in restaurants. And forced calorie counts to be listed on menus. Then they took on salt.[2]

The real question is not "Should you eat salt or not?" It's "What *kind* of salt should you eat?"

Good News for Salt Lovers

You need salt to live, and to continue living. No doubt about it...

- A human embryo develops in salty amniotic fluid.

- Your body consists of three distinct fluid systems, all salty — blood plasma, lymphatic fluid, and extracellular fluid.

- Salt carries nutrients across cell membranes into your cells.

- Salt keeps calcium and other minerals soluble in your blood.

- Salt helps regulate muscle contractions.

- The mainstay of fluid replacement therapy for treatment of dehydration — or as an IV therapy to prevent hypovolemic shock due to blood loss — is a saline solution of 0.9% sodium chloride.

- Salt helps regulate blood pressure and fluid volume.

- In hot temperatures, salt regulates your fluid balance.

- It helps stimulate your nerves by increasing conductivity in nerve cells, for communication and information processing.

You can't live without salt in your body.

You're unable to digest food without it. Your heart needs it to function. So do your adrenals. Your liver and kidneys cannot work without salt.

You sweat salt. Your tears are salty. Your blood is salty.

So I trust you'll look past conventional medicine's blindness in pressing for low-salt diets.

Is Low-Salt Really Better?

The idea that salt consumption causes high blood pressure in the first place is a relatively recent belief — based, in fact, on questionable conclusions from a handful of studies.

Repeated studies failed to show a major causal link between salt intake and high blood pressure. *In fact, some research points in the opposite direction.*[3]

A huge government study on thousands of people concluded that minerals — especially potassium and magnesium — are better at lowering blood pressure than salt.[4]

Even the CDC's own data over the space of 30 years showed that adequate mineral intake acts to keep your blood pressure low.[5]

A low-salt diet supposedly reduces your risk of heart attacks and strokes. But where's the evidence? I've seen compelling evidence that shows you ***increase*** your risk of a heart attack on a *low*-salt diet.[6]

Why an increase?

Because low-salt diets can create or worsen nutritional deficiencies. And you know you need vitamins and minerals for good heart health.

So I take conventional medicine's low-salt advice with a grain of salt — and I suggest you do, too. This should come as good news if you enjoy salty foods.

But yet, it's worth considering what type of salt is best for your health.

Choose "Living" Salt for Life

Regular table salt is a highly processed product that's devoid of nutrients and minerals — like most other processed foods.

Due to extensive processing, which either destroys nutrients with high temperatures or strips them out, it lacks the nutrients found naturally in unrefined salts such as sea salt.

I advise switching to natural sea salt as your replacement for "traditional" table salt.

Think of unrefined salt as a whole, living food, because it is. It provides up to 82 vital trace minerals that promote your best possible life function and cellular health.

Even in tiny amounts, these minerals rally to regulate your body's systems. They restock your electrolytes and balance your acid/alkaline levels.

Say Good-Bye to Traditional Table Salt

Your best way to replace processed table salt with unrefined sea salt is to eat whole organic vegetables, fruits, and meats you cook yourself, and then add your own sea salt to taste.

Here's a list of high-sodium prepared foods, with lower sodium alternatives to substitute. Choose these options — and add your own healthy replacement for processed table salt.

Sources of Added Salt	Substitute Instead
Canned / frozen vegetables	Fresh vegetables
Soups	Homemade soup
Ready-to-eat cereals	Shredded wheat, puffed rice, oatmeal, low-sodium cereals
Celery salt, garlic salt	Caraway seeds, pepper, garlic, parsley, sesame, thyme, lemon, other spices
Salad dressings	Homemade dressings
Steak sauces, sauces, Prepared mustard, ketchup	Lemon, spices
Crackers, potato chips, Corn chips	Salt-free matzoh, crackers,
Club soda	Seltzer water, juices

Bacon, ham, salami	Nitrite-free sandwich meats
Fast food	Salad, sandwiches

You can purchase sea salt in health-food stores and many mainstream grocery stores.

Still Worried about High Blood Pressure?

Since studies show poor outcomes for people low in minerals, here are some ways to increase your dietary intake of the most critical ones.

Magnesium — Helpful for healthy heart function and normal blood pressure. Dark green leafy veggies like spinach are rich in magnesium because chlorophyll molecules contain magnesium. Beans, peas, nuts, seeds, and seafood also provide magnesium. You should strive to eat enough magnesium-rich foods to get 500-1,000 mg. of magnesium daily.

Potassium — Maintains normal fluid and electrolyte balance, and promotes normal muscle function. Helps optimize blood pressure levels.[7]

Foods rich in potassium include orange-colored fruits and veggies like apricots, cantaloupe, oranges, nectarines, peaches, sweet potatoes, and butternut and acorn squash. Other foods rich in potassium are black and kidney beans, spinach, Swiss chard, artichokes, bananas, kiwi, fish, meat, poultry, and milk. You should strive to get your potassium from a healthy diet.

Calcium — Populations with low calcium intake have higher blood pressure. But it's not been proven that popping extra calcium supplements will automatically lower your blood pressure.

---

[1] Neuman W. "Citing Hazard - New York Says Hold the Salt." *The New York Times.* Jan 10, 2010.

[2] "Chemistry Essays – Saline & Fluids in the Body." UKESSAYS.

[3] "Salt Your Way to Health," Brownstein, David, MD, www.celticseasalt.com (Reprinted from the Winter 2006 issue of *A Grain of Salt.*

[4] ibid.

[5] ibid.

[6] ibid.

[7] "Lower Your Blood Pressure with Potassium-Rich Foods," *Vancouver Sun,* 02/11/10.

Chapter 15

Are Some Eggs Healthier than Others?

Think about what a hen's stress level is doing to the nutrition of the eggs you eat.

You know what stress can do to you as your cortisol levels go up. Cortisol is the "fight or flight" hormone that reacts to danger and to stress. It usually drops back down once your stress levels return to normal.

But when stress remains high, your cortisol level remains high. This can lower your immunity against disease. It prevents you from absorbing nutrients and may cause you to get sick. Over the long term, it can affect your DNA.

Animals can react the same way. When hens are cramped together in an unnatural environment, they have excess cortisol their whole lives.

Hens can't absorb nutrients under these conditions. *And* their diet is unnatural. It consists of grain products, plant protein products, processed grain by-products, roughage products, and forage products.[1] Notice how it's all "products" and "by-products" instead of just the name of a real food. This is why so little nutrition passes along into the egg.

After a while, it affects a hen's DNA.[2] Inferior genetic material is passed along into the egg. So when you buy conventional eggs, they have little of the nutrition you expect.

But hens that have the run of a pasture live in a natural, native environment. Their behavior remains instinctual. And they eat the way nature intended. Fresh grass every day, plenty of insects and grubs. Their diet is rich in vitamins, minerals, and a natural source of protein.

Cage-free, pastured eggs give you:[3]

- Two-thirds more vitamin A.
- Three to four times more omega-3 fatty acids.
- Three times more vitamin E.
- Seven times more beta-carotene.
- Four to six times the vitamin D.

I came across a chart comparing eggs from 14 farms in the U.S. to battery-caged birds. Here's a summary of what was found:[4]

All values are per 100 grams of egg	Vitamin E (mg.)	Vitamin A (IU)	Beta-Carotene (mcg.)	Omega-3s (mg.)	Cholesterol (mg.)	Saturated Fat (g)
Eggs from Confined Birds (per USDA Nutrient Database)	0.97	487	10	0.22	423	3.1
Eggs from Non-Confined Birds (Mother Earth News, 2007)	3.73	791.86	79.03	0.66	277	2.4

More Space Equals Less Disease

The World Health Organization (WHO) was also concerned about the health of your eggs. They wanted to know if a hen's living conditions had any impact on the risk of salmonella.

Salmonella is the most common illness you can get from food. In the U.S., more than 1.4 million people are infected every year.

WHO discovered you've got a greater chance of salmonella when you buy conventional eggs from battery-caged hens.

When the number of chickens living together is reduced by one-fourth, your chance of contracting salmonella is cut in half.[5] More space per hen, and your chances are even lower.

I've read many more similar studies from the European Union, where battery cages were made illegal in 2012.

Almost 24% of farms with battery-caged hens test positive for salmonella compared to 6.5% in flocks that are free to roam.[6]

And the European Food Safety Authority (EFSA) wrote, "Without exception... there was significantly higher risk of salmonella infection in hens confined in cages."

The EFSA found battery-cage systems have 25 times greater odds of salmonella contamination than cage-free environments.[7]

Making Sense of the Labels

It can be confusing to shop for eggs. So I hope I've made it a little easier by recommending "cage-free" or "pastured" rather than conventional eggs.

But you may come across a few other choices when you shop for eggs. So here's a short breakdown of what else you might find.

1. Free-Range: Free-range may also mean cage-free and pastured, but not necessarily. There's a wide variety of interpretation by farmers. The USDA defines free-range as "Allowed access to the outside." Chickens do have a door, so they can get outside. But chickens may never learn to go out. They get sunlight, exercise, and fresh air. Free-range eggs have better nutrition than conventional eggs.

2. Vegetarian: Vegetarian eggs come from cage-free hens. They may be pastured, but they're only fed vegetarian feed. This isn't a normal diet for chickens. If they're let outside, chickens will naturally eat bugs, worms, and other non-vegetarian fare. Vegetarian eggs have better nutrition than conventional eggs.

3. Omega-3 Eggs: Omega-3 eggs may come from cage-free hens. They may be pastured. Chickens are fed more flax and canola seed to increase the omega-3 content of the egg. But you get far less than what you find in a small piece of salmon or fish oil supplement. Omega-3 eggs have better nutrition than conventional eggs.

4. Organic: Organic eggs come from cage-free hens fed organic, vegetarian feed. Neither the hens nor their feed are subjected to antibiotics, hormones, pesticides, or herbicides. Organic eggs have better nutrition than conventional eggs. Look for a "USDA Organic" symbol as shown here.

5. Certified Humane Raised and Handled: This means the eggs come from cage-free chickens that are raised and treated humanely. Look for a "Certified Humane" symbol as shown here.

Your Best Source for Cage-Free Eggs

At our office, all of us are getting our eggs from a local farmer. I thank A.N. and her family. My foundation, Wellness and Research Foundation, is assisting her so she can convert her farm to organic.

Her chickens are cage-free and pastured. The hens go outside and eat grass, grubs, and worms. At night, they're brought in so they're safe from predators.

She supplements their feed with flax seed to increase the omega-3 content. The hens are in the sun, so vitamin D is high. The nutrition is superior, and the taste is much richer. The minute you taste an egg like this, you swear you'll never eat any other.

It may be worth it to you to know where your eggs are coming from. Do a little investigation into your supplier or farmer. Visit their farm if it's local. Or call them up and ask questions. Make sure the eggs you buy come from hens that are cage-free and pastured.

I suggest you look for a local source like I did.

- Search for cage-free or pastured eggs in your area. Search for farmer's markets where you may find local farmers who carry them.

- Or look for them at your local grocery store or a health-food store that carries eggs. Most local grocery stores carry at least one selection of cage-free eggs. But look for pastured eggs at a grocery dedicated to health such as Whole Foods Market.

---

[1] Long C, and Alterman T. "Meet Real Free-Range Eggs." Mother Earth News. October/November 2007.

[2] Bureau, C., Hennequet-Antier, C., Couty, M., Guemene, D. "Gene array analysis of adrenal glands in broiler chickens following ACTH treatment," *BMC Genom-*

ics. 2009; 10: 430.

[3] Karsten, H. et al. "Pasture-ized Poultry." Penn State Research Encyclopedia 2003;24(2).

[4] "Egg Chart" *Mother Earth News.* 2007.

[5] "Risk assessments of Salmonella in eggs and broiler chickens." World Health Organization Food and Agriculture Organization of the United Nations 2002.

[6] Snow, LC., Davies, RH., et al. "Survey of the prevalence of Salmonella species on commercial laying farms in the United Kingdom." *The Veterinary Record* 2007;161:471-476.

[7] "Report of the Task Force on Zoonoses Data Collection on the Analysis of the baseline study on the prevalence of Salmonella in holdings of laying hen flocks of Gallus gallus" EFSA.2007 Feb.

Chapter 16

I Admit, I Forgot about Bananas

It got me before I could swat it.

Now I had the biggest welt I ever got from a bug bite. I knew it was going to itch like crazy — the mosquitoes here are huge.

I showed my guide and laughed a bit. The tall, lean Ugandan said, "Wait..."

He fished a banana out of his pack, pulled off a strip of the peel and handed it to me.

I have to admit I forgot about bananas.

I rubbed the inside of the peel on the giant bite. It never did itch. And today the angry bump is almost completely gone.

Simple things like that are among the reasons I love to travel to remote places. It reminds me that nature usually provides the remedy in the same area there's a problem. So along with mosquito bites you can get cuts, rashes, bruises and other skin reactions, and banana peels are good for all of them.

But Ugandans don't only use them as medicine. They eat more bananas per person than anyone else. Five hundred pounds for each person every year. No wonder they always have them around.

They even make banana beer they call "lubisi." I haven't tried it yet, but when I find some I'll let you know how it tastes.

The First Crop

You might say the banana is the original superfood. It *is* probably the first domesticated crop. In fact, the history of the banana might make us rewrite the history of the world.

I think the story of our history is one we're still learning. And our children will probably get to know a different story than the one we know.

Bananas come from Southeast Asia, and botanical evidence tells us that everywhere else they grow, they were brought there by humans.

We know this because the bananas outside of Asia are "polyploidy," meaning they're a hybrid of two or more other kinds of bananas. And they are incapable of growing on their own. Someone has to cultivate them.

The ones that still have seeds and don't need to be actively cultivated are rare. And they're only in Asia. The rest are infertile "parthenocarpic clones." They don't make seeds because they have extra numbers of chromosomes.

Yet these hybrid bananas that need people to help them grow are all over Africa. They're all over the Caribbean islands. They're in Central and South America. And they were in the New World before the Europeans came.

So it's probable that someone traveled to the Americas hundreds of years before the Europeans.

In fact, bananas were introduced in Africa according to a certain route that started a thousand years BC in what is now Nigeria. We can trace the progression because the people who cultivated bananas replaced the hunter-gatherers. So if you trace that route... you'd have to rewrite the history of humans leaving Africa, too.

But it still leaves the question, where did they get the original banana in the western coast of Africa? We don't know because the people who went there, like the Phoenicians and the Romans, didn't have bananas.

So it was someone else.

Maybe someone from India went all the way around the Horn? Maybe the Chinese? Someone brought them there.

Same thing in South America. They diverged from the other cultivars of bananas 5,000 years ago. But the kinds that grow there can't grow on their own. Someone took them to South America a very long time before Columbus.

It's interesting to me because I've seen people who live high in the mountains of Peru, who look exactly like Pakistanis. And there are fierce warrior tribes in Peru whose people look Polynesian, while other Peruvians look Japanese.

So there had to be many waves of human migration to the Americas that occurred in many places at many times.

But... Why Bananas?

What makes the banana so special that people would choose it as the one plant to take with them across the ocean to a new world?

As it turns out, bananas have a lot of benefit for your brain, heart, and stomach. They even fight cancer.

For instance, you may have noticed that it can just plain make you feel good to eat a banana. Part of the reason could be that bananas have dopamine in them.[1]

Dopamine is a brain chemical that enhances learning, memory, and motivation, and even helps with attention and sleep. It's also the key to experiencing pleasure and maintaining an overall sense of well-being and a good mood.

Plus bananas have tryptophan, serotonin and norepinephrine, which all help alleviate depression. And bananas help you produce nitric oxide, which lowers your blood pressure and helps you relax.

Bananas can also give you feel-good effects similar to dark chocolate and a warm cup of tea. They have gallocatechins,[2] antioxidants that also help give green tea and chocolate their benefits.

A lot of athletes eat bananas because they give you a pick-me-up. Part of the reason is probably because bananas contain a good mix of all three natural sugars — fructose, sucrose and glucose — plus fiber, so the energy lasts.

But they also have potassium. This mineral is an electrolyte, which means your cells need it to work right. Potassium regulates the heartbeat and function of the muscles.

It also nourishes your brain so you can think clearly throughout the day. Potassium channels play a key role in maintaining the electrical conductivity in your brain. So it's involved in higher brain function like memory and learning.

Plus, bananas have choline, the main ingredient in the brain chemical acetylcholine, which you need for all the basics like thought, memory and sleep. It even controls how you move. Your muscles receive commands from your brain via acetylcholine. That means your sense of balance and stability is controlled by this key transmitter.

Bananas can also protect you in several important ways. The first is that bananas guard your stomach by triggering mucus production. This gives you a protective barrier against stomach acids. They also have protease inhibitors, which can break down the harmful stomach bacteria that cause ulcers.

Banana extract is so powerful that researchers were able to use it to prevent malignant cancer in animal studies. Giving the animals banana extract alone raised the survival rate of the animals from zero to 30%.[3]

You could think of bananas as the original superfood. They have almost every essential nutrient including B vitamins, vitamin A, vitamin C, calcium, magnesium, and selenium.

Is That a Banana?

What we think of as a banana "tree" is really a very big herb. The biggest flowering herb in the world. And the banana is a huge berry.

You'll probably only ever see three kinds of banana that you can buy and eat. There are "red" bananas (which are really brown), baby bananas (like a mini yellow banana) and the typical yellow banana, which is a Cavendish.

They are all peel-and-eat, as opposed to a plantain, a kind of banana that needs to be cooked before you eat it.

When I went to India, I noticed that there's no difference between a banana and a plantain. They just call one a cooking banana, and the other a "dessert" banana.

We don't cook with bananas too much in the West, except to make breads or muffins. But that changes what you're eating into a high-glycemic food, which I don't recommend. I like banana as is, for the most part.

But you can make a sweet treat by roasting bananas. All you have to do is cut a banana in half lengthwise. Place the halves cut sides up on a coated cookie pan and bake at 450° for four minutes.

Sprinkle a bit of brown sugar on them, or, to make them even tastier, roast a few walnuts and lightly press them into the cut side of the banana on top of the sugar. Then bake for three more minutes.

If I want a frozen treat, I'll grab one banana, dip it in plain yogurt, then roll it in finely chopped coconut. Afterwards I put it in the freezer and eat it whenever I want a quick snack.

If you buy a lot of bananas and they get overripe, just peel them and put them in a ziplock bag and freeze them. A plain, ripened, frozen banana tastes a lot like banana-flavored frozen yogurt — but without the added sugar. Try it for yourself.

[1] Kanazawa, K, Sakakibara, H. "High Content of Dopamine, a Strong Antioxidant, in Cavendish Banana" *J. Agric. Food Chem.*, 2000, 48 (3), pp 844–848.

[2] Someyaa, S. Yumiko Yoshikib, Y, Okubob, K. "Antioxidant compounds from bananas." *Food Chemistry.* November 2002; Volume 79, Issue 3, Pages 351-354.

[3] Guha M, Basuray S, Sinha K. "Preventive effect of ripe banana in the diet on Ehrlich's ascitic carcinoma cell induced malignant ascites in mice." *Nutrition Research*, August 2003. Volume 23, Issue 8, Pages 1081-1088.

Chapter 17

Easy Way Out of the Big Fat Mess

Did you hear that Norway ran out of butter?

The news media made fun of the "diet craze" that caused the shortage. It seems someone has convinced Norwegians to go on a "high-fat diet" and take in fewer carbs and more protein and fat.

If that's how they eat, I think Norway just moved up the list of places I want to visit.

Dietary Fat		
Unsaturatede Fat	**Saturated Fat**	**Trans Fat**
Almonds	Beef	Cookies
Vegetabeles	Butter	Donuts
Fish	Pizza	Cakes
Olives	Ice Cream	Fries
Olive Oil	Lard	Hydrogenated Oil
Benefits		
Works in conjunction with saturated fats to prevent heart attacks and strokes	Works in conjunction with unsaturated fats to prevent heart attacks and strokes	None

The sad part is that the mainstream considers it a "diet" when people eat what, in evolutionary terms, is a healthy amount of fat.

Because the truth is, we don't eat a high-fat diet. We eat less fat than our ancestors did. And yet we're the ones with obesity, heart disease, high cholesterol, clogged arteries and high blood pressure.

If you want to live better and disease-free, you should forget about the modern recommendations to eat like a rabbit.

Instead, eat the fat-rich foods you were born to eat. You have a natural

328 | HEALTH CONFIDENTIAL

desire for them. Dropping weight will come easier and faster, and you will wake up charged with energy that will last the whole day.

I've helped hundreds of people use this approach. I've watched them make a remarkable transition. They are becoming leaner, healthier and disease free.

Unfortunately the modern medical establishment has been nagging you for 30 years to drop foods with fat from the list of what you eat. They claim that fat — one of three main nutrients the human body needs to survive and thrive — is bad for you.

Big Fat Benefits

But modern medicine didn't think it through. Because if they did, they would have realized that taking one of your three macronutrients and telling you not to eat it anymore is a universally bad idea.

A minority of doctors including myself have been advising the contrary. Because you need this nutrient to give you six essential benefits:

1. **More energy:** It supplies more than twice the calories per gram of carbohydrate, and produces zero insulin response, meaning you don't turn it into body fat.
2. **A healthy body temperature.**
3. **Injury protection:** It shields your vital organs from many different kinds of trauma.
4. **More nutrients:** It helps you absorb and transport vitamins A, D, E and K, plus other nutrients and minerals.
5. **Tastier and more satisfying food:** It makes food feel better in your mouth and taste better, and it gives you that "full" feeling that controls how much food you eat at one time.
6. **Faster brain, stronger heart:** Your body must have two types of it to survive, but you can't make them yourself. They contribute to a stronger heart, sharper brain and even clear hearing.

Despite all the benefits to your brain and body, many people took the advice given to them by "experts," their doctors, and the ads on TV. They cut out the dietary fat.

We stopped eating foods like steak and eggs, and started eating more grains and other carbohydrates. Many of which had unnatural, man-made trans fat.

And as a population, we became exceptionally diseased. Our bodies have responded to the fact that we eat 25% less fat than we used to. And that adaptive response has been a disaster.

The rate of diabetes is 10 times higher than it was just a few years ago. Heart-related diseases that were rare in the early twentieth century now kill more people than anything else.

Thirty years ago there wasn't one state that had an obesity rate over 20%. Last year, there was only one state that had an obesity rate UNDER 20%. This is not a genetic problem.

Saturated Fats vs. Trans Fats		
	Saturated Fats	**Trans Fats**
Cell Membranes	Essential for healthy function	Interfere with healthy function
Hormones	Enhance hormone production	Interfere with hormone production
Inflammation	Suppress	Encourage
Heart Disease	Lower Lp(a) - Raise "good" cholesterol	Raise Lp(a) - Lower "good" cholesterol
Omega-3 Fatty Acids	Put in tissues and conserve	Reduce levels in tissues
Diabetes	Do not inhibit insulin receptors	Inhibit insulin receptors
Immune System	Enhance	Depress
Prostalandins	Encourage production and balance	Depress production; cause imbalance

The good news is that fixing this "fat-free" mess is not as hard as you might have imagined. Follow my two simple rules for selecting your food, and you will be able to eat better-tasting meals, reduce your risk of disease, feel more satisfied and stay lean.

Rule 1) Make Quality Protein the Centerpiece to Every Meal. Humans are not meant to eat grains or processed foods. Our bodies don't recognize things like corn and bread as sources of food. They have incomplete proteins and too many unhealthy fats in the wrong ratio.

So skip the grains and potatoes. Eat a large variety of protein instead. Plan your meals around which kind of protein you'll be eating. Eat everything you can try, from grass-fed buffalo to elk to beef.

Why grass-fed? The unnatural living condition of animals in the modern food industry produces diseased animal fat. All of the herbicides, pesticides, toxins and hormones that the animal has been exposed to collect in the fat.

And modern farming techniques prevent the animals from getting normal exercise and they feed a diet of grains instead of grasses. This makes for an obese animal with the wrong kind of fat. It has an unnatural and unhealthy concentration of omega-6 fatty acids that cause heart disease.

Grass-fed, pasture-raised animals have nutrient-rich, naturally produced fat. Also, the meat has a higher concentration of the healthy and essential polyunsaturated fat omega-3, and less omega-6, just like nature intended. Trim the fat how you like, but don't trim it all off. You need it.

Your protein list should also include wild-caught fish. Stay away from farm-raised fish as it will have high levels of a destructive fat called arachidonic acid.

And don't forget eggs, nuts and beans. They have healthy fats, too.

Rule 2) Avoid Processed Meats. Processed meats like bacon, sausage, hot dogs and lunch meat contain chemicals, preservatives, and additives. Or they're smoked or cured, which gives them twice as many nitrates. Nitrates cause plaque to build up in your arteries.[1]

Smoked or cured meat like sausage and bologna also contains high levels of benzo (A) pyrene. This is a cancer-causing chemical in cigarette smoke.[2]

Instead, eat meat from animals that have been raised in their natural environment and are free from processing. Like pasture-raised meat. In grass-fed beef alone there's:

- **More Omega-3s.** Grass-fed beef has 2 to 10 times more ome-ga-3s than grain-fed.[3]
- **Healthier ratio** of omega-3s to omega-6s.[4]
- **More CLA.** Two to five times more than the grain-fed variety.[5,6]
- **More Vitamin E.** Grass-fed beef has three to six times more vitamin E than grain-fed.[7]
- **More Carotenoids:** Up to four times more beta-carotene than grain-fed beef.[8]
- **More B Vitamins, CoQ10, and Zinc:** These vitamins collect in the healthy fat around the organs. In grain-fed beef, the fat is full of toxins and hormones.

So, do what I do. Throw a big, juicy grass-fed steak or lamb chop on the grill and enjoy. But remember, for meat to be its healthiest, it should be cooked as little as possible. Quickly sear the meat on both sides, leaving the healthy fat intact and the inside rare.

---

[1] Paikabc, DC., Wendel, TD., Freeman, HP. "Cured meat consumption and hypertension: an analysis from NHANES III (1988-94)." 2005; 25(12):1049-1060.

[2] Rhee, KS., Bratzler, LJ., "Benzo(A)Pyrene in Smoked Meat Products." *Journal of Food Science.* 2006 Aug; 35(2):146-149.

[3,4] The "Scientific Research" section of Eat Wild. www.eatwild.com. Retrieved Jan 24, 2012.

[5] Dhiman, T.R., G.R. Anand, L.D. Satter, Pariza, M.W. "Conjugated Linolenic Acid Content of Milk from Cows Fed Different Diets." *J Dairy Sci* 1999; 82, (10): 2146-56.

[6] French P, Stanton C, Lawless F, O'Riordan E, Monahan F, Caffrey P, Moloney, A. "Fatty Acid Composition, Including Conjugated Linolenic Acid, of Intramuscular Fat from Steers Offered Grazed Grass, Grass Silage, or Concentrate-Based Diets." *J Anim Sci* 2003;78, (11): 2849-55.

[7] Smith, G. "Dietary Supplementation of Vitamin E to Cattle to Improve Shelf-Life and Case-Life for Domestic and International Markets." Colorado State University.

[8] Priolo A, et al. "Persistence of carotenoid pigments in the blood of concentrate-finished grazing sheep: its significance for the traceability of grass-feeding." *J Anim Sci* 2003;81(2): 360-7.

PART 4

NATURAL CURES TRUMP
THE PRESCRIPTION PAD

Chapter 1

My Discovery in Peru Could Make Omega-3 Supplements Obsolete

I discovered an oil in Peru that has more heart-healthy omega-3s than any substance on earth — even wild Alaskan salmon.[1]

This oil — which comes from nuts, not fish — has a mild nutty flavor; almost like almonds. It's so light and delicious, you could literally drink it right out of the bottle. Mixed with balsamic vinegar, it makes a wonderful salad dressing. It's not available in the U.S., but I'm working to import it. If I'm successful, it will be a major breakthrough for health and nutrition.

Now don't get me wrong — I'm still a strong advocate of eating fish if you can find unpolluted ones. Or you may want to take cod liver oil for the right mix of healthy fats and fat-soluble vitamins. It may be the best option you currently have. I have less faith in individual omega-3 supplements. They just don't occur as isolated compounds by themselves in nature.

Yet you need to find some source for omega-3s. I write a lot about them because they are so vital to your health. Your heart, brain and all the cells in your body rely on them to function well. Problem is, the amount of these essential fatty acids in your food keeps shrinking. Why?

Because our food supply has been altered. Salmon and steak are no longer the "wonder foods" that they once were. Most salmon and almost all cattle have been cut off from their traditional diets. They are fed unnatural diets of corn and soy. It causes inflammation and changes their physiology. Their flesh lacks the omega-3s it once had. But your body's need for omega-3s has not changed. Little did I know that I would find a solution to this problem growing wild on a hillside deep in the Amazon rainforest...

I Held the Key to Native Heart Health in the Palm of My Hand

My trip to Peru turned out to be much more of an adventure than I imagined. As you may know, I set out to investigate rumors of a special kind of maca, a plant that boosts energy levels, strengthens your immune system and improves oxygen delivery. But along the way I made a totally unexpected yet extraordinary discovery...

It was midday on my seventh day in Peru. I could see the excitement in J.C.'s smile. (J.C. had been to my organic gardens in Florida the month before and invited me to visit him while in Peru. He is an enterprising organic expert. If it grows in the Amazon, J.C. knows about it.)

I listened closely when J.C. announced, "Here it is..."

I followed his gaze to a bushy plant I had never seen before. It looked unremarkable, distinguished only by a green star-shaped fruit. But I knew by his reaction I had stumbled upon something exceptional.

He cracked open a flower and placed the seeds in my hand. "This is the Sacha Inchi plant," he said. "It's been used by the indigenous people of the Peruvian Amazon for thousands of years."

It turns out that the Sacha Inchi is an incredible rich non-animal source of omega-3s and was once a staple of the ancient Incas. I don't know how it has remained a secret for so long. Very soon you will be hearing much more about it.

These Rich Omega-3s Could Turn the Tables on Heart Disease — Even Cancer

A shortage of omega-3 fatty acids has been linked to:[2]

- Dyslexia;
- Depression;
- Weight Gain;
- Heart Disease;
- Violence;
- Memory Problems;
- Allergies;

- Diabetes;
- Eczema.

The list goes on and on. Now we can add cancer to the list. According to a recent study published in the *Journal of the American Medical Association*,[3] researchers found that high amounts of fatty acids significantly decreases the risk of certain types of cancers in women.

But all cancers appear preventable when you get an adequate supply of omega-3s.[4] Make sure you keep your diet rich in omega-3s. Your best food sources are wild, cold-water fish, grass-fed red meat, eggs, olives and olive oil, nuts, and avocados.

Your best current supplement source is cod liver oil. Be sure to get a brand that has been tested to be free of mercury and PCBs. One teaspoon a day with food is a good starting dose.

---

[1] O'Brien, D. "Studies Tip Scales." *The Baltimore Sun*. Oct. 18, 2006.

[2] "Omega-3 is Essential to the Human Body." Mercola.com. 3/16/02.

[3] Alicja Wolk, DMSc; Susanna C. Larsson, MSc; Jan-Erik Johansson, MD, PhD; Peter Ekman, MD, PhD. "Long-term Fatty Fish Consumption and Renal Cell Carcinoma Incidence in Women," *Journal of the American Medical Association* 2006;296:1371-1376. l. 296

[4] Ternan, C. "Omega-3 Fatty Acids: An Essential Contribution." The Nutrition Source. Harvard T.H. Chan School of Public Health. September 18, 2012.

Chapter 2

How to Boost Your "Master Antioxidant"

Cutting-edge research is revealing the power of a "master antioxidant" — a tripeptide molecule called **glutathione** (GSH). Those with the highest levels of GSH are the ones who routinely live past 100. GSH may prevent a host of chronic diseases like arthritis, high blood pressure, heart disease, cancer and diabetes — just to name a few.

Best of all, boosting your levels of GSH is easy. I'll give you an effective strategy that may add decades to your life. I'll tell you exactly how to get the most powerful forms of GSH and how much to take.

GSH Increases Life Span by 30-38%

When Dr. Calvin Lang and scientists at the University of Louisville gave mosquitoes a GSH booster, their levels went up by 50% to 100%. And, their life spans increased by a remarkable 30% to 38%.[1] Doctors at the Montreal General Hospital Research Institute in Canada then repeated the experiment with mice.[2] They were able to duplicate the results — boosting levels of GSH and increasing life spans.

Their success prompted others to investigate the effects of GSH in humans. Dr. Helle Andersen and her colleagues at Odense University in Denmark compared levels of GSH in centenarians (age 100 to 105) and people age 60 to 79 and found that GSH was higher in the centenarians. And among the centenarian group, those who were the most active had the very highest GSH.[3]

In another study, Dr. Lang followed women aged 60 to 103 for five years. He concluded that, "high blood glutathione concentrations... are characteristic of long-lived women."[4]

GSH Super-Charges Your Immune System and Prevents Chronic Disease

In the same way that high levels of GSH increase life spans, low levels of GSH show a direct link to chronic degenerative diseases. Here's just a partial list:

- Heart Disease;
- Arthritis;
- High Blood Pressure;
- Diabetes;
- Cancer;
- Macular Degeneration;
- Cataracts;
- Renal Failure;
- Leukemia;
- Hearing Loss;
- Obstructive Lung Disease (COPD).

While Dr. Lang found that low levels of GSH dramatically increase your risk of chronic disease, Dr. Mara Julius from the University of Michigan — in a study of 33 people over age 60 — found that high levels of GSH were associated with fewer illnesses. Her patients reported a greater sense of well-being along with lower blood pressure, lower cholesterol and reduced body fat.[5]

Four Simple Strategies for Boosting Your Own Levels of GSH

You can pump up your levels of GSH in 4 ways:

- GSH Containing Foods;
- GSH Boosting Nutritional Supplements;
- GSH Precursors;
- GSH Containing Supplements.

The most natural way to get more GSH is eating foods high in glutathione. These include horseradish, broccoli, cauliflower, cabbage, kale, and Brussels sprouts.

These nutritional supplements will also boost your GSH:

- Alpha-Lipoic Acid (ALA);
- Melatonin;
- Bilberry;
- Grape Seed Extract;
- Turmeric.

There are also two reliable GSH precursors — substances that stimulate the production of GSH. These are **whey protein**,[6] commonly found in protein powders and **N-acetyl cysteine**[7] (in a dose of 1,800 mg. to 2,400 mg. a day) — both are available at your local nutrition and/or health food stores.

Finally, you can take GSH supplements (1 to 2 grams per day). The latest reports show that up to 80% of most GSH supplements are absorbed and used by your body.

For best results, I recommend using a combination of all four ways to boost GSH.

---

[1] Richie JP, et al. Correction of a glutathione deficiency in the aging mosquito increases its longevity. *Proc Soc Exp Biol Med.* 1987 Jan;184(1):113-7.

[2] Bounous G, et al. "Immunoenhancing property of dietary whey protein in mice: role of glutathione." Clin Invest Med. 1989 Jun;12(3):154-61.

[3] Andersen HR, Lower Activity of Superoxide Dismutase and High Activity of Glutathione Reductase in Erythrocytes from Centenarians, Age and Aging, 1998;27:643-648.

[4] Lang CA, Mills BJ, Lang HL, et al. "High blood glutathione levels accompany excellent physical and mental health in women ages 60 to 103 years." J Lab Clin Med. 2002 Dec; 140(6):413-7.

[5] Julius M, Lang CA, Gleiberman L, et al. "Glutathione and morbidity in a community-based sample of elderly." Journal of Clinical Epidemiology. 1994 Sep;47(9): 1021-6.

[6] Bounous G, et al. The influence of dietary why protein on tissue glutathione and the diseases of aging. *Clin Invest Med.* 1989a Dec;12(6):343-9.

[7] Schaller M. Oxidant-Antioxidant Balance in Granulocytes During ARDS-Effect of N-Acetyl cysteine, *Chest*, Jan 1996;109(1):163-166.

Chapter 3

Anti-Aging Vegetable Compound Protects Your Skin

If you love staying out in the sunshine but worry when that tan turns into a burn, there's a groundbreaking study you should know about. It blows another hole in the modern medical myth that sunshine's bad for you — and that sunscreens full of toxic chemicals are your best and only defense.

There's no question that if you get sunburns often, you're risking lasting damage to your skin, including melanoma, the most dangerous kind of skin cancer. But it turns out that Nature's got a weapon against sunburn that may outperform any sunscreen on the market. It halts the processes that lead to sunburn by nearly 80%.[1] And unlike the commercial skin care products, it's completely safe and natural.

It unleashes your body's natural healing power so that spending time in the sun won't hurt you. It lasts for days, long after it's been washed away. Even better — it works *without blocking the sun's rays*.

You can spend a relaxing day at the beach, play a full eighteen holes on the golf course, or just putter around the garden without worry of having to slather artificial chemicals on your skin — all the while reaping the health benefits of sunlight. And to find the source of the most powerful new ally in skin cancer prevention, you don't have to look any further than the produce section at your local supermarket.

Meet Sulforaphane: Nature's Powerful Cancer Fighter

Broccoli's the simple vegetable that might cut into the $5 billion-a-year sunscreen industry's profits someday.

There's a naturally occurring chemical compound in broccoli called *sulforaphane*. It's a potent antioxidant and cancer-fighter scientists stumbled on fifteen years ago. It's in kale, cabbage, cauliflower, turnips, even Brussels sprouts. (Your mother was right when she told you to eat your Brussels sprouts.)

Since it was first discovered, there's been a mountain of clinical research proving sulforaphane's power as an ironclad defense against many kinds of cancer, including cancers of the breast and prostate.[2] But until recently, studies focused on it as something you'd get in foods or as a supplement. It hadn't occurred to anyone to look at how sulforaphane might work if you used it like a lotion.

So a team of researchers at John Hopkins University did just that. They started out with three-day-old broccoli sprouts, because the sprouts of the plant have 30-50 times more sulforaphane than the mature broccoli we're used to seeing at the grocery store.

The Johns Hopkins team made a lotion with the broccoli sprout extract and applied it to the skin just like sunscreen, testing it on the skin of mice and on human volunteers. One of the keys to this particular study was that they exposed the skin to high intensity ultraviolet radiation for up to *three days*.

And that's when something amazing happened. In the human volunteers, those who hadn't been given lotion developed sunburns, including reddening and inflammation. But the other group saw a 40% reduction in sunburn on average, and nearly *80%* in one case.

What's more the lotion's healing power lasted long after it had already been fully absorbed by the skin. In other words, the broccoli extract lotion practically eliminated sunburn under extreme conditions.

So how does it work?

Turn on Your "Sun-Protecting" Gene

The Johns Hopkins researchers found that rather than "coating" the top layer of your skin like commercial sunscreen, their broccoli sprout lotion actually goes straight into your skin cells. From there it fires up a number of processes that maintain robust skin health.

Overexposure to sunlight causes sunburn because the sun's rays interact with oxygen to create molecules that can eventually damage the DNA in your skin cells. Over time, this causes them to die or become cancerous.

Sulforaphane has the power to guard DNA by turning on a set of skin-protection genes, like a key in an ignition. Once activated, they release chemicals called "phase 2 enzymes." These enzymes neutralize the molecules that damage DNA. They also reduce inflammation, another painful symptom of sunburn.

So you can see how differently it works from sunscreen. It lets the sunlight in while sparking your skin's natural healing power. Think of it as a kind of skin cream that works from the inside out.

Since it works without blocking the sun's rays, broccoli extract lotion has the potential to protect you from overexposure without robbing your body of the sun's many health benefits.

Your Body Needs Sunlight

No matter what the medical establishment and the sunscreen industry say, your body has a physical need for sunlight. You probably already know that your skin reacts to sunlight by making vitamin D. But you may not know just how beneficial vitamin D really is. Here's just a sample of its clinically proven power. Vitamin D:

- Elevates mood and boosts mental performance.
- Prevents many types of cancers, including prostate, breast and ovarian.
- Reduces the risk of melanoma.
- Halts and even reverses the effects of bone diseases like rickets, osteomalacia and osteoporosis.
- Relieves depression and lessens the symptoms of schizophrenia.
- Enhances the function of your pancreas.
- Increases insulin sensitivity and prevents diabetes.
- Promotes weight loss.

- Provides more restful sleep.

- Lends energy, vitality, and stamina.

- Lowers blood pressure.

- Brings high blood sugar levels down.

- Lowers the amount of bad cholesterol in your blood.

- Increases white blood cell activity and strengthens immunity.

It will probably be a while before broccoli extract lotion becomes available to the general public. (Among other things, they still need to figure out how to keep it from breaking down before it makes its way onto store shelves.)

Four Steps to "Sun Living"

In the meantime, there's plenty you can do to take advantage of the sun's health-promoting power and protect yourself. Here are four simple steps you can take right now.

1) *Stop* using sunscreen.

Most people don't know this — even many dermatologists — but sunscreen offers no real protection against skin cancers from overexposure to the sun. In fact, it can actually *cause* cancer. Here's a short list of some of the artificial, carcinogenic compounds widely used by the sunscreen industry:

Cancer-causing chemicals in commercial sunscreens

Chemical	
PABA (also known as octyl-dimethy and padimate-O)	When exposed to sunlight, it attacks DNA and causes genetic mutation.
Octyl-methoxycinnamate (OMC)	Toxic too and can kills cells.
Octyl-dimethyl-PABA (OD-PABA) Benzophenone-3 (Bp-3) Homosalate (HMS) Octyl-methoxycinnamate (OMC) 4-methyl-benzylidene camphor (4-MBC).	Mimic estrogens, causing disruption of real hormone and stimulate cancer cells to grow.

What's more, there's never been any evidence that sunscreens prevent the most serious kinds of skin cancer. The science backs me up on this. A recent study published in the prestigious journal *Lancet* found that while sunscreen may protect against two of the three most common skin cancers, it has not been conclusively shown to protect against melanoma, the most lethal type.[3]

2) Get your skin-healthy nutrients, especially antioxidants.

There's no question that overexposure to sunlight can cause free-radical damage to your skin. The good news is antioxidants are powerful free-radical "scavengers." They not only prevent skin damage, they can actually reverse the effects of aging from long-term sun exposure.

For your skin these three supplements in particular are important: vitamin C — 1000 mg., CoQ10 — 100 mg., and vitamin E — 400 IEU. They're inexpensive and readily available online or in health food stores.

You can also ramp up the antioxidant content in your diet. Look for foods rich in vitamins E, C, and A. Here are a few of the best foods for your skin:

Food	Vitamin Levels
Citrus fruit — oranges, grapefruit, tangerines, etc.	Up to 70 mg/serving of vitamin C — builds collagen, reduces inflammation, protects cells
Cantaloupe	29 mg/serving of vitamin C
Guava	165 mg/serving of vitamin C
Kiwifruit	162 mg/serving of vitamin C
Eggs	140 micrograms (mcg)/serving vitamin A — powerful antioxidant that helps maintain healthy cells
Plain Yogurt	35 mcg/serving of vitamin A
Chicken liver	11,000 mcg/serving of vitamin A
Almonds	11 IU/serving of vitamin E — beneficial to skin health, prevents skin cell damage
Peanut butter	6 IU/serving of vitamin E

Cooked spinach	2.5 IU/serving of vitamin E
Beef	3.4 mg/serving Coenzyme Q10 — important antioxidant and a building block of the body's tissues
Sardines	7.3 mg/serving of CoQ10

And by the way, even without the extract, you can still get those phase 2 enzymes by eating broccoli or broccoli sprouts, which, as I mentioned, are now widely available in many supermarkets.

As always, I encourage you to try to buy organic, free-range, grass-fed, and minimally processed kinds of these foods whenever you can.

3) Get outside and enjoy the sun every day you can.

A recent study published in *Anticancer Research* found that just by getting a little sunlight every day — about 20 minutes for fair-skinned folks, and two to four times that much for those with dark skin — you can reduce the risk of *16 types of cancer in both men and women.*[4]

4) Try natural lotions that *truly* promote skin health

Look for all-natural lotions with vitamins E or C. Vitamin C is especially good for your skin. It's been clinically proven to protect you from overexposure to both UV-A and UV-B rays, prevents age spots, and a reduction in inflammation in the skin.[5]

To learn more about the natural power of sunlight check out my book, *Your Best Health Under the Sun.* You'll find over 250 pages of useful information to help you live a longer, healthier life.

---

[1] Talalay, et al. "Sulforaphane mobilizes cellular defenses that protect skin against damage by UV Radiation." *Proceedings of the National Academy of Sciences.* 2007. 104(44): 17500-17505.

[2] Verhoeven, DT, Verhagen H, Goldbohm RA, et al. "A review of mechanisms underlying anticarcinogenicity by brassica vegetables." Chem Biol Interact. 1997 Feb 28; 103(2):79-129.

[3] Lautenschlager, et al. "Photoprotection," *Lancet.* 2007. 370(9586):528-537.

[4] Grant WB, Garland CF. "The association of solar ultraviolet B (UVB) with reducing risk of cancer: multifactorial ecologic analysis of geographic variation in age-adjusted cancer mortality rates." Anticancer Research. 2006 Jul-Aug; 26(4A):2687-99.

[5] Farris PK. (2005) "Topical vitamin C: a useful agent for treating photoaging and other dermatological conditions." *Dermatologic Surgery.* 31(7pt2): 814-17.

Chapter 4

The Original Cancer "Medicine"

Vitamin E is the Rodney Dangerfield of the vitamin world — it gets no respect.

You may have heard that vitamin E is not "safe." Or not to take vitamin E because it might raise your risk of lung cancer, it thins your blood, or it even increases your risk of death…

But studies show vitamin E protects you from at least 10 different kinds of cancer.

And we don't need any new inventions or drugs to prevent cancer. All we have to do is recreate our native environment.

You see, cancer was almost unknown in the ancient world.

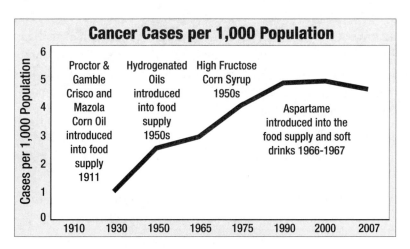

In a study completed just recently and published in the journal *Nature*, researchers looked at tissue samples from hundreds of Egyptian mummies. There should have been evidence of cancer in all of them, according to modern cancer statistics. And mummification would have preserved any sign of tumors.

But instead of finding cancer in nearly every mummy, they found only a single case. The hundreds of other mummies showed no sign of cancer at all.[1]

These results would be impossible if cancer were not an entirely modern plague. Statistically, it could not happen.

And it wasn't because Egyptians didn't live long enough to get cancer. The mummies had evidence of age-related problems like brittle bones and hardened arteries.

Even as recently as 1930, cancer rates were 460% lower than they are today.

But with the development of modern farming practices that strip our food of its nutrients like vitamin E, cancer rates have shot up.

The Oldest Cancer Fighter Is New Again

Vitamin E protects you because it stands guard on the outer layer (the membrane) of all your cells. It's your cells' first line of defense against attacks from things like pollution, toxins, and other free-radical damage that makes them older and weaker.

As an anti-aging doctor, I've always thought of vitamin E as the original anti-aging "medicine" — the original antioxidant. In fact, did you know that the ORAC scale, which was developed to measure the antioxidant power of foods, is based on comparing foods to the antioxidant effects of vitamin E?

The ORAC scale measures the "trolox equivalent" of foods, and trolox is a vitamin E derivative used as the benchmark to measure free-radical fighting power.

Vitamin E works to prevent cancer partly because your immune cells rely on it. They must have it to keep you from getting sick.[2]

But vitamin E's biggest effect is that it puts a cold stop to free-radical attacks on cell membranes, which can cause carcinogenesis, or formation of cancers.[3] That's why vitamin E is the standard for comparing antioxidant power.

Vitamin E blocks the formation of carcinogens, especially nitrosamines. These are cancer-causing compounds that can come from smoke (cigarette, chimney or industrial), and can also form in the stomach from nitrites in the cured (processed and preserved) meats typical of the Western diet.

The newest research is on prostate cancer. Prostate cancer may be caused by a specific kind of stem cell in the prostate. We are learning that one of the reasons why prostate cancer seems to come back is that most prostate treatments get the tumors but not these stem cells.

A new study found that the gamma-tocotrienol form of vitamin E not only stops prostate cancer cells from forming, it also keeps any cancer cells from invading. And, vitamin E also sensitizes cancerous cells so that other treatments can kill them.[4]

And there are hundreds more studies on vitamin E's effectiveness against cancer. Here are just a few:

- One study done just a few months ago looked at about 1,000 people and found that high intake of vitamin E reduced the risk of pancreatic cancer by 40%.[5]

- The Nurses Health Study looked at 83,234 women over 14 years. It found that pre-menopausal women with a family history of breast cancer who took in the most vitamin E had 43% fewer cases of breast cancer.[6]

- A study just completed in *Cancer Prevention Research* took animals with lung cancer and then gave them vitamin E. Researchers found that the delta-tocopherol form of vitamin E strongly inhibited tumor growth.[7] In people, studies have shown that higher levels of vitamin E protect against lung cancer.[8]

- The Harvard School of Public Health did a huge study on supplements and the risk of colon cancer. The study looked at over 676,000 people and followed them from seven to 20 years. They found that taking in more than 200 mg. of vitamin E a day from both food and supplements reduced the risk of getting colon cancer by 22%.[9]

- And a study I read that hasn't even been published yet showed that high intake of vitamin E is correlated with greater survival for all people who have gliomas (spine or brain tumors).[9]

- Vitamin E's benefits can even cross generations. The same study reports that mothers who took vitamin E and other antioxidants throughout their pregnancies had children with fewer incidences of glioma.[10]

Many other studies point out that people with cancers of the cervix, colon, stomach, rectum, liver, and pancreas all have low levels of vitamin E.

As it turns out, vitamin E is becoming essential in the fight against cancer. In fact, they even use vitamin E to protect people from the effects of some chemical breast and lung cancer treatments.

This makes vitamin E *the most important* fat-soluble antioxidant you have.

Eight Is Enough to Fight Cancer

What you may not know is that vitamin E is not just a single vitamin.

It's really a group of at least eight "vitamers," all with vitamin E activity, named tocochromanols.

Four of those are called tocopherols and four are tocotrienols. They're all antioxidants, and each has its own unique health properties.

You may have heard of the alpha tocopherol. It's the one you'll see on most vitamin supplements. It's also the one your body has the most of, but be careful... you don't want to start getting huge doses of it.

Not only is it the tocopherol with the least heart benefit, but when you take too much of it, you cause a decreased absorption of gamma-tocopherol. Gamma has been shown to have a lot of benefit for your heart and blood vessels.

Also, tocotrienols have benefits that tocopherols don't have. They help lower your triglycerides and your blood pressure.

Tocotrienols also lower your cholesterol by "attacking" a cholesterol-creating enzyme called HMG-CoA.[11]

Tocotrienols also work in your blood in other ways. A new study by researchers looking to help people's brains shows that tocotrienols in natural vitamin E supplements build up inside the blood and protect your brain.[12]

What this means for you is that you need this important form of vitamin E to support normal, natural heart and blood function.

So, how do you get vitamin E that has the right amount of tocopherols and also contains tocotrienols?

Source #1) Oils — You can find high concentrations of tocotrienols in oils like palm, coconut and wheat germ. You should be able to pick these up at a health food store or specialty grocer. Keep in mind that soybean oil and sunflower oil have NO tocotrienols. In fact, the only sunflower (also called safflower) oil you would ever want to consume is the cold, polyunsaturated kind that you store in the fridge. This has the healthy fats.

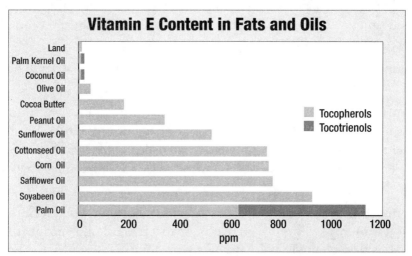

Personally, my favorite oil is annatto. I first encountered it in the Andes Mountains. After you ascend the Andes from the east and start down into the Amazon basin, you find annatto growing in the foothills before you get to the dense rainforest.

The natives there recognize annatto as a powerful health tonic, and even use it as a dye. This is because annatto has compounds with a unique reddish-orange color that are chemically similar to beta-carotene — which gives carrots their color.

So, it's not surprising that beta-carotene-filled foods like cranberries and carrots have tocotrienols, too.

Annatto oil is full of tocotrienols, especially the delta tocotrienol, and has almost no tocopherols.

Source #2) Eggs and Avocados — Eggs and avocados are almost perfect foods. Whether it's vitamins, proteins, minerals or nutrients, they're a great source for all of them.

Source#3) Nuts — I've heard nutritionists claim that walnuts have vitamin E, but they have very little. Pecans and Brazil nuts have a good amount, but the kings of vitamin E are hazel nuts and almonds. One handful a day will significantly boost your intake of vitamin E.

Source #4) Plants — Alfalfa leaves have a lot of vitamin E, but the seeds and sprouts do not. You can get dehydrated leaves at most health food stores. Asparagus, Brussels sprouts, parsley, spinach, and broccoli also have vitamin E.

Source #5) Fruit — Black currants, blackberries and the avocado pear all have vitamin E, as do dried sultana grapes — raisins!

Source #6) Grass-Fed Beef — Do you know why all those nutritionists tell you that beef doesn't have a lot of vitamin E? Because the only beef they know about — commercial, grain-fed beef — doesn't have a lot of vitamin E. Grass-fed beef, on the other hand, has four times as much.[13]

Source #7) Supplements — Remember, getting your vitamin E from natural sources will give you a mix of tocotrienols and tocopherols. Plus, your vitamin E will have all its micronutrients, co-factors and minerals, just like nature intended.

But most people are unlikely to eat a wide enough variety of foods to get enough vitamin E, so you can supplement.

- You'll want to get a mix of tocopherols and tocotrienols,
- Don't take too much alpha tocopherol. I recommend 200 IU (about 20 mg.).

- Take tocotrienols a few hours apart from other sources of vitamin E so that the alpha-tocopherol doesn't lessen their benefits.

---

[1] David R, Zimmerman M. "Cancer: an old disease, a new disease or something in between?" *Nature Reviews Cancer.* Oct. 2010;728-733.

[2] Pekmezci, D. "Vitamin E and immunity." *Vitam. Horm.* 2011;86:179-215.

[3] Marnett L. "Lipid peroxidation-DNA damage by malondialdehyde." *Mutat. Res.* Mar. 8, 1999;424(1-2):83-95.

[4] Luk S, et al. "Gamma-tocotrienol as an effective agent in targeting prostate cancer stem cell-like population." *Int. J. Cancer* May 1, 2011;128(9):2182-91.

[5] Bravi F, Polesel J, Bosetti C. et al. "Dietary intake of selected micronutrients and the risk of pancreatic cancer: an Italian case-control study." *Ann. Oncol.* Jan. 2011;22(1):202-6.

[6] Zhong S, et al. "Dietary carotenoids and vitamins A, C, and E and risk of breast cancer." *J. Natl. Cancer Inst.* 1999;91:547-556.

[7] LiG, Lee M, Liu A, et al. "{delta}-Tocopherol Is More Active than {alpha}- or {gamma}-Tocopherol in Inhibiting Lung Tumorigenesis In Vivo." *Cancer Prev. Res* (Phila). Mar. 2011;4(3):404-13.

[8] Ratnasinghe, D, et al. "Serum tocopherols, selenium and lung cancer risk among tin miners in China." *Cancer Causes Control.* Feb. 2000;11(2):129-35.

[9] Park Y, et al. "Intakes of vitamins A, C, and E and use of multiple vitamin supplements and risk of colon cancer: a pooled analysis of prospective cohort studies." *Cancer Causes Control.* Nov. 2010;21(11):1745-57.

[10] Sheweita S, Sheikh B. "Can Dietary Antioxidants Reduce the Incidence of Brain Tumors?" *Curr. Drug Metab.* Mar. 25, 2011.

[11] Schaffer S, Müller W, Eckert G. "Tocotrienols: Constitutional Effects in Aging and Disease," *J. Nutr.* 2005; 135:151-154.

[12] Khanna, Savita, Parinandi, Narasimham L, Kotha, Sainath R, et al. "Nanomolar vitamin E alpha-tocotrienol inhibits glutamate-induced activation of phospholipase A2 and causes neuroprotection." *Journal of Neurochemistry.* March 2010;112(5):1249–1260.

[13] A.U. "Dietary supplementation of vitamin E to cattle improve shelf life and case of beef for domestic international markets." G.C. Smith Colorado State University, Fort Collins, Colorado 80523-1171.

Chapter 5

The 93,000-Mile-Long Organ You've Never Heard Of

There's an organ in your body that most people don't even know about. Yet it's so important that in one way or another, it can be linked to most heart-related diseases like high blood pressure and heart disease.

It's a living, intelligent and reactive system. It protects the vessels of every other organ system, even your eyes and your lymph nodes. Your blood brain barrier is part of it, too.

This organ is called the *endothelial cell barrier*, or ECB for short.

It's a dynamic system that also regulates the flow of almost every biologically active molecule in your body.

You could think of it as a relative of the largest organ in your body, your skin. It shields you from attacks on the outside, and your ECB does a similar job on the inside.

When it's working well, your ECB:

- Keeps your blood pressure low.
- Regulates vascular system growth.
- Stops blood clots.
- Allows vitamins and other nutrients to reach your organs.
- Protects your blood and lymph vessels.
- Synthesizes, converts, and activates hormones.
- Normalizes blood supply to your organs.
- Activates microbe-killing white blood cells.
- Reduces inflammation.

- Suppresses heart-damaging genes.
- Reduces swelling, pain, and stiffness.[1]

But the ECB is becoming weakened and dysfunctional in most Americans. One of the reasons is your ECB's worst enemy, inflammation.

When any part of your ECB becomes inflamed, it's vulnerable to all kinds of damage.

For example, part of your ECB system is the lining of your blood vessels. Inside these delicate tubes, inflammation leads to the formation of scar tissue. These cracks and rough, bumpy patches act like a net in your bloodstream. They catch all kinds of bad stuff that would normally pass right through. That includes triglycerides, waste from cellular metabolism, and even good things like cholesterol, fat and calcium.

These become arterial plaque, the main cause of atherosclerosis, or hardening of the arteries, which can cause a heart attack.

Another cause of ECB inflammation may surprise you. It's infections and allergens.

Your ECB is under constant attack from foreign invaders. You know that your body responds to these kinds of attacks by unleashing an army of white blood cells to surround and destroy them.

But what most people don't know is that as they attack harmful bacteria and other microorganisms, white blood cells also release a class of hormones called "**cytokines**."

Cytokines kick your immune system into high alert, signaling for "reinforcements" of white blood cells to help combat diseases.

Unfortunately, they also cause an inflammatory response across your entire body — especially in your ECB system.

This is why people who don't floss regularly are at greater risk for atherosclerosis and heart attack. The bacteria that colonize the area below your gum line unleash a continuous, low-level flow of toxins into your bloodstream.

If they're not cleared out, your immune system responds, causing the inflammation that can eventually lead to ECB damage.

It turns out that the presence of cytokines is directly linked to the risk of fatal heart attack. German researchers looked at over 150 patients suffering from chronic heart failure. They found that high concentrations of cytokines in the bloodstream were the strongest predictor of death.[2]

Fortunately, you can fight the buildup of cytokines and help keep your ECB system clean and free of inflammation and damage — safely and naturally — in four easy steps:

Step 1) Crush cytokines with CoQ10. It's the number one antioxidant for fighting inflammation in your gums. There are two reasons for this. The first is that CoQ10 is one of the most powerful antioxidants we know of. And studies show that antioxidants dramatically lower cytokines in inflamed gum tissue.[3]

The other reason is that inflammatory cytokines can cause dysfunction in the energy-producing centers of critical immune cells called PBMCs (peripheral blood mononuclear cells).

Two kinds of PMBCs you may have heard of are kinds of white blood cells called "T-cells" and "natural killer" cells.

The engines that power these immune defenders need as much energy as possible to fight off infectious diseases. And the fuel they use for energy is CoQ10.

PMBCs from people with gum disease are known to be deficient in CoQ10.

To reduce cytokine production and stop this from contributing to heart disease, I recommend that everyone take CoQ10 regularly as a constant source of new energy for your cells. Especially the new form of CoQ10 called ubiquinol, that's eight times more potent than regular CoQ10.

Step 2) Shut down inflammation with omega-3. I can't think of a fresher, more potent source of omega-3s than Sacha Inchi nut oil. The omega-3s in Sacha Inchi oil turn off excess inflammation like flipping the "off" switch. Recent science backs me up on this.

The latest research into omega-3s uncovered their two most powerful inflammation fighting compounds: resolvins and protectins. Groundbreaking studies show these omega-3 components go to work almost immediately to relieve inflammation.[4,5]

They've also been shown to drastically reduce the levels of pro-inflammatory factors like cytokines.[6]

The potent omega-3s in Sacha Inchi are easy to digest and fully absorbed by your body. Its quick response time means it creates direct benefits you can feel right away.

Step 3) Reverse inflammation with foods high in antioxidants (high ORAC values). The ORAC scale was designed to help compare the antioxidant power of different foods. The higher the ORAC value of a food, the more power it has to stop inflammation.

In one study, they measured high levels of inflammatory cytokines in the brains of aging animals. Then they gave the animals the high-ORAC superfood spirulina and watched in amazement as it dramatically lowered their cytokine levels.[7]

Other high-ORAC foods include acerola cherries, elderberries, pecans and walnuts, and the herbs sage and basil. And don't forget ginger root and the spices turmeric, cinnamon, and clove.

One of the most powerful antioxidants you can get that will drive down cytokine levels is resveratrol. It's found naturally in grapes, blueberries, and cranberries, but it's difficult if not impossible to get enough from food alone. A 50 mg. supplement per day is a good antioxidant dose.

Step 4) Stamp out cytokines with a secret from China. They call it Golden Thread in the East, but in the West, we would call the herbal extract berberine, an anti-inflammatory.

Berberine (BBR) is a flavonoid from the root of the *coptis chinensis* plant. Two of its main uses are to treat skin inflammation, and to reverse inflammation in your ECB. But scientists didn't know why it worked until they discovered that berberine squelches your body's production of inflammatory cytokines.[8]

As you can see from the graphic, it helps your body fight many causes of ECB irritation and inflammation, including high triglycerides and excess fat, and improves your ECB system function.

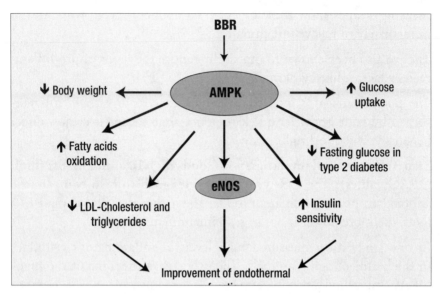

Berberine is also known to reduce inflammatory symptoms of arthritis. That's because it stops your body from producing COX-2, an enzyme responsible for causing pain and inflammation.

You can find the dried roots of coptis chinensis at most Asian specialty stores. They even have the dried root powder available online. There is also some berberine in turmeric, barberry and its cousin, the Oregon grape.

To supplement with capsules, take from 200 to 500 mg. of berberine extract per day.

[1] Bassenge E. "Endothelial function in different organs." *Prog Cardiovasc Dis.* 1996 Nov-Dec;39(3):209-28.
[2] Rauchhaus, et al. "Plasma cytokine parameters and mortality in patients with chronic heart failure." *Circulation.* 2000. 102:3060-3067.
[3] Chae HS, Park HJ, Hwang HR, et al. "The effect of antioxidants on the production of pro-inflammatory cytokines and orthodontic tooth movement." *Mol Cells.* 2011 May 12. [Epub ahead of print]
[4] Ariel A, et al. "The docosatriene protectin D1." J *Biol Chem.* 2005 Dec 30;280(52):43079-86.
[5] Chiang N, et al. "Cell-cell interaction of omega-3 fatty acid." *Methods Mol Biol.* 2006;341:227-50.
[6] James MJ, et al. "Dietary inflammatory mediator production." *Am J Clin Nutr.*

2000 Jan;71:343S-8S.

7 Gemma C, Mesches M, Sepesi B, et al. "Diets Enriched in Foods with High Antioxidant Activity Reverse Age-Induced Decreases in Cerebellar β-Adrenergic Function and Increases in Proinflammatory Cytokines." *Journal of Neuroscience,* July 2002; 22(14): 6116120.

8 Enka R, et al. "Differential effect of Rhizoma coptidis and its main alkaloid compound berberine on TNF-α induced NFκB translocation in human keratinocytes." *Journal of Ethnopharmacology.* January 2007;Volume 109, Issue 1, 3;Pages 170-175.

Chapter 6

We Don't Get Enough of This Vitamin

The national campaign to keep us out of the sun has finally caught up with us. The result?

A new study from the prestigious Archives of Internal Medicine found that an astounding three out of four Americans don't get enough vitamin D.

Here's why you should care:

Low vitamin D levels don't just cause rickets in children and weaken bones in adults. They are strongly linked to cancer, heart disease, and many other serious health problems.

The study shows that vitamin D levels dropped 20% from 1994 to 2004 on average. The number of people who have a clinical deficiency of vitamin D tripled, and those who are below the healthy level of vitamin D jumped by almost 50%.[1]

Given our obsession with staying out of the sun — Nature's way of creating vitamin D in our bodies — and the dramatic drop in vitamin D nutrients in our foods, it's no wonder that this has become a national epidemic.

Plus, the government has kept its recommended levels for vitamin D supplements way too low for far too long. Its current recommendation is to take:

- 200 IU per day from birth to 50 years old;
- 400 IU per day for aged adults 51 to 70;
- And 600 IU per day for those 71 and older.

The study's authors recommend taking 1,000 IU or more a day of vitamin D supplements on top of increasing your exposure to the sun. The government, however, is dragging its feet and says it may take up to a year to recommend new guidelines.

Don't wait. This report will show you how to safely increase your vitamin D levels and avoid the risks of vitamin D deficiency.

Don't Fear the Sun — It's Nature's Cancer Fighter

Your body needs exposure to the sun to produce vitamin D. An *Anticancer Research* study found that just by getting a little sunlight every day — about 20 minutes for fair-skinned people and two to four times that much for those with dark skin — could reduce the risk of *16 types of cancer.*[2]

Numerous studies prove the cancer-destroying properties of vitamin D. In fact, it causes melanoma cells to self-destruct.[3]

One group of scientists at the University of New Mexico found that exposure to the sun helped cancer patients to *recover* from already established melanoma. So much so, their rate of survival doubled![4]

But with their stern warnings and dire predictions, you won't hear many dermatologists — or the $6 billion sunscreen industry — voicing this evidence. Just like the great "cholesterol con" — that tricked so many into fearing cholesterol and swallowing toxic "statin" drugs — their "fear of the sun" campaign is just as ridiculous.

The real research suggests that the best way to avoid deadly melanoma is to spend more time in the sun. For instance, dozens of studies show that people who work inside — like office workers — have a much higher risk of melanoma than those who work outside — like construction workers and lifeguards.[5]

To underscore this point, melanoma commonly occurs in areas that don't receive any sunlight at all — like the palms of your hands, the soles of your feet, under your arms, beneath your fingernails — even inside your nose.

Enjoy the Sun and Protect Yourself Naturally

First, some common sense: Avoid sunburn. It hurts and damages your skin. Second, stop using chemical-based sunscreens — like the ones

362 | HEALTH CONFIDENTIAL

you get at the drugstore. The chemicals can actually be carcinogenic. If you like, you can find sunscreens available on the Internet that are natural and chemical free.

Most importantly, it's critical that you boost your body's natural defenses. Our change in diet has left us defenseless against the sun's normally health-enhancing rays. Thanks to commercial farming and processing, the nutrients we need to prevent skin cancer are increasingly absent from our food. That's why we require supplements to get the nutrients we need.

Here are my favorite supplements to help:

Cod Liver Oil — The lack of healthy omega-3 fatty acids in our diet is one of the primary factors contributing to the rise of skin cancer. Grains, sugars and processed foods — even commercial beef are full of omega-6 fatty acids. Not only are these inflammatory, but they prevent your skin from fighting the sun's UV rays.

A tablespoon of cod liver oil a day will replenish your omega-3 levels and keep your skin looking young and fresh. It will also give you a boost of vitamin D in its most natural form.

Astaxanthin is a carotenoid found in shrimp, lobsters, salmon, trout and algae. It gives them their red/pinkish color. (Carotenoids are nutrients that protect plants and animals from UV radiation.)

Astaxanthin is hundreds of times more powerful than most carotenoids and multiplies the effects of vitamin C and E, increasing their antioxidant activity.[6] This is one of the best supplements to prevent skin cancer. During periods of prolonged exposure, you can't beat it. It's available as a capsule. I recommend 2 mg. a day with meals.

Alpha-Lipoic Acid — ALA is a powerful antioxidant that works at all levels — including your skin. Not only does it protect skin cells from free radicals, it protects their mitochondria (the power plant of every cell) and pumps up your cancer defense mechanisms.

It also preserves collagen and prevents the damage associated with aging skin, making your skin more youthful and vibrant. I recommend 200 mg. to 400 mg. daily.

Vitamin C — A lack of vitamin C makes your skin vulnerable to damage from the sun's rays. And we have recently started getting far less vitamin C in our diets.

I recommend 3,000 mg. per day if you're currently in good health. This will give you enough to produce the collagen required for strong blood vessels and heart disease prevention.

Pregnant women should get at least 6,000 mg. per day — and in times of stress or sickness, you can take up to 20,000 mg. A powdered form may be more convenient for larger doses.

Vitamin D — Finally, take a good vitamin D supplement. I recommend 1,000 to 2,000 IU daily, *particularly during the winter or if you live in cold, damp climates with little sunlight.*

---

[1] Ginde, A. *Archives of Internal Medicine*, March 23, 2009; vol 169: 626-632.

[2] Grant WB et al., "The association of solar ultraviolet B (UVB) with reducing risk of cancer: multifactorial ecologic analysis of geographic variation in age-adjusted cancer mortality rates," *Anticancer Research*, 2006; 26:2687-2700.

[3] Danielsson C, et al. (1998). Differential apoptotic response of human melanoma cells to 1alpha,25-dihydroxyvitamin D3 and its analogues. *Cell Death Differ.* 5:946.

[4] Berwick M, Armstrong BK, Ben-Porat L, Fine J, Kricker A, Eberle C, Barnhill R. Sun exposure and mortality from melanoma. *J Natl Cancer Inst.* 2005 Feb 2;97(3):195-9.

[5] Elwood JM, Gallagher RP, et al. "Cutaneous melanoma in relation to intermittent and constant sun exposure -- the Western Canada Melanoma Study." *Int J Cancer* 1985;35:427

[6] "What are the health benefits of natural Astaxanthin?" Astaxanthin by SeaQuarius Skin Care. Nov 11, 2014.

Chapter 7

Blood Pressure Meds for All?

I just finished reading the *British Medical Journal,* and there was an article by a group of researchers telling doctors they should put everyone over 40 on blood pressure drugs — even if they don't have high blood pressure![1]

According to the study's authors, "Guidelines on the use of blood pressure lowering drugs can be simplified so that drugs are offered to people with all levels of blood pressure. Our results indicate the importance of lowering blood pressure in everyone over a certain age, rather than measuring it in everyone and treating it in some."

Can you imagine? Taking drugs every day, when you're in perfect health? This is a sign of things to come. Drug companies aren't satisfied with controlling medical schools, the media and the FDA. Now they want you — all of us — to take a drug every day whether we need it or not.

Do You Have These Symptoms?
It Could Be Your Blood Pressure Meds

Make no mistake; blood pressure meds put you in an early grave. Just look at the side effects of the most popular pills.

Beta Blockers, the most common treatment for hypertension and chest pain, work by reducing nerve signals to the heart and blood vessels thus lowering blood pressure. But, it comes at a high price. Including:

- Fatigue;
- Lowered Sex Drive;
- Dizziness;
- Depression;

- Nausea;
- Impotence.

But what's really worrisome are the long-term effects they have on overall cardiovascular health.

They raise your triglyceride levels — the "bad fats" that clog your arteries — and lower your HDL levels — the "good" cholesterol your body needs for optimal health. Not exactly the ideal cure for heart disease.

Calcium Channel Blockers have similar side effects. They work by preventing calcium from going into heart and blood vessel muscle cells (thus causing the cells to relax) which lowers blood pressure.

And, like beta blockers, a number of studies have found that people on them ran a much higher risk of heart attack than those on other medications — as much as 60%.[2]

Angiotensin-Converting Enzyme (ACE) Inhibitors actually block the production of a hormone that causes blood vessels to narrow, frequently causing severe reactions including heart fibrillation, kidney failure and death.[3]

Angiotensin II receptor blockers allow blood vessels to widen by preventing a hormone called angiotensin from affecting vessels. Side effects are as minor as dizziness, diarrhea or back pain to as severe as kidney and liver failure. Pregnant women take note — angiotensin II receptor blockers can cause birth defects.[4]

Nitrate drugs, in the short term, open up your blood vessels allowing for better flow. But over time they destroy the sensitive lining of your blood vessels, called the endothelium. This leads to damage of your cardiovascular system (aren't these drugs supposed to heal it?).

A recent Japanese study found that people taking nitrate drugs were 2.4 times more likely to suffer heart attacks than those who didn't.[5] And the damage caused to the endothelium made those heart attacks more severe.

Finally, there are **Diuretics.** They work by causing the kidneys to remove more sodium and water from the body. This helps the blood vessel walls to relax, resulting in lower blood pressure. Far safer (and cheaper) than the other drugs, but they are no less dangerous.

Common side effects of diuretics include:

- Weakness;
- Muscle cramps;
- Sensitivity to light;
- Diarrhea;
- Dehydration;
- Joint pain;
- Decreased sexual desire;
- Vomiting.

Are they kidding?

The truth is that you may not need blood pressure drugs — even if you have high blood pressure. I see this all the time.

Patients come into my office looking wrecked and demoralized, drugged up on blood pressure meds like beta blockers and ACE inhibitors.

Most folks don't realize these things make you fat — you literally blow up like a balloon. They can even cause heart failure.

Worried about high blood pressure? I'll show you what I've been using with my patients for years and the results are amazing. Here's what you do: check your blood pressure; start the simple strategies I mention below and then test again a few months later. You'll see what I mean.

Steer Clear of Dangerous Pills

Case in point: One of my patients, Roxanne, had been on an ACE inhibitor for four years. She had gained 10 pounds and was tired all the time. And at 140/85, her blood pressure was still on the high side, even on the drugs.

I told her to stop taking the blood pressure pills immediately. They weren't working anyway. And I put her on a simple nutrient. After nine months, her blood pressure was back to a healthy 118/80.

Plus, she told me she had more energy and was already working on losing the weight she had gained.

Roxanne's story isn't unique. Blood pressure pills typically make you weak and tired. Some patients have nasty side effects like depression, impotence, joint pain, and even kidney and liver damage.

What's worse is that blood pressure meds don't even work for the majority who take them. Only 42.9% of patients ever see acceptable blood pressure levels.[6]

Another study published in the *Archives of Internal Medicine* reveals just how worthless they are. In the group given the placebo, 30% lowered their blood pressure below the set goal. Apparently, just doing nothing will help close to a third of those with high blood pressure.[7]

Of course, I wouldn't advocate that you do nothing if you have high blood pressure — it does raise your chances of heart disease, heart attack, and stroke. But you can treat your high blood pressure effectively without exposing yourself to the side effects that come with these drugs.

Get the One Nutrient That Eliminates Hypertension

The first thing I instruct my patients with high blood pressure to do is take 50 mg. of ubiquinol CoQ10 every day. It's the only thing I told Roxanne to take. She made no other changes and watched her blood pressure return to healthy levels.

A team at the University of Texas found that CoQ10 is so effective, it enabled them to safely take patients off blood pressure medications.[8]

A meta-analysis of studies that looked at CoQ10 and hypertension revealed that CoQ10 can lower systolic blood pressure by up to 17 mm Hg and diastolic blood pressure by up to 10 mm Hg without side effects.[9]

If you only do one thing for healthy blood pressure, take CoQ10.

But there are other steps you can — and should — take. If you can lower your blood pressure naturally, your chance of heart disease, heart attack, and stroke go back to normal. It's as if you never had high blood pressure in the first place.

Control your stress. Here's a great meditation exercise that I recommend to my patients. It's a yoga technique called Stimulating Breath. It involves rapid breaths to flood your body with oxygen.

- Keep your mouth closed and breathe through your nose.

- Take short, quick breaths — as many as three or four a second, if possible.
- Remember to engage your diaphragm (the large muscle at the top of your belly).
- Breathe this way for fifteen seconds to start. (Stop sooner if you begin to feel dizzy.)
- Then allow your breathing to return to normal.
- Each time you practice this technique, go for a little longer. Gradually work your way up to one minute.

Most people feel on top of the world after doing the Stimulating Breath exercise.

Exercise. For quick results, try my PACE™ program.

It takes less than 15 minutes a day to do. And in addition to blood pressure benefits, it increases your lung volume, strengthens your heart, and gets you in great shape. And trimming excess fat is a great way to lower your blood pressure. Try this PACE™ workout on for size.

Warm-Up	Set 1		Set 2		Set 3	
	Exertion	Recovery	Exertion	Recovery	Exertion	Recovery
5 min (Stretching)	20-meter sprint	2–4 min	40-meter sprint	2–4 min	50-meter sprint	3–5 min

Set 4		Set 5	
Exertion	Recovery	Exertion	Recovery
60-meter sprint	3–5 min	100-meter sprint	*

You should be panting at the end of each exertion period, but you should not be exhausted throughout the workout. Gradually increase the intensity with each workout, and watch your blood pressure plummet.

Mother Nature's Super Blood Pressure Reducers

Plus, there are several foods and supplements you can take that help you lower your blood pressure naturally. If your blood pressure is very high (140/90 according to the American Heart Association) try some of these remedies:

Cod Liver Oil. Long recommended by our parents and grandparents, cod liver oil has been found in clinical studies to lower blood pressure induced by stress-elevated levels of cortisol, the body's primary stress hormone.[10] A separate study found that the vitamin D in cod liver oil promotes absorption of calcium and magnesium, thereby lowering blood pressure.[11]

Sesame Oil. In a 2003 study, people who weren't responding to their blood pressure pills were asked to simply cook with sesame oil. In 60 days, the patient's average blood pressure fell into the normal range.[12]

The combination of the heart-healthy polyunsaturated oil and the unique compound sesamin found in sesame oil causes the blood vessels to relax. This prevents pressure spikes.

Dark Chocolate. A German study found that just 6.3 grams of chocolate (the size of about two Hershey's kisses) was enough to lower blood pressure two to three points.[13] Look for dark chocolate that is at least 70% cacao.

Garlic. Garlic is an excellent heart-healthy supplement. Another German study showed that garlic reduces diastolic blood pressure, cholesterol, and triglycerides.[14]

I prefer to use a clove of raw garlic every day. Sometimes my patients prefer to take a garlic supplement. If you use a supplement, be sure that it contains at least 3,600 mcg of the active ingredient allicin.

Hawthorn Berry. Hawthorn is an herb used for centuries as a cardiac tonic. A recent study proved hawthorn's effect on high blood pressure. Participants either took hawthorn extract, magnesium, or a placebo. The study lasted for 10 weeks. The hawthorn group had a promising reduction in diastolic blood pressure. Hawthorn also reduced anxiety better than the magnesium and placebo.[15] I recommend taking 1,000 mg. of hawthorn extract daily.

Magnesium. Magnesium helps keep blood vessels relaxed and prevents blood clots. The average American takes in half as much magnesium as they did just 50 years ago. Today's fruits and vegetables have lower levels of magnesium. You'd have to eat eight of today's apples to get the same amount as one apple gave you 50 years ago.

Magnesium is your blood's own natural calcium-channel blocker. Why take a drug when this overlooked mineral can have the same effect? Take 600 mg. of magnesium daily.

I've used hawthorn berry and magnesium in my practice with great results. They are the key ingredients in my Blood Pressure Support supplement.

[1] Law MR, Morris JK, Wald NJ. "Use of blood pressure lowering drugs in the prevention of cardiovascular disease…," *BMJ* 2009; 338:b1665.

[2] Psaty et al., "The risk of myocardial infarction associated with anti-hypertensive drug therapies," Journal of the American Medical Association, 1995, 274(8):620-625.

[3] Tinerello D, MS, RD, CD/N. "Potassium in Heart Disease." Wellness Research Foundation.

[4] Mayo Clinic Staff. "Diseases and Conditions High blood pressure (hypertension)." Mayo Clinic. Sept. 6, 2014.

[5] Circulation Supplement II, Circulation, 2002, 106(19): Preliminary Abstract 1494.

[6] Rosenfeldt FL, Haas SJ, Krum H, Hadj A, Ng K, Leong J-Y, Watts GF. Coenzyme Q10 in the treatment of hypertension: a meta-analysis of the clinical trials. *J Human Hypertension* 21: 297-306, 2007.

[7] *Redwine K, Howard L, Simpson P, et al. "Effect of Placebo on Ambulatory Blood Pressure Monitoring in Children."* Pediatr Nephrol. 2012 Oct; 27(10): 1937-1942.

[8] Walker A., et al., Promising hypotensive effect of hawthorn extract: a randomized double-blind pilot study of mild, essential hypertension. **Phytother Res** 2002 Feb; 16(1): 48-54.

[9] P. Langsjoena, et al. Treatment of essential hypertension with Coenzyme Q10. Molecular Aspects of Medicine. Volume 15, Supplement 1,1994, Pages s265-s272.

10 Codde JP, Beilin LJ. Dietary fish oil prevents dexamethasone induced hypertension in the rat. *Clin Sci.*(Lond) 1985;69:691-9.

[11] Vilaseca J, Salas A, Guarner F, Rodriguez R, Martinez M, Malagelada JR. Dietary fish oil reduces progression of chronic inflammatory lesions in a rat model of granulomatous colitis. Gut 1990;31:539-44.

[12] "Sesame Oil Benefits Blood Pressure." WebMD. April 28, 2003.

[13] Allday E. "DAILY DOSE: Small amounts of dark chocolate lower blood pressure, study says." *San Francisco Chronicle.* July 4, 2007.

[14] Auer W. et al., Hypertension and hyperlipidaemia: garlic helps in mild cases. *Br J*

Clin Pract Suppl 1990 Aug; 69: 3-6.

[15] Walker A., et al., Promising hypotensive effect of hawthorn extract: a randomized double-blind pilot study of mild, essential hypertension. *Phytother Res* 2002 Feb; 16(1): 48-54.

Chapter 8

If This Were a Drug, They Would Give It the Nobel Prize

What if there were a drug that dramatically reduced the risk of heart disease, cancer, and diabetes?

A drug that prevented 17 different types of deadly internal cancers, and helped reduce overall cancer risk by 77 per cent.

It would be front-page news. You'd be hearing about it every day.

Well, there is such a thing, but it's not a drug.

It also lowers the risk of type 1 and type 2 diabetes, and helps prevent autoimmune disorders like MS and rheumatoid arthritis.

This "non-drug" has no side effects, and you can get it absolutely free. And, the more you get of it, the better you feel.

I'm talking about vitamin D.

It's the only vitamin you can get from sunshine. The only vitamin that is also a hormone.

And it's the vitamin we, here in the United States, are most deficient in.

Have you ever noticed how much better you feel after walking in the sun? It can brighten your spirits, can give you a great tan, and may just save your life.

Most doctors don't realize the sun can prevent disease. They want you to avoid sunshine at all costs. But following their advice actually puts you at a higher risk level for heart disease and cancer.

For years, most doctors failed to make the connection between prostate cancer and sunlight. But, back in 1990, Professor Gary Schwartz,

PhD, of Wake Forest University, connected the dots. He discovered that people with too little vitamin D were the ones most likely to get prostate cancer.

And these people lived primarily in the north!

He found that men living in the south, where there was plenty of sun year round, were 20 – 40% less likely to get prostate cancer than men living in the north.[1]

The World May Have Changed, but Our Genetic Makeup Hasn't

We used to get all the sun we wanted. Our ancestors lived in the sun for millions of years. They lived outdoors every moment of their lives. They were naked, near the equator, in tropical environments, and they didn't use sunscreen.

Things began to change with the Industrial Revolution. People began migrating to the cities and working indoors in factories. They were no longer working outdoors in the sunlight. Then in the late nineteenth century the lightbulb was invented, and people worked indoors for longer hours under artificial light.

The Real Truth Is We Aren't Getting Enough Vitamin D

Ongoing research confirms these findings. For example:

1. National Cancer Institute confirms that people living in sunnier places get less prostate cancer. Men with more exposure to the sun have up to 50% less risk than those with the lowest sun exposure.[3]

2. Prostate cancer patients consistently show a vitamin D deficiency.[4]

3. A recent study published in the *International Journal of Health Geographics* detailed a higher incidence of prostate cancer in northern U.S. They suspect lower levels of vitamin D to be the cause.[5]

This boosted living standards for many, but this migration indoors altered our native relationship with the sun forever.[6]

And while the world around us may have changed, your genetic make-up hasn't. You still need sunlight and vitamin D to stay healthy and prevent disease.

Vitamin D is one of the most potent health-boosting substances in your body.

Vitamin D helps:

- Boost your mood and mental performance.
- Prevent prostate, breast, ovarian, and many other cancers.
- Reduce your risk of skin cancer.
- Prevent and treat bone diseases.
- Prevent diabetes.

Vitamin D may be the single most important nutrient in your body. And we can all get plenty of it free just by spending some time in the sun. But you want to be sure that you get safe sun exposure.

Sunlight Reduces Cancer Risk. More Sun Equals Less Disease

A study in the *Journal of Cancer Research* showed for the first time that vitamin D can stop human cancer cells from growing. Researchers then used vitamin D to block malignant melanoma tumors from taking up shop in human cells.

Their experiment worked. And, since then, scores of clinical studies have confirmed the same thing. That vitamin D can inhibit skin, colon, breast, and other cancers.

Despite today's "avoid-the-sun" mentality, we now face a growing epidemic of cancers. Today, heart disease, cancer, hypertension, and diabetes are common, while they were very rare just a century ago.

Unfortunately, a powerful minority has a financial stake in having you fear the sun. For them, a return to common sense leaves them unemployed. Anyone who opposes this "fear-the-sun" view is viewed as a dangerous radical.

If you don't advocate wearing sunscreen, well, you're a danger to not only yourself but your children, too.

The real truth is the "sun police" actually put your health at risk, while acting under the guise of safety.

Sunlight is the best source of vitamin D available. But because of the fear we all have today of the sun, there is an epidemic of vitamin D deficiency.

There's a link between less exposure to the sun and vitamin D deficiency. Low levels of Vitamin D are also associated with other diseases like fibromyalgia and autoimmune diseases like multiple sclerosis and arthritis.

Research also shows that vitamin D lowers the risk of the deadliest trio of killers — heart disease, cancer, and diabetes.

By altering many of the natural ways we lived our lives over hundreds of years, we've created new diseases. Prostate cancer is now becoming ubiquitous in all cultures.

Five Ways Vitamin D Helps Reduce Your Risk of Getting Cancer

The sun triggers your body's ability to make vitamin D. Here are five ways it helps your body reduce the risk of getting cancer.

1. Converts tumor cells into normal cells. Cancer cells divide rapidly in your body but don't differentiate themselves into specific cells. Vitamin D helps this process, restoring the cancer cells to productive cells and inhibiting cancer growth.

2. Prevents cancer cells from multiplying. Cancer cells can't reproduce and spread to new tissue when introduced to vitamin D.[7] Laboratory and animal studies show that vitamin D prevents cancer cells from multiplying and also tells them when to die.

3. Keeps cancer from spreading. Vitamin D promotes normal cell growth. As a result, it helps prevent cancer cells from spreading.

4. Suppresses genes responsible for cell proliferation. Research shows that vitamin D can suppress genes prone to mutation and likely to form cancerous growths.[8]

5. Inhibits formation of new blood vessels that feed tumors. During the creation of new blood vessels, new vessels begin to branch off existing vessels. This is bad news if they're cancerous. For any tumor to have a chance to grow, there must be formation of new blood vessels to feed it. Vitamin D inhibits formation of these vessels naturally, starving the tumor of the nutrients it needs to grow.

How to Get Enough Vitamin D in Northern Climates

Vitamin D is vital to your health. Be sure and get enough of this valuable nutrient every day. It could save your life. Here are three ways I recommend you get your full share of vitamin D:

1. Get some sun. The easiest, most reliable way to get it is simply by getting out in the sun for 10 to 15 minutes a couple days a week. It's free, and will make you feel great. Depending upon where you live, this might not be possible. And simply taking a multivitamin won't give you enough Vitamin D, either. So I recommend taking a vitamin D supplement every day.

2. Eat foods with high vitamin D. Best sources are small fish like herring, sardines, and anchovies. Stay away from the larger fish that are higher up on the food chain, as the mercury content may be too high to safely eat.

3. Take some cod liver oil. Besides sunlight, the best natural source of vitamin D is cod liver oil. Just a single teaspoon contains 1,360 IU of vitamin D. Check out just how powerful cod liver oil is compared to some other pretty good sources of vitamin D:

Food Sources of Vitamin D

Food	Serving	Vitamin D IU's
Cod Liver Oil	1 Tablespoon	1,360
Salmon, cooked	3-1/2 ounces	360
Mackerel, cooked	3-1/2 ounces	345
Tuna fish, canned in oil	3 ounces	200
Sardines, canned in oil	1-3/4 ounces	250
Orange juice, fortified	8 ounces	100
Milk, organic, from grass-fed cows and fortified	1 cup	98
Cereal, fortified	¾ to 1 cup	40
Egg (vitamin D is found in egg yolks)	1 egg	20

Liver, beef, cooked	3-1/2 ounces	15
Cheese, Swiss	1 ounce	12

4. Take 5,000 IU of a good form of Vitamin D. *What makes a good form of Vitamin D? Vitamin D3. Our bodies may be conditioned to produce less Vitamin D during the winter months, when sunlight is less readily available for many. However, that's when other seasonal stresses come into play.*

Don't rely on your multivitamin to give you enough Vitamin D3. It only has 200 to 400 IU. There is a movement to increase the RDA, but it hasn't been approved yet. A Vitamin D3 supplement will help keep your body strong all year long.

---

[1] Hanchette, CL Schwartz GG. (1992) "Geographic patterns of prostate cancer mortality. Evidence for a protective effect of ultraviolet radiation." *Cancer*, 70(12): 2861-9.

[2] Schwartz, GG, Hanchette, CL, "UV, latitude, and spatial trends in prostate cancer mortality: all sunlight is not the same (United States)." *Cancer Causes Control*, 2006 Oct;17(8):1091-101.

[3] Luscombe, CJ, et al. (2001). "Exposure to ultra-violet radiation; association with susceptibility and age at presentation with prostate cancer." *Lancet*, 358:641-2.

[4] Ibid.

[5] St-Hilaire S, et al. "Correlations Between Meteorological Parameters and Prostate Cancer." *International Journal of Health Geographics* 2010, 9:19.

[6] DeLuca HF, Ostrem V. (1986). "The Relationship Between the Vitamin D System and Cancer." *Adv Exp Med Biol.* 206:413.

[7] Studzinski GP, Moore DC, (1996). "Vitamin D and the retardation of tumor progression." In Watson RR, Mufti SI, editors, Nutrition and cancer. Boca Raton:CRC Press p. 257-82.

[8] Maruyam R, et al. "Comparative genome analysis identifies the vitamin D receptor gene as a direct target of p53-mediated transcriptional activation." *Cancer Research* 2006; 66(9): 4574-83.

Chapter 9

The Sun IS Your Sunscreen

Corporations would have you believe the sun is a cancer-causing ball of radiation threatening our planet.

But the fact is, the sun protects you from cancer. It enhances your health and is vital to your well-being.

One of the most important ways the sun protects you is through your skin, which makes vitamin D from its ultraviolet type B rays. And it's vitamin D that keeps you from getting not just skin cancer, but more than a dozen others.

Here's the proof in black and white:

- A study by the journal *Anticancer Research* says very clearly that the more you make vitamin D from UVB rays, the lower your chances are of dying from *15 kinds of cancer*.[1]

- Another study in the *American Journal of Clinical Nutrition* found that vitamin D can lower the chance you'll get cancer by 77%.[2]

- The *European Journal of Cancer* looked at cancer rates all over the world. Their study says plainly that vitamin D production in the skin decreases the likelihood you'll get any of these cancers: stomach, colorectal, liver and gallbladder, pancreas, lung, breast, prostate, bladder and kidney cancers.[3]

- A study done for the journal *Nature* shows that the active form of vitamin D (calcitriol or D3), and its derivative vitamin D2, both cause skin cancer cells to die.[4]

- And did you know that people who work outside like construction workers, roofers and lifeguards have a much lower risk of skin cancer than those who work inside?[5]

I could go on…

Meanwhile, if you followed conventional medical advice, you'd be putting sunscreen all over your body.

But sunscreen lowers your body's ability to make vitamin D by up to 95%.

I'm going to show you how to let the sun work with your body to prevent cancer. Keep reading to find out what's really in sunscreens, when you should use sun protection and safe ways to help prevent sunburns.

We Were Made to Live under the Sun

If you've been to a doctor, turned on the television, been on the Internet, or read a magazine lately, you've probably heard some form of this message:

"The sun causes cancer. If you're going outside, wear sunscreen no matter what. No excuses."

Does it seem as though scientists think nature must be wrong? I get the feeling they think millennia of trial and error resulted in a mistake with our survival. And even worse, that we need some kind of intervention — some synthetic chemicals — to make it right again.

The truth is, your body already has everything it needs to properly protect itself from the sun's UV rays. The real problem isn't the sun. It's that you might not spend enough time outdoors to trigger these natural defenses.

Let me explain…

Your native ancestors survived outdoors just fine. They lived and worked in the sun's rays every day. They didn't use sunscreen and they didn't burn themselves to a crisp or die off from diseases caused by the sun.

Why? Because our bodies are designed perfectly to live in our natural environment.

When you're out in the sun, your body itself takes action. Besides making vitamin D, which I talked about earlier, your body also starts to produce another natural protectant. A built-in sun block called melanin.

Melanin is what causes your skin to darken or tan. And with just a little bit of sunshine every day — 20 minutes if you have light skin and up to three times longer if your skin is darker — you're stimulating melanin production.

By slowly developing this basic darkening, you allow yourself even more time in the sun without risk of burning.

Sunscreen — a Toxic Skin Cocktail

Corporations and modern doctors want you to put on sunscreen to block UVB rays. We've already seen how this affects vitamin D production. But sunscreen has another effect. It delivers chemicals and known carcinogens into your skin — chemicals that are banned in other countries.

One of the main chemicals used in sunscreens to filter out UVB light is octyl methoxycinnamate (OMC).

OMC can be found in 90% of sunscreens on the market even though studies found it can kill mouse cells — even at extremely low doses. And it becomes even more toxic when it's exposed to sunlight.

Other harmful chemicals include benzophenone and avobenzone.

These attack the cells in your body causing premature aging. They are also estrogen mimics that can create hormonal imbalances, cause allergic reactions and skin irritation, and are known to promote the onset of breast cancer.[6]

And there's plenty more. Below is a chart of some of the common chemicals found in sunscreen that you should avoid.

Chemical	Health Risks
Parabens	Endocrine disruptor. Mimics estrogen, upsets hormonal balances, and can cause reproductive cancer in men and women.
PABA (may be listed as octyl-dimethyl or padimate-O)	Attacks DNA and causes genetic mutation when exposed to sunlight.
Mineral oil, paraffin, petrolatum	Coats skin like plastic and clogs pores, traps toxins in, slows skin cell growth, disrupts normal hormone function, suspected of causing cancer.

Sodium laurel, lauryl sulfate, sodium laureth sulfate (sometimes listed as "from coconut" or "coconut derived")	Combined with other chemicals, it becomes nitrosamine, a powerful cancer-causing agent; penetrates your skin's moisture barrier, allowing other dangerous chemicals to enter your bloodstream.
Phenol carbolic acid	Circulatory collapse, paralysis, convulsions, coma, death from respiratory failure.
Acrylamide	Breast cancer.
Toluene (may be listed as benzoic, benzyl, or butylated hydroxtoluene)	Anemia, low blood cell count, liver and kidney damage, birth defects.
Propylene glycol	Dermatitis, kidney and liver abnormalities, prevents skin growth, causes irritation.
PEG, polysorbates, laureth, ethoxylated alcohol	Potent carcinogens containing dioxane.

It's Tough to Get Enough

The problem is that even if you have the best intentions, there are a dozen other obstacles in the modern world besides sunscreen that keep you from getting enough sunshine:

1. We wear clothing.

2. We don't migrate with the sun.

3. We don't live near the equator.

4. We work inside during the day.

5. We drive cars that block the sun.

And during the winter months, it's not uncommon — even if you live in a warm, sunny climate like I do in South Florida — to get less sunshine just because the days are shorter.

When that happens, you produce less melanin, and become more sensitive to the sun when you are exposed.

You'll need to be careful until melanin production kicks in again and can help prevent your skin from burning.

Fortunately, there are ways you can help defend your skin until you can get more sunshine without chemical sunscreens.

1. One way to help your skin is to boost the three nutrients your body uses to produce its master antioxidant, SOD (*superoxide dismutase*). SOD is your best defense against harmful molecules that attack your skin.

The best food for this job is blueberries. You probably know blueberries are good for your brain, and that they have beta- carotene and lots of vitamins. But the real power of the blueberry is that it has all three co-factors for SOD — copper, zinc and manganese. Eat a cup of blueberries every day, especially during the winter, and you'll be doing your skin a big favor.

2. Another excellent skin-defender is any food that has the omega-3 EPA. In one study of using omega-3 to reduce ultraviolet radiation sensitivity, researchers found that EPA supplementation reduces sensitivity to UV rays by 36%. And the chemical changes to skin induced by UV radiation exposure were cut in half.[7] The study concluded: "Longer-term [EPA] supplementation might reduce skin cancer in humans."

The best sources for EPA are small, cold-water fish like herring, mackerel, anchovies and sardines. Eggs and grass-fed beef also are good sources. Grass-fed beef has double the omega-3s of grain-fed beef.

In addition, you can get omega-3s in some plant-based sources like Sacha Inchi nuts, butternuts, walnuts and chia seeds. But these omega-3s are in the form of alpha linolenic acid, which then has to be converted to EPA in the body.

3. If you are going to be out in the sun for a long time, and you haven't had a chance to let your body generate enough melanin to darken you up a bit, you should use a natural sunscreen. Choose one made from natural ingredients like zinc oxide. It's been used all over the world for over 75 years as a safe sunscreen. And unlike chemical sunscreens that absorb ultraviolet light, zinc oxide sits on top of your skin to reflect and scatter UV rays.

Zinc oxide works even better when you add shea butter. That way, your pores won't clog and you'll add extra moisture to keep your skin smooth.

However, it can be very hard to find a sunscreen with the right mix of protection and nutrients. This is why I've been working with my team of experts to create a natural sunscreen with the benefits of zinc oxide and shea butter that's completely safe. It has no chemical fragrances or dyes, leaves no white residue and moisturizes at the same time.

It's perfect for a day at the beach, fishing, tennis or any outdoor activity.

---

[1] Grant, W.B. et al., "The association of solar ultraviolet B (UVB) with reducing risk of cancer: multifactorial ecologic analysis of geographic variation in age-adjusted cancer mortality rates," *Anticancer Research* 2006; 26:2687-2700

[2] Lappe, J.M., et al., "Vitamin D and calcium supplementation reduces cancer risk: results of a randomized trial," *Am. J. Clin. Nutr.* June 2007;85(6):1586-91

[3] Tuohimaa, P., et al., "Does solar exposure, as indicated by the non-melanoma skin cancers, protect from solid cancers: vitamin D as a possible explanation," *Eur. J. Cancer* July 2007;43(11):1701-12

[4] Danielsson, C., et al., "Differential apoptotic response of human melanoma cells to 1alpha,25-dihydroxyvitamin D3 and its analogues," *Cell Death Differ.* 1998; 5:946

[5] Elwood, J.M., Gallagher R.P., et al., "Cutaneous Melanoma in Relation to Intermittent and Constant Sun Exposure — The Western Canada Melanoma Study," *Int. J. Cancer* 1985;35:427

[6] Hanson, K., et al., "Sunscreen enhancement of UV-induced reactive oxygen species in the skin," *Free Radical Biology & Medicine* 2006

[7] Rhodes, Lesley E., et al., "Effect of eicosapentaenoic acid, an omega-3 polyunsaturated fatty acid, on UVR-related cancer risk in humans," *Carcinogenesis* March 2003; 24 (5): 919-925

Chapter 10

Decades in the Dark

After over 20 Years of Deceit, New Evidence That Dermatologists and Sunscreen Makers Are Making Us All Disease Magnets

Bad but widely accepted advice just might be killing you slowly if you buy into what they say about the dangers of our native sun.

They want you to avoid sunshine... slather on chemical sunscreen if you go outside... stay indoors during peak sun hours... wear long-sleeved shirts and sunglasses even when it's not sunny... and strive to cut your sun exposure to none.

Abide by these instructions and it could spell disaster for your health. By following their "no safe level of sun exposure" rule, you'll put yourself at higher risk for deadly cancers, heart disease and more.

It's time to set the record straight. *Real science* supports more, not less, sun exposure. If you know how to safely take advantage of the sun, you'll live a happier, longer life for it. You'll see how to enjoy the warm, golden, mood-lifting rays of the sun once again.

The True Crisis Is a Deficiency of Vitamin D

When the sun's rays strike your skin, an amazing hormonal reaction begins. Your skin absorbs the light and uses it to make vitamin D3. Think of it as the human version of photosynthesis.

Next your liver and kidneys metabolize the vitamin D3 into an active hormone called 1, 25- dihydroxyvitamin D3. It's quite a mouthful, but this substance plays an important role in almost every system of your body. For example:

1. Vitamin D helps build healthy bones. Vitamin D deficiencies contribute to osteoporosis, other bone-weakening conditions, and unhealthy teeth.

2. Vitamin D helps keep the immune system tuned. Vitamin D deficiencies promote a number of painful autoimmune

conditions like rheumatoid arthritis and lupus.

3. Vitamin D helps keep your circulatory system healthy. People with heart disease commonly have a vitamin D deficiency.

4. Vitamin D helps keep cells healthy. There is a link between higher rates of several deadly cancers and vitamin D deficiency.

Sunlight is the best source of vitamin D available. Because of the dire warning about the sun, many doctors recommend you avoid sunlight. This well-meant advice about sun avoidance is creating an epidemic of vitamin D deficiency.[1]

Twenty percent of children and adults up to age 50 don't get enough vitamin D every day. After 50, deficiencies affect as much as 95% of the population.

Let the Evidence Shine through — You Need More Vitamin D

Many studies show that vitamin D provides a myriad of specific health benefits like:

- Research reported in the *American Journal of Clinical Nutrition* correlated widespread vitamin D deficiency with osteoporosis, increased cancer risks, heart disease, rheumatoid arthritis, multiple sclerosis and diabetes. Increased, but safe, sun exposure is a way to counteract vitamin D deficiency.[2]

- Studies show that vitamin D reduces the risks of colon cancer, breast cancer, prostate cancer, and ovarian cancer. Your risk of mortality from each of these deadly cancers falls as your vitamin D levels rise.[3]

- More research shows that adequate vitamin D levels help to control blood pressure levels in patients with high blood pressure. It also helps control blood glucose levels in patients with adult-onset diabetes.[4]

The most natural and effective way to get adequate vitamin D levels is from sunshine. You want to be sure you get enough sunlight, that you get safe sun exposure, and that you know how to give your vitamin D levels a boost when sun exposure isn't enough.

Sunshine — Get What You Need to Prevent Deadly Disease

The big concern most people have about sun exposure is skin cancer. The vast majority of skin cancers are basal cell and squamous cell carcinomas. Both of these cancers need attention and you want to avoid them, but they are not deadly cancers.

The third type of skin cancer — melanoma — is very serious and can be deadly. However, safe sun exposure can help protect you against this skin cancer. Research shows that people who get regular sun exposure as part of their jobs are less likely to get melanoma skin cancer than people who work inside all the time.[5]

So, let me give the rules of safe sun exposure to you in three basic steps.

1. Expose as much of your skin as possible. A swimsuit is perfect. And go without sunglasses.

2. Depending on your pigmentation, go out in the sun for at least 10 to 20 minutes, two or three times a week. If you are fair-skinned, your body can make enough vitamin D in just minutes. If you have darker skin or a deep tan, it will take longer for you to get the vitamin D you need.

3. Do not allow your skin to burn. This is very important. A sunburn will damage your skin, can contribute to all three types of skin cancer and cause aging changes in your skin. You want to get your vitamin D safely. That means getting out of the sun or putting on protective clothing before you burn.

If you live in the southern states, then this is all you need to know to keep your vitamin D levels high year round. However, if you live anywhere north of Georgia, then you need to give your body a vitamin D boost in the winter months. The low angle of the sun during those months prevents the vitamin D synthesis that your body needs.

How to Get Your Vitamin D in the Winter

Between late fall and early spring, if you live in a northern state, there just isn't enough UV light reaching you to make adequate vitamin D. The government recommended amount of vitamin D every day is 400 IU. Yet research shows that your body will use 3000 IU in a day, as long as it is the natural form of vitamin D, cholecalciferol.[6] When you choose a supplement, avoid the man-made form of vitamin D, erclocalciferol.

Short of sunshine, the best natural source of vitamin D is cod liver oil. A single tablespoon of cod liver oil contains 1360 I U of natural vitamin D. In the table below, you can see other sources of natural vitamin D and how they match up to cod liver oil.

Food Source	Amount	Vitamin D
Cod Liver Oil	1 tablespoon	1360 IU
Sardines (canned)	3.5 ounces	270 IU
Salmon (cooked)	3.5 ounces	360 IU
Tuna (canned)	3 ounces	200 IU
Egg (yolk)	1 egg	25 IU
Beef Liver (cooked)	3.5 ounces	15 IU
Swiss Cheese	1 ounces	12 IU

Make cod liver oil a part of your daily supplement routine each and every winter and make safe sun exposure a habit all year round. Make sure you get a brand that is free of mercury and PCBs.

---

[1] Raloff, Janet. "Understanding Vitamin D Deficiency," *Science News* 2005; 167(18).

[2] Holick ME. "Sunlight and Vitamin D for Bone Health and Prevention of Autoimmune Diseases, Cancers, and Cardiovascular Disease," *AJCN* 2004; 80(6): 16785883.

[3] Garland CF, et al. 'The Role of Vitamin D in Cancer Prevention," *AJPH* 2005; 12/27/2005

[4] Zittermann A. "Vitamin D and Disease Prevention with Special Reference to Cardiovascular Disease," *Prog Biophys Mol Bic* 2005; 92(1): 39-48.

[5] Nelemans PJ, Groenendal H, Kiemeney LA, et al. "Effect of Intermittent Exposure to Sunlight on Melanoma Risk Among Indoor Workers and Sun Sensitive individuals." *Environmental Health Perspectives* 1993; 101(3): 252-55.

[6] Heany RP, et al. "Human Serum 25-hydroxycholecalciferol response to extended oral dosing with cholecalciferol," *AmNutr* 2003; 77(1); 204-10.

PART 5

THE FORGOTTEN KEYS TO HEART HEALTH

Chapter 1

A Healthy Heart Plan for Women

My female patients routinely ask me how to keep their hearts healthy. That shouldn't be a surprise to you. While many have the notion that it's mostly men who have to worry about heart problems, in fact since 1984 more American women have died from heart disease than men.[1,2]

Heart disease is both the number one killer and the leading cause of disability for women in the United States.[3] Out of every four women, one will die of heart disease. And two thirds of women who have had a heart attack never fully recover.[4]

These frightening facts should be all the inspiration you need to better your heart's health. But if you turn to the solutions the big pharmaceutical companies push, you'll end up with a doctor advising you to take statin drugs to lower cholesterol, beta and alpha blockers to lower your blood pressure, anticoagulants to prevent blood clots, or nitrates to increase blood flow.

Statin drugs can cause kidney and liver failure. Beta blockers de-condition your heart. And anticoagulants can cause uncontrollable bleeding.

Not only are these drugs dangerous, they also fail to treat the major causes of heart disease. While cholesterol and high blood pressure can be factors in heart disease, what you really need to pay attention to are the heart threats C-reactive protein, homocysteine, and triglycerides.

I've developed a four-point plan to *safely* help women protect their hearts.

- Testing;

- Healthy Eating;
- Heart-strengthening Exercise;
- Recognizing Trouble.

I'll show you how to put it into action.

Get Screened for Safety's Sake

In order to protect your heart, screening is key. First, ask your doctor for a test that examines the C-reactive protein (or CRP) levels in your blood. When there's inflammation in your body as a result of an injury or an infection, your liver secretes CRP in your blood. An excess of CRP leads to inflamed arteries.

Those with the highest levels of CRP are more than twice as likely to suffer from heart disease, heart attack and stroke, whether their cholesterol is high or low.[4] Knowing your CRP levels is one way to tell your risk for heart attacks and cancer.

Second, get checked for the homocysteine level in your blood. Too much homocysteine in your blood prevents your blood vessels from dilating properly, which can cause both heart attacks and strokes.

Third, have your triglycerides checked. Doctors routinely test for triglyceride levels, but they often don't have a clear idea of how to treat high triglycerides or even how much of a risk factor they are, especially in women.For women in our Wellness Center, reduction of triglycerides has made a huge difference.

Fourth, have your blood pressure examined. High blood pressure is an even more serious risk factor for women before menopause than after, as recent studies have shown.[5]

Diabetes can lead to heart disease, so you should have your blood sugar checked with a fasting glucose test. A new study indicates that heightened blood sugar levels increase your risk for heart disease.[6]

Here's a test you can do in a matter of minutes to get a better picture of what kind of shape your heart is in.[7] The lower your score, the more you need to take action to strengthen your heart.

Scoring the Duke Activity Status Index

Can You...	Yes, with no difficulty. (score)
Take care of yourself, that is, eating, dressing, bathing, and using the toilet?	2.75
Walk indoors, such as around your house?	1.75
Walk a block or two on level ground?	2.75
Climb a flight of stairs or walk up a hill?	5.50
Run a short distamce?	8.00
Do light work around the house like dusting or washing dishes?	2.70
Do moderate work around the house like vacuuming, sweeping floors, carrying in groceries?	3.50
Do heavy work around the house like scrubbing floors, or lifting or moving heavy furniture?	8.00
Do yard work like raking leaves, weeding or pushing a power mower?	4.50
Have sexual relations?	5.25
Participate in moderate recreational activies, like golf, bowling, dancing, doubles tennis, or throwing baseball or football?	6.00
Participate in strenuous sports like swimming, singles tennis, football, basketball or skiing?	7.50
Total Score No points for "yes, with some difficuty," :No, I can't do this," or "I don't do this for other reasons." Adding the point values for all questions above scores the DASI.	

Eat Wisely for Heart Health

Your kitchen is the best place for fighting the battle against heart disease. A high-fiber diet rich in fruits, whole grains, legumes, vegetables, and nuts can help you combat inflammation of the arteries. Barley, beans, and oats are the best for soluble fiber.[8]

Despite what you may have heard about the "dangers" of red meat, it doesn't raise your cholesterol levels. In fact, a recent study proved that eating lean meat helps reduce LDL and raise HDL levels, the "good" cholesterol that fights plaque. Treat yourself to grass-fed red meat, which is higher in omega-3 fatty acids.

If you like Italian or Asian cuisine, you're in luck. Garlic and ginger are excellent for thinning your blood and inhibiting clots.

In terms of foods to avoid, reduce your intake of blood sugar boosting foods, ones that rank low on the Glycemic Index. I have seen great success with a low glycemic diet for diabetes and reducing high triglycerides levels.

Eliminate artery-clogging trans fats from your diet. Breaded and fried foods such as french fries and chicken, commercially baked crackers and cookies, and *anything* with hydrogenated or partially hydrogenated soybean oil needs to go.

As I am constantly reminding my patients, the average American diet is far too high in starch. Starches in foods such as potatoes, rice, and wheat-based products build up plaque in your arteries. Lower your intake for your heart's sake.

You should supplement your healthy meals with vitamin B2 (25 mg.), B6 (25 mg.), B12 (500 mcg.) and folate (800 mcg.), which will help lower the level of homocysteine in your blood.

Zinc is a mighty tool for reducing plaque buildup in your blood vessels. While it's present in foods such as red meat, fish, and oysters, I recommend you take 30-60 daily as a supplement.

And you can reduce you CRP levels with L-arginine, folic acid, taurine, vitamin E and vitamin C.

Finally, take 100 mg. of CoQ10 every day for overall heart health. In one study, approximately 87% of the patients had significant improvement for their various cardiac problems with CoQ10 therapy.[9]

Exercise the Smart Way

You'll be happy to know you don't have to exercise for a long period of time to keep your heart pumping vigorously. In fact, endurance exercising makes your heart smaller and reduces the capacity of your heart to respond quickly to sudden demands on it.

What you need to focus on is short-duration exercise that alternates between intensity and rest. Twenty minutes every other day is good. When you first start training, it will take you time to build up your conditioning. Once you get in better shape, you can start taking breaks in between bursts of intensity.

When you begin short-duration training, start with 10 minutes of exercise, followed by five minutes rest, then another 10 minutes of exercise. You can then gradually reduce the amount of time exercising into smaller units, until you are exercising for five minutes or less at a time, with two-minute intervals in between bursts.

Any kind of exercise that gets your heart and lungs going will do, be it biking, running, dancing, or working out on elliptical machines. As long as you keep making the exercise more challenging, your heart will keep expanding its capacity.

Recognizing Trouble is the Key to Survival

Taking care of your heart isn't just a matter of prevention. If, God forbid, you ever suspect you might be in danger of having a heart attack, getting help can make a huge difference. Be aware signs of heart trouble, which don't always involve the abrupt pain you might have seen in the movies or on TV.

If you feel any of the following for five minutes or longer, get help quickly by calling 911:

- Shortness of breath;
- Uncomfortable pressure in your chest;
- Discomfort in the arms, back, neck, jaw, or stomach;
- Nausea, especially when accompanied by vomiting;
- Lightheadedness;
- Cold sweats.[10]

Also, keep in mind that women are more prone than men to experience dizziness, nausea, and anxiety as symptoms of a heart attack.[11]

Keep Your Smile Bright for a Healthy Heart

You're old enough that I don't have to tell you to brush your teeth, or not to smoke. Smoking is widely known as a major risk factor in heart disease. But did you know that gum disease affects your circulation, and that infrequent brushing can lead to plaque buildup in your arteries? Have a heart and be sure to brush and floss twice a day.

---

[1] "Heart Breakers: Heart disease and women." *Community*. February 19, 2008.

[2] "Go Red For Women Day Is Feb. 15." February 15, 2005.

[3] "What Is the Heart Truth?" accessed April 29, 2008.

[4] Zoler, M. "Obesity is the Cause of Most U.S. Liver Damage: Risk of Disease Fourfold Higher in Obese…" *Family Practice News*. July 1, 2004.

[5] Grady D. "In Heart Disease, the Focus Shifts to Women." *The New York Times*. April 18, 2006.

[6] Reinberg S. "High Blood Sugar Boosts Women's Heart Disease Risk." *HealthDay*. January 21, 2008.

[7] "Outcomes in Cardiopulmonary Rehabilitation, Scoring the Duke Activity Status Index." cardiosource.com, accessed April 29, 2008.

[8] "Guide to a Healthy Heart: Improve Your Cholesterol Levels." Accessed April 29, 2008.

[9] Gordon, et al. "High-density lipoprotein as a protective factor against coronary heart disease. The Framingham Study." *Am J Med* 1997 May; 62(5); 707-714

[10] "Warning Signs of a Heart Attack?" American Heart Association. October 20, 2012.

11 "Symptoms of Heart Attack in Women." Accessed May 16, 2008.

Chapter 2

The One Critical Thing You Can Do to Protect Your Blood Vessels

You can eat right… you can exercise. But despite doing all of these things, *you still haven't done the number one thing that will protect your blood vessels.*

And that's critically important if you want to live a long and healthy life.

When you're young, your blood vessels are thick and flexible. They provide blood flow to your heart — keeping it pumping strong. And they deliver oxygen-rich blood to every single organ in your body.

But by the time you've hit your 40s, chances are slim that your arteries have the elasticity they had in their youth.

It's important to keep your arteries firm and flexible — so your heart and lungs can deliver oxygen-rich blood to your extremities, heart and brain.

You can take the *single most important step* toward keeping your blood vessels strong, elastic and performing their job for years to come.

It's not cholesterol. It's not triglycerides or calcium deposits.

This Substance Is Floating in Your Bloodstream

For the past 20 years, I've noticed something interesting. Many of my heart patients have something in common: high blood levels of a simple, typically harmless amino acid: homocysteine.

I say "typically harmless" because when levels are normal, it's not a problem. However, when you have too much of it in your body it can affect the health of your arteries.

But there's good news.

I've had success treating my patients with key nutrients that quickly reduce excess homocysteine. Many patients show an increase in their arterial health within a matter of weeks.

And here's the great news: even if you *already have* high levels of it racing through your blood, it can be easily addressed — as long as you get these nutrients in the right ratio.

It's a surefire way to support your blood vessels, and today I'm going to share it with you. First, let me tell you about...

A Strong Link to Cardiovascular Health

It's important to keep homocysteine at bay to keep your arteries strong, healthy and flexible, and to support your cardiovascular health. In fact, there are a number of studies showing just that:

- In a study published in the journal *Arteriosclerosis, Thrombosis, and Vascular Biology,* researchers found that for every 10% increase in the blood level of homocysteine, there was an almost equal rise in the risk of developing serious arterial problems![1]

- Research from the Physicians' Health Study, which tracked 15,000 male physicians, found that those with low levels of it had overall better heart health than those with higher levels.[2]

- A study published in the *New England Journal of Medicine* confirms these findings. They discovered that high levels of this simple amino acid are the strongest predictor of death. More so than any other measured factor — *including cholesterol.*[3]

I've seen at least 20 more studies like this, indicating a strong link between high levels of this amino acid and overall cardiovascular health.

<u>Bottom line:</u> Maintaining low levels of homocysteine is critical to support the health of your heart and arteries.

Homocysteine Was Never a Problem — Until Now

There was a time when high levels homocysteine weren't a problem. Here's why:

Almost everything our ancestors ate gave them the life-giving, heart-protecting nutrients they needed to stay healthy and strong. Their food was pure… untainted by the hands of man and modern technology. Their diet automatically gave them all the critical nutrients needed to flush out excess buildups of homocysteine.

Today's world is a whole different story.

Now, most of our food is heavily processed and stripped of the powerful nutrients your body needs to heal and protect itself from disease. What's more, even unprocessed foods like fruits and veggies are severely lacking in essential vitamins and minerals.

That's because of advances in technology like high-yield over-farming, genetic modification, hybrid crops and commercial fertilizers. The net result is nutritionally impotent food that fails to give your body what it needs.

For example, you'd have to eat 10 servings of vegetables to equal just one serving from 50 years ago!

That's why homocysteine has become such a big problem in today's world. Without the critical nutrients that were once abundant in our food supply, your body is powerless. It can't stop this amino acid from building up to dangerously high levels.

Busting the Cholesterol Myth

It always surprises me to see how many doctors let this potentially harmful amino acid — homocysteine — slip by unnoticed.

That's because mainstream medicine is still hell-bent on lowering cholesterol.

But you know what?

Low cholesterol doesn't mean healthy veins and cardiovascular system. Just take a look at some of the research that debunks this myth:

- Research done at the Department of Cardiovascular Medicine at Yale University found that nearly *twice* as many people with low cholesterol developed seriously poor cardiovascular health compared to those with high cholesterol.[4]

- One of the most well-known and publicized heart studies is the Framingham study. The findings are nearly identical to the Yale study. *Half of the subjects developed extremely poor heart health despite having low cholesterol.*[5]

The truth is there's a sea of research that proves homocysteine is an important predictor of cardiovascular health.

For instance, in Norway, doctors studied a group of men for six years. They found that those with lower levels of homocysteine had better cardiovascular health.[6]

Another study found that men with low levels of it were less likely to have serious heart problems.[7]

When taken together, all this research suggests one thing: homocysteine is a better predictor of cardiovascular health than cholesterol.

Every doctor learns about this amino acid oover the course of his or her medical training. So it's a mystery why most don't give it a second thought, since the benefits of lowering it have been documented repeatedly in clinical studies.

Good news is, all you need are three, all-natural, everyday nutrients to sweep out any excess of this amino acid from your bloodstream.

Guard Your Blood Vessels with Three Simple Nutrients

You should get your blood levels checked. You could have high homocysteine levels and not know it.

There are no symptoms. Fortunately, a simple blood test can give you an accurate reading. I always tell my patients to keep their homocysteine level at seven or below to maintain arterial health.

If your levels are high, don't panic. There's an easy way to lower your homocysteine levels: B vitamins. B vitamins are the "missing" link your body needs to get rid of this potentially harmful amino acid.

Researchers at the National Institute on Aging (NIA) found that those who took B vitamins saw their homocysteine levels drop. But those who didn't take them saw their levels actually increase.[8] This confirms what I've seen in my heart patients in the last 20 years.

Vitamin B-6. B-6 is one of the most overlooked supplements. Over 60 different bodily enzymes rely on B-6 to do their job properly.

You can get B-6 from the following foods:

Food	Quantity	B-6 (mg.)
Chicken breast	3 ounces	0.6
Pork Loin	3 ounces	0.4
Banana	1 medium size	0.6
Watermelon	1 cup	0.23
Black beans	1 cup (boiled)	0.12
Spinach	½ cup	0.22

I recommend getting at least 50 mg. of B-6 daily for your heart health.

Vitamin B-12. A study from Oxford in England found that 500 micrograms of B-12 lowers homocysteine.[9]

Lean meats — particularly grass-fed beef — and organ meats are a great source of B-12. Here's a list of other good sources:

Food	B-12 (mcg.)
Mollusks, clams, cooked, 3 oz	84.1
Liver, beef, braised, 1 slice	47.9
Trout, rainbow, wild, cooked, 3 oz	5.4
Salmon, sockeye, cooked, 3 oz	4.9
Beef, top sirloin, lean, choice, broiled, 3 oz	2.4
Haddock, cooked, 3 oz	1.2
Tuna, white, canned in water, drained solids, 3 oz	1.0
Milk, 1 cup	.9

Vitamin B-9. You probably know vitamin B-9 better as folate or folic acid. Folate is the nutrient found in food, while folic acid is the supplement form. It's a key B vitamin for heart health.

Folic acid lowers levels of toxic substances that irritate the heart's lining. Less endothelial irritations equates to a reduction in cardiac events.

One study found that "folic acid supplementation significantly improved endothelial dysfunction..." [10]

The best natural sources of folate are vegetables. Vegetables with the highest folate content are dark, leafy greens like spinach, kale and romaine lettuce. But, your body only absorbs half of the folate you consume. So taking folic acid as a supplement is a good idea. I recommend taking 800 mcg. a day.

And there's one other supplement I recommend to lower your homocysteine levels. It's called **trimethylglycine (TMG).**

When researchers at the University of New South Wales studied people with genetically elevated homocysteine, they discovered that adding TMG to a regimen of B vitamins kept homocysteine levels at 25% of the pre-TMG levels.[11]

I recommend getting 1,000 mg. of trimethylglycine each day.

---

[1] Verhoef P, et al. "Plasma total homocysteine, B vitamins, and risk of coronary atherosclerosis." *Arteriosclerosis, Thrombosis, and Vascular Biology.* 17:989-995, 1997.

[2] Dean W, MD. "Homocysteine Risks Include Stroke, Heart Disease and Other Health Concerns." *Anti-Aging and Life Extension Medicine.*

[3] Nygard O, et al. "Plasma homocysteine levels and mortality in patients with coronary artery disease." *New Engl J Med.* 1997, 337:230-6.

[4] Krumholz HM, Seeman TE, Merrill SS, et al. "Lack of association between cholesterol and coronary heart disease mortality and morbidity and all-cause mortality in persons older than 70 years." *Journal of the American Medical Association.* 1994 Nov; 272(17): 1335-1340.

[5] Gordon T, Castelli WP, Hjortland MC et al. "High density lipoprotein as a positive factor against coronary heart disease:The Framingham Study." *American Journal of Medicine.* 1997 May; 62(5): 707-714.

[6] Nygard O, Nordrehaug J, Refsum H, et al. "Plasma homocysteine levels and mortality in patients with coronary artery disease." *New Engl J Med.* 1997, 337: 230-6.

[7] Wald NJ, Watt HC, Law MR, Weir DG, McPartlin J, Scott JM. "Homocysteine and ischemic heart disease: results of a prospective study with implications regarding prevention." *Arch Intern Med.* 1998; 158:862-7.

[8] Hodis HN, Mack WJ, Dustin L, et al. "High-dose B vitamin supplementation

and progression of subclinical atherosclerosis: a randomized controlled trial." *Stroke.* 2009 Mar;40(3):730-6. 10.1161/STROKEAHA 108.526798. Epup 2008 Dec 31.

[9] Clark R, Armitage J. "Vitamin supplements and cardiovascular risk: review of the randomized trials of homocysteine-lowering vitamin supplements." *Semin Thromb Hemost.* 2000;26(3):341-8.

[10] Title LM, Cummings PM, Giddens K, et al. "Effect of folic acid and antioxidant vitamins on endothelial dysfunction in patients with coronary artery disease." *J Am Coll Cardiol.* 2000 Sep;36(3):758-65.

[11] Frankel P, PhD, Mitchell T. "Vitamin B6 And Homocysteine." *Life Extension Magazine.* July 1997.

Chapter 3

Are You Slowly Roasting Your Heart and Blood Vessels?

There may be a fire inside you.

But it's not the inspirational kind. It's a damaging fire sparked by swollen and inflamed tissues inside your heart and your blood vessels.

Even worse, this "silent killer" doesn't give you any clues or symptoms. It just burns. It can smolder inside your body for decades, causing irreversible damage and making you more vulnerable to heart attack and stroke.

In *The Doctor's Heart Cure*, I pointed out that this kind of silent inflammation is the root cause of heart disease. Now it's been directly linked to cancer, asthma, Alzheimer's, kidney failure, stroke, obesity, and more.

I'll explain where this silent killer comes from and the simple steps you can take to get it under control.

New Study Shows the Destructive Power of Inflammation

A group of researchers studied people and followed their habits for 16 years. Their goal: to find the number one risk factor for dying in both men and women.

Many risk factors were considered. These included:

- Age;
- Gender;
- Weight;
- Smoking history;
- Physical activity level;

- Heart disease history;
- Lung function;
- And a whole lot more…

The results? ***The biggest contributor to death was inflammation.***[1]

At first glance, inflammation seems harmless. It's your body's immediate response whenever you get a cut, burn, or infection.

The REAL Cause of Heart Disease

The biggest myth fueled by mainstream medicine is the cholesterol myth — that cholesterol is the major cause of heart disease.

This simply isn't so. I've been saying it for years. And I've proven it in my own practice with heart patients who were "undiagnosable," despite being on cholesterol-lowering and a slew of other unnecessary drugs.

The good news is many doctors are starting to wise up. The main culprit behind heart disease is inflammation.

Dr. Paul Ridker of Harvard University puts it this way: *"We have to think of heart disease as an inflammatory disease, just as we think of rheumatoid arthritis as an inflammatory disease."*

If you'd like to get a good idea of your heart health, ask your doctor to do a blood screen of C-reactive protein (CRP).

CRP is released by the liver when your body experiences inflammation.

Normally, your blood contains no CRP. Elevated levels indicate a problem.

The *British Journal of Urology* published a study that examined the levels of almost 400 people. They found that once the CRP levels reached twice the normal level, the participants were 150% more likely to suffer heart attack![2]

Another study found that risk of heart attack increased 6- to 7-fold in patients with elevated CRP.[3]

Here's the bottom line…

Maintaining healthy levels of good and bad cholesterol is important. But even more important is keeping inflammation and your CRP levels at bay.

Immune system cells collect at the site of the problem in order to guard against infection and speed recovery.

This is perfectly normal and harmless. The problem starts when you experience a *chronic* state of inflammation. And it's more common than you may imagine. There are triggers in your environment that get into your body and irritate your blood vessels to the point of injury.

Cigarette smoke, vegetable oils, and the poor nutrient quality of the food we eat all contribute to small tears and injuries to your heart and blood vessels — injuries that cause a tidal wave of inflammation.

When a Good Thing Goes Bad

If your blood vessels are always inflamed, you're in trouble.

In response to the inflammation, your body uses oxidized LDL, the so-called "bad" cholesterol, to "patch" the crack or tear in your blood vessel wall.

Over time, chronic inflammation causes small lesions in the arterial walls leading to the heart and brain. These lesions, or bumps, are formed when plaque and other deposits "stick" to the walls of your blood vessels instead of simply flowing through as is normally the case with smooth, healthy arteries.

This buildup leads to clogging and hardening of the arteries. And that spells big trouble for your health.

Arteries are the main food source for your vital organs. This includes your heart, your brain, and kidneys. As the arteries harden, blood can't get to the organs as easily. The end result is life-threatening disease.

But that's not all…

Because inflammation affects your entire system, it's also directly linked to asthma, obesity, and even depression. That's why it's become such a hot topic these days.

Successfully reducing inflammation in your body means preventing and, in some cases, even reversing a wide array of diseases.

Should You Be Worried?

The tricky thing about inflammation is there are many things that can trigger it.

A big factor is the environment we live in.

For example, the foods we eat, chemicals we expose ourselves to, and environmental considerations all contribute to chronic inflammation.

Here are some common triggers:

- Processed foods;
- Foods containing dyes or chemicals;
- Foods that have been sprayed with pesticides;
- Food additives like glutamate and aspartic acid;
- Heavy metals like aluminum and mercury;
- Excess of omega-6 fatty acids (commonly found in vegetable oils);
- Cooking food at high-heat temperatures.

Aside from that, infections, bacteria, and even constant cuts or bruises can all contribute to chronic inflammation.

So what can you do?

For starters, get your C-reactive protein (CRP) levels checked. CRP is produced in the liver in response to inflammation. Under normal circumstances, your blood has zero CRP. Elevated levels mean trouble somewhere in your body.

If your levels do come back high, the first thing you can do is exercise. This is one of the best ways to lower CRP. Studies clearly show that people who went from couch slouching to exercising lowered their CRP as much as 30%.[4]

But make sure you exercise efficiently, as I describe in my PACE™ program. Your body was not designed for long duration type exercises such as aerobics or long-distance running. In fact, this type of exercise has been shown time and time again to *increase* inflammation.[5]

Eating right should also be a priority.

The best diet to follow is one similar to our ancestors' diet. Eat small meals that start with a moderate portion of high-quality protein such as grass-fed beef, poultry, or fish, balanced with copious amounts of pesticide-free vegetables and fruit.

Include monounsaturated fats such as those found in nuts, avocados, olive oil, and grapeseed oil. Eat grains and sweets only in very small quantities.

Fight This "Silent Killer" with These Three Natural All-Stars

Our ancestors never really had to worry about chronic inflammation. Much less all the modern disease we have today as a result. They had access to nature's three most powerful inflammation fighters. The same ones you can use today to take control:

Omega-3s — Fish oil is best. Numerous studies prove the omega-3 fatty acids from fish oil are incredibly effective at reducing inflammation and levels of C-reactive protein. Choose wild-caught Alaskan salmon. If not, get a good supplement. Take at least 1,000 mg. per day for maximum benefit.

Vitamin D — It's not well-known, but vitamin D is one of nature's most potent anti-inflammatories. You can get it free, simply by spending some time in the sun. Fifteen to 20 minutes a day should do the trick. If that's not possible, take a supplement. You'll see it at your grocery store or health-food store labeled as vitamin D3 (cholecalciferol). Aim for 1,000 to 2,000 IU per day.

Flavonoids — Flavonoids are powerful antioxidants that have a remarkable ability to suppress inflammation. They're found abundantly in fruits and vegetables. Good sources include plums, blueberries, and pomegranates. Dark-green leafy veggies such as spinach and dark lettuces are great too. Resveratrol is also a flavonoid that suppresses inflammation. You'll find it in red wine. Southern French and Italian wines are best, as they have the highest resveratrol content.

1 Newman AB, Sachs MC, Arnold AM, Fried LP, et al. "Total and cause-specific mortality in the cardiovascular health study." *J Gerontol A Biol Sci Med Sci.* 2009 Dec;64(12):1251-61. Epub 2009 Sep 1.

2 Mendall M, et al. "C-reactive protein and its relation to cardiovascular risk factor." *British Journal of Urology.* 1996; 312:1061-1065.

3 St-Pierre AC, Bergeron J, Pirro M, et al. "Effect of plasma C-reactive protein levels in modulating the risk of coronary heart disease associated with small, dense, low-density lipoproteins in men (The Quebec Cardiovascular Study)." *Am J Cardiol.* 2003 Mar 1;91(5):555-58.

4 Church T, Barlow CE, Earnest CP, et.al. "Association between cardiorespiratory fitness and C-reactive protein in men." *Arteriosclerosis and Thrombosis: Journal of Vascular Biology.*2002 Nov 1;22(11):1869-1879.

5 Siegel A, Stec JJ, Lipinska, I, et al. "Effect of Marathon Running on Inflammatory and Hemostatic Markers." *Amer Jour Card.* 2001;88(8):918-920.

PART 6

ELIMINATE THE THREAT
OF DEADLY TOXINS

Chapter 1

Rid Your Body of Today's Toxins

Did you know that, when tested, newborn babies have an average of 200 industrial chemicals and pollutants already present in their blood?[1]

Then, as we make our way through life, toxins enter our body through the air we breathe, the water we drink, the food we eat, and even through our skin.

The world we were designed to live in millions of years ago has changed. And our bodies haven't adapted quickly enough to flush out the countless man-made chemicals, toxins and pollutants that are now present in our everyday lives.

But getting rid of these toxins will help you live a longer, disease-free life. You can reduce or eliminate numerous problems such as chronic pain, digestive troubles, depression, and even poor eyesight. Detoxifying your body can boost your immune system, clear your mind, balance your hormones, and much more.

The good news is there are steps you can take to cleanse your body.

In particular, you want to make sure you pay attention to two key organs when detoxifying: the colon and the liver.

Your Body's Toxins

"Silver" dental fillings and farm-raised fish both contain mercury. Problems can be severe — permanent damage to the central nervous system, kidneys, liver, and digestive tract. It causes irreversible hormonal imbalances and is extremely harmful to the unborn.

Fertilizer and pesticides from the agricultural industry have a huge impact on groundwater quality.1 They are known to have a dangerous effect on the nervous system, immune system, and major organs like the liver and kidneys. They can also cause problems with growth and neurological development in children.

Drinking water can contain lead from old lead and even newer brass pipes.2 Too much exposure to lead can lead to high blood pressure, kidney damage, and neurological damage.

A study of even the most popular brands of bottled water found dangerous chemicals and bacteria such as chloroform, phthalate, and arsenic.3 All are known to cause cancer and even death.

Pesticides sprayed on conventional fruits and vegetables are the same family of pesticides used for nerve gas in WWII.4 These pesticides have dangerous effects on the brain, nervous system, immune system and vital organs.

Cleanse Your Colon and Prevent Disease from Spreading

When your colon doesn't function properly, you feel it. It can cause aching muscles, joint pain, fatigue, bloating, diarrhea, constipation, headaches, dull eyes, poor skin, spots, and depression. And the inflammation from it can spread through your body and get into your blood. Over time, this can lead to serious health problems, including heart disease and cancer.

In short, having a toxic digestive system is one of the main reasons people are chronically ill.

When toxins stress your large intestine, it protects itself by producing extra mucus. The mucus sticks to the sludge produced by a low fiber, Western diet; creates a build-up and narrows the colon.

This build-up is the perfect breeding ground for all kinds of harmful bacteria and parasites. It also rubs and pushes against the walls of your colon, making them irritated and inflamed.

An effective colon cleanse can release years of toxic build-up and reduce your risk of developing chronic diseases such as irritable bowel syndrome. And it will prevent the toxins from overloading your colon, digestive system, and blood stream.

Detox Your Colon the Safe, Natural Way

Many natural herbs can safely cleanse your colon without harsh chemicals. But here are the ones I recommend.

- **Cascara Sagrada** — This plant extract helps to stimulate the muscles of the colon to contract, helping to push waste and toxins out of your body. It also helps tone and strengthen the colon, which can then bring bowel function back to normal.

- **Marshmallow root** — This root acts as a natural adhesive. When it is exposed to water, as it is when entering the intestinal tract, it provides a very soothing and protective coating to the irritated intestinal lining.

- **Flax seed** — Contains high levels of omega-3 fatty acids. These fats help calm inflammation as well as provide a source of fiber and lignans, which promote intestinal health.

- **Rhubarb** — Stimulates bowel function and acts as an astringent. This helps neutralize the effects of the toxins and slows the growth of bacteria that may be in the colon. It also helps tone and tightens the muscles of the intestinal wall, adding strength and improving function.

You can find all of these herbal remedies in most health food stores. They also come in premixed blends. Some also contain fiber such as psyllium, which is also very effective.

Don't Forget This Vital Organ When Detoxifying

When toxins overload the liver, it stores the toxins instead of processing them out of the system. Over time, this can cause liver damage and a host of other health problems.

Your liver is also vital for the metabolism of your hormones. If it is not functioning properly, your hormones go out of whack. For instance, in women, an imbalance can cause infertility, PMS, irregular periods, headaches, migraines, and more.

The liver also plays a part in eye health. Your eyes get nourishment from your blood in order to see properly. If the liver fails to do its job of filtering toxins out of your blood, your eyes feel the effects.

Keep Your Liver Healthy with These Proven Methods

Here are the natural liver-cleansing remedies that I have found work well.

- **Milk thistle** — For liver detox, milk thistle is my first choice. Milk thistle is the plant *Silybum marianum*. I have been able to document its capacity to heal damaged livers by measuring serum liver enzymes. I recommend 200 mg. in capsule form twice a day. Look for dried extract with a minimum of 80% silymarin, the active ingredient for liver cleansing.

- **Alfalfa** — This herb cleanses the blood and liver. It can also lower cholesterol. It's a good source of protein, vitamins A, D, E, B-6, and K, calcium, magnesium, chlorophyll, phosphorus, iron, potassium, trace minerals, and several digestive enzymes.

- **Dandelion** — This root stimulates bile production and acts as a diuretic for excess water produced by a diseased liver. Asian and Western physicians alike use dandelion to treat hepatitis, jaundice, swelling of the liver, and deficient bile secretion.

- **Burdock Root** — This ancient remedy is a diuretic and a diaphoretic. This means it increases urine and perspiration production. These actions exercise and strengthen these natural purging systems.

- **Sarsaparilla** — This is one of my favorite teas. Its benefits are many, including blood detox, and it tastes great. Native Americans cherish it as a restorative tonic.

Try mixing your own blend of these herbs. You can also look for a premixed blend with as many of these ingredients as you can find on the label.

Flush Toxic Metals Out of Your Body with the 'Claw'

A key concept to remember when it comes to detox is *chelation*. The word chelate comes from the Greek word *chele*, which means claw. And it describes the process by which a molecule from a nutrient (or chemical) surrounds and binds (or grabs like a claw) to metal toxins such as mercury, lead, and arsenic, and carries them out of your body through your kidneys and out in your urine.

Chances are you have some level of exposure to heavy metals. Believe it or not, arsenic and lead are among the most common forms of heavy metal toxicity.[5] These poisons are used in the manufacturing processes of things like pesticides, glass, wood preservatives, fertilizers, paint, batteries, plumbing, and ink. Not to mention hobby paints, hair coloring, and cosmetics.

In some cases, doctors will use a synthetic solution or chemical called ethylenediaminetetraacetic acid (EDTA) through injection. But this can sometimes cause side effects including headache, rash, and high blood pressure. And in some cases, it can remove vital minerals from your body along with the toxins.[6]

There are some safer, more natural methods of chelation that I would recommend for removing toxic metals from your body.

- You can take chlorella, a form of dried algae. You can find it in most health food stores. Take one 500 mg. capsule per day initially. Some people are sensitive to chlorella. If you start experiencing nausea or burping, it means your body can't tolerate it and you should go for another option.

  If you don't have a sensitivity, work up slowly over one to two weeks to a dose of one teaspoon (ten tablets or capsules) per day until your levels come down.

- Fresh cilantro has also been shown to remove mercury from the body. About a teaspoon a day should work.

- Garlic is also a good option. Three cloves of fresh garlic per day should help.

Try a Detox Method That Was Natural to Our Ancestors

Fasting is as old as humankind. Despite what you might often hear in the media, fasting is quite safe. Our body is resilient. So not eating for a day or two won't hurt it.

In fact, this was common for our hunter-gatherer ancestors who didn't always have food at their disposal. Only modern times have made food constantly available.

Fasting turns on your "auto cleaning" mode — it speeds your body's detoxification process. When food no longer enters your body, your body turns to its fat reserves for fuel or energy. And when these fat reserves are used while fasting, they release the toxins from the fatty acids into your system and then flush them out of your body through your liver, colon, kidneys, lungs, and skin.

There are a number of different types of fasting methods for detoxification. The truest form is water fasting. You simply eat or drink nothing but water for one to three days. Make sure you get plenty of water during a fast.

Juice fasting is another option. I don't recommend packaged juices. To enjoy the benefits of a juice fast, you should really make your own juice. For a detoxifying fast, drink only citrus juice. Drink as much as you want along with as much water as you want.

Work Up a Good Sweat and Get Rid of Impurities

Sweating is the most efficient way to detox. And a trip to the sauna or steam bath, or even a good workout can get you sweating.

Your skin is your largest organ, and 30% of your body's waste passes through it. A sauna, for example, increases the detoxifying capacity of the skin by opening pores and flushing impurities from the body.

Exercise is efficient because it not only gets you sweating to rid your body of waste, but it also builds muscle and burns fat at the same time.

The Ultimate Detox in Four Easy Steps

There are many ways you can put together an effective detox program using the methods I explained. But here's one that I have used myself and have recommended to my patients. You can do it over a weekend.

Day 1: Get up an hour early and perform brief but intense bouts of exercise to give your heart and lungs a workout and to start sweating. Follow this with a hot shower, as hot as you can tolerate for at least 10 minutes, followed by a cool rinse. Eat your normal diet. Repeat the exercise and heat therapy before going to bed.

Day 2: Eat nothing. Drink only plenty of water. Do a light workout followed by a warm shower.

Day 3: Eat only tomatoes, fresh made vegetable juices and wild salmon. Treat yourself to a steam room or sauna. Begin herbal detox for your blood, liver and colon as described above.

Day 4: Return to your normal diet and exercise. Continue the herbal detox for your blood, liver, and colon for six more days.

Try doing a detox every three or four months and you will be pleasantly surprised at how amazing you will feel.

---

[1] "Body of Burden — The Pollution in Newborns." Environmental Working Group. July 14, 2005.

[2] Sircus M. "The Poisoning of America's Water Supplies." *Natural News*. July 3, 2008.

[3] Sircus M. "The Poisoning of America's Water Supplies." *Natural News*. July 3, 2008.

[4] Sherman, C. "Tracing Pesticides in Children From Ingestion to Elimination." *NaturalNews.com*. 3/28/08

[5] ibid.

[6] "Heavy Metal Toxicity." Life Extension. 6/12/03.

Chapter 2

The Living Link Missing from Our Diets

For millions of years, our ancestors hunted for meat and gathered fruits, nuts and other plant foods. They followed the food supply, so there was no kitchen sink to wash it in. Instead, they brushed the dirt off the foods they gathered. Or rinsed it in a nearby stream.

Today, factory farms add thousands of tons of pesticides and herbicides to our food. Even if we wash our fruits and vegetables thoroughly, we run the risk of slowly poisoning ourselves.

This modern dilemma means that our ancestors received a benefit from their food that we don't. I think of that benefit as "living foods" — the good bacteria that inhabit our guts.

Living foods aid digestion. They hold dangerous bacteria in check. And recent research has revealed an amazing variety of other benefits. Here are just a few of the health benefits connected to these living foods:

- They support normal growth in infants.[1]
- They help protect against early childhood infections.[2]
- They improve your body's defenses against food-borne toxins.[3]
- They may be useful in the treatment of ulcers.[4]
- They can reduce the discomfort of diseases such as irritable bowel syndrome.[5]
- They can reduce the damaging effects of alcoholism.[6]

We have these healthy bacteria growing in our guts, too. But many of us have far fewer than we need.

I'll show you why you need living foods. How an entire industry has misled consumers about them. And how you can enjoy the healthy benefits living foods offer.

Protection from Disease-Causing Bacteria

There wasn't much interest in the good bacteria in our guts until the early 20th century. Then a Russian scientist named Metchnikoff had an idea. He believed that replacing the "bad" bacteria in our systems with "good" bacteria could slow aging.

Mechnikoff's early theories were a little off. But his work led to many discoveries about the bacteria living in our digestive systems. In the 1970s, these living foods were named "probiotics."

I like that term. It directly counters modern medicine's dependency on "antibiotics," which focuses on killing biological organisms rather than on supplying them.

The word "bacteria" makes most people think of germs and infection. But trillions of *good* bacteria live in our digestive systems. These good bacteria promote better health in several ways.

Your intestinal wall is like a parking lot with billions and billions of individual "parking spaces." Many disease-causing bacteria can only make you sick if they find an open space on the intestinal lining.

If good bacteria have taken up all the available parking spots, the bad bacteria can't adhere to the intestinal lining. Instead they pass through the gut. And you don't get sick.

If bad bacteria take over, they can migrate throughout your body and cause a host of diseases that you would never associate with your gut.

There's a good reason bacteria thrive in our intestines. There's plenty of food. Probiotic bacteria compete against bad bacteria for this food supply.

Your digestion works a lot like natural decomposition. And that's a perfect environment for bacteria. Bacteria don't have complex digestive systems. So they take advantage of the free meals available in our intestines.

But probiotics give us plenty in return. Because they're more efficient feeders than many harmful bacteria, they can crowd bad bacteria out .[7]And a U.K. study found that probiotics lower the toxin levels of a bacteria that causes a form of colitis.[8]

Add these to the benefits I mentioned earlier, and you can see how probiotics promote good health.

But don't run out and fill your fridge with cultured yogurt products. Because most of the so-called probiotic foods on your grocer's shelf aren't that useful. In fact, neither are most of the probiotic supplements I've seen.

And a pair of product tests help explain why.

Make Sure Your Probiotic Gets
Past These Two Obstacles to Be Effective

In 2003, ConsumerLab.com tested 25 probiotic products. Some were supplements. Others were foods with bacteria added. Nine products failed their tests. Almost a third contained "too few live bacteria to be effective."

ConsumerLab.com's second round of tests didn't do much better. In their 2006 study, five of the 13 products they tested flunked.

But there's still a problem. Even if a product contains "enough" bacteria, those bacteria still have to survive two attacks in your body.

First, they have to survive your stomach acid. Then, they have to face the bile salts in your upper intestine. Up until now, survival rates have been less than exciting.

The food industry has spent a fortune on special coatings to protect probiotics from stomach acid. But a research paper presented at the Israel Institute of Technology found they're not having great success.

They tested three of the most common coating processes. They found the coating process itself killed up to 60% of the bacteria.[9] So, even if the bacteria make it through your stomach, most of them could already be dead.

Getting through your stomach is a challenge. But even the latest double-coating process is no match for bile salts. The new process worked well with stomach acid. But researchers found the double-coated capsules didn't provide any extra protection against bile salts.[10]

What this all boils down to is that most probiotic products simply don't deliver on their promises. And even those promises are being called into question.

Yogurt giant Dannon Corp. recently agreed to settle a $300 million class-action lawsuit out of court. The reason for the suit? Evidence that health claims for Dannon's probiotic yogurt products may not be true.

Dannon says it stands behind its claims. But the fact they're settling the suit seems to say something else. And this isn't the first time they've been called out on probiotic claims.

The U.K.'s Advertising Standards Authority (ASA) asked Danone, Dannon's parent company, to pull "misleading" ads in both 2006 and 2008. Danone also ran afoul of the ASA in 2003. Then it was for ads for its "Shape" yogurt product.

Danone isn't alone. The U.S. National Advertising Division claimed General Mills was running misleading ads for its Yoplait "Yo-Plus" product. General Mills pulled the ads in December 2008.

So you're faced with a dilemma. Probiotics are good for you. But getting enough of them can be a challenge. And you may not be getting what you think you are anyway.

What do you do?

Getting Probiotics' Benefits

There are several ways to get more of these healthy living foods into your diet.

The first is to grow your own organic fruits and vegetables. Fresh, organic produce from your own garden doesn't require the scrubbing that factory-farmed veggies do. And you'll have the bonus of tastier meals.

I've been growing my own organic garden for years, and I rarely get sick. In fact, I've been known to just pluck a tomato off the vine, dust if off, slice it up and eat it. No washing required.

If you don't have room or time for your own organic garden, buy organic when you shop. Your local farmer's market is a great place to find organic fruits and veggies. You should still wash this produce. But, like homegrown, it doesn't need the kind of thorough cleaning commercial produce does.

Plus you can give the healthy bacteria in your gut a better chance of surviving. Simply cut out the foods that bad bacteria thrive on.

Sugar and refined carbohydrates are bad bacteria's favorite meal. These "foods" aren't natural to your body anyway. So giving them up — or even cutting down — offers a whole range of health benefits, including weight loss.

A lab in Europe has been quietly breeding new strains of good bacteria. These bacteria are highly resistant to both stomach acid and bile salts. But they're not genetically engineered, and there's no coating involved.

So far, the research has been very promising. But I'm not going to jump on board until I know that these living foods live up to their promise. If they do, you can be sure I'll let you know.

---

[1] Scalabrin DM, et al. "Growth and Tolerance of Healthy Term Infants Receiving Hydrolyzed Infant Formulas Supplemented With Lactobacillus rhamnosus GG..." *Clin Pediatr.* 2009 Mar 4.

[2] Rautava S, et al. "Specific probiotics in reducing the risk of acute infections in infancy - a randomised, double-blind, placebo-controlled study." *Br J Nutr.* 2008 Nov 6:1-5. [Epub ahead of print]

[3] Gratz S, et al. "Lactobacillus rhamnosus strain GG reduces aflatoxin B1 transport, metabolism, and toxicity in Caco-2 Cells." *Appl Environ Microbiol.* 2007 Jun;73(12):3958-64.

[4] Lam EK, et al. "Probiotic Lactobacillus rhamnosus GG enhances gastric ulcer healing in rats." *Eur J Pharmacol.* 2007 Jun 22;565(1-3):171-9.

[5] Gawronska A, et al. "A randomized double-blind placebo-controlled trial of Lactobacillus GG for abdominal pain disorders in children." *Aliment Pharmacol Ther.* 2007 Jan 15;25(2):177-84.

[6] Forsyth CB, et al. "Lactobacillus GG treatment ameliorates alcohol-induced intestinal oxidative stress, gut leakiness, and liver injury in a rat model of alcoholic steatohepatitis." *Alcohol.* 2009 Mar;43(2):163-72.

[7] Wilson KH, Perini F. "Role of competition for nutrients in suppression of Clostridium difficile by the colonic microflora." *Infect Immun.* 1988 Oct;56(10):2610-4.

[8] Plummer S, et al. "Clostridium difficile pilot study: effects of probiotic supplementation on the incidence of C. difficile diarrhoea." *Int Microbiol.* 2004 Mar;7(1):59-62.

[9] Semyonov D. "Dry Microencapsulation and Enteric Coating of Probiotic Bacteria." M.Sc Thesis, Department of Biotechnology and Food Engineering, Israel Institute of Technology.

[10] Ding WK, Shah NP. "An improved method of microencapsulation of probiotic bacteria for their stability in acidic and bile conditions during storage." *J Food Sci.* 2009 Mar;74(2):M53-61.

Chapter 3

How to Beat the Hidden Effects of Modern Stress

I want to talk to you now about something that can benefit every part of your body from your heart to your brain and even your sex hormones. Most doctors won't tell you about it, but when it's working right, you'll:

- Feel more energized.

- Have a positive frame of mind.

- Concentrate better.

- Sleep soundly.

- Eliminate mood swings.

- Think more clearly.

- Have fewer food cravings.

- Maintain a healthy weight.

The problem is, the modern world causes you to overuse it. Your ancestors had only brief periods of stress, lasting a few minutes at a time. Today, you are constantly being assaulted by stressors that can last for days, or years.

But your body wasn't built for that. The system your body uses to deal with stress — your adrenal system — didn't evolve to be in a constant state of "fight or flight."

And that's why we have the modern problem of what I call "adrenal burnout."

The solution to adrenal burnout involves returning to some of the practices of your ancestors, and I'll tell you what those are in a bit. But first, let me ask you: Does your day go something like this?

- You don't really seem to "wake up" until midmorning, even though you've been awake since early.
- You get a little sleepy and "foggy" in the early afternoon.
- You have a burst of energy around and after dinner.
- You get sleepy around 9, but you resist going to bed.
- You experience a kind of second wind, but then can't get to sleep until after midnight.

In between you crave salty foods. You don't have much energy throughout the day. You're a little lightheaded when you stand up, get up from your desk, or get out of your car. Your muscles feel weaker than they used to. You sigh a lot.

If this sounds anything like what you experience each day, you're not alone. Far from it.

Stress Response Breakdown

The sad part is, if you feel this way and you go to mainstream medicine to try and solve the problem, most doctors have no idea what's wrong. They won't be able to tell you that your stress response has gone haywire because of our modern environment.

Let me explain.

It's healthy for your body to go through the occasional ups and downs of daily stress responses. They're normal and you may not even know they're happening. In fact, your body is constantly having these kinds of responses based on your environment. Everything your body does is an evolutionarily-designed decision by your body to make you more survivable.

This worked well for thousands of years in our native environment. Stressors usually were very brief. If they lasted hours or days, that was the exception, and the body was built to count that as an exception.

But your physiology came from a different world, and now the stressors and our physiological reactions are mismatched. The environment has changed so quickly over the last 100 years that your body hasn't caught up.

The "fight or flight" alarm system used to get activated only for short periods of time. You would release stress hormones like adrenaline, norepinephrine and cortisol, and when the attack or challenge ended your hormones would have time to re-balance themselves.

Today stresses not only last longer, but we prolong them in our minds. Our brains are too powerful for our own good. We worry, we try to plan… we have stressors that can last for weeks, months, even years. A good example is a 30-year mortgage. That's 30 years of anxiety right there.

Stress hormones are meant to protect our lives. And in life or death situations you don't need to build muscle, eat, or have sexual thoughts. So these hormones are "catabolic." They burn up emergency energy, and turn off long-term maintenance and rebuilding functions. Your body uses all its resources to focus on the problem at hand until it's over.

But it's never over in today's world. Every time you perceive a threat, get perturbed or angry, take in too much caffeine, or are rushing from one daily event to the next, your adrenals receive a signal from the brain to make extra stress hormones.

This chronic catabolism is not only the biggest cause of premature aging and cardiovascular disease but it makes it almost impossible for you to have normal hormone and energy levels.

Doctors Don't Recognize the Problem

What's worse is that if you go to your doctor, chances are he or she won't know what's happening. In medical school, they are only taught to look for extreme adrenal malfunction. Either Addison's disease, which is when the adrenal glands don't produce enough cortisol, or Cushing's syndrome, which is when they make too much.

They check adrenal function by testing ACTH levels. But only the top and bottom 2% are considered abnormal. Everything in the middle is considered "normal." Yet adrenal burnout happens to 15% of people on either end of the testing.

That means your adrenal glands could be working far from normally, but most mainstream doctors won't even recognize that you have a problem.

The good news is, your ancient ancestors have shown us the way to overcome it all. You can completely reverse adrenal burnout in four easy steps, and have all the energy, enthusiasm and relaxed, confident happiness you were built for.

Step 1) Eat for energy: Our modern diet has replaced nutritious, healthy protein and fats with worthless grains and starchy carbohydrates. Your body's not designed to recognize them as food.

And all those "low fat" foods flying off store shelves just make it worse. The advertising and labels seem to promise that they're better for you because they're "fat free." But they're basically the original food with the fat removed and with refined sugar added.

Refined sugar stimulates your adrenal glands to unnaturally release a cascade of the hormones that adversely affected you in the first place.[1]

Protein, on the other hand, is an essential form of fuel. So when you eat protein your body uses this energy source to function at its best. Your body also uses the good fats you get from eating protein-rich foods to deliver nutrients to your organs.

Going back to the protein-based way your ancestors ate is essential for balance within your body. Here are three tips on how to eat for increased energy:

- Focus all your meals around high-quality animal protein. You should eat a large variety, and plan your meals around which kind of protein you'll be eating.

- Fruits and vegetables, not grains, should make up your carbohydrates. And the more variety you can get the better. Eating seasonally grown produce is a good idea, because it'll be local and not frozen or imported from long distances.

- Watch what you snack on. Make your snacks natural. Berries, nuts, and other treats like pumpkin seeds.

Step 2) Turn back the clock: In a groundbreaking study, researchers took muscle samples from young adults and older adults. The older group exerted themselves intensely three times per week.

Here's what happened.

Before exercise training, the older adults were 59% weaker than the younger adults. After several weeks, the older individuals were able to improve muscle strength by approximately 50%.

But here's something even more remarkable: After exercise training, their muscle tissue was re-energized from a cellular level. In fact, *most of the genes that express aging were reversed back to younger levels!*[2]

This study gives us new insight into the role of exertion and keeping the vitality of youth. Because strong muscles maintain adrenal production.

But there's a catch: long, drawn-out endurance exercise will only drain your energy and further wear out your adrenal glands. Instead, I recommend PACE™ workouts.

Endurance Exercises – Aerobics and Cardio	P.A.C.E.
Shrinks muscle mass	Builds muscle
Diminishes your lung capacity	Increases your lung capacity
Reduces your secondary sexual features. Men, you'll losr your broad shoulders and deep voice. Women, you'll lose your breast tissue and curvy figure.	Enhamces secondary sexual features—builds a desirable attractive figure.
High rate of injury	Low rate of injurey
Lowers your overall energy levels	Raises energy levels—eipes fatigue forever!
Tales 60 to 90 minutes, 5 times a week	Takes 12 to 20 minutes, 3–4 times a week
Hard to stick with	Easy to stick with

In fact, my new POWER Fit program shows you both how and what to eat, and when, and how to work out to rebuild the lean, energetic body you were meant to have. Look for it soon.

You can get specific workouts, resources and information about PACE™ at my website. The best part is, PACE™ only takes 12 minutes a day.

Step 3) Use nature's pharmacy: I call DHEA the "anti-stress hormone." It is the most abundant product of the adrenal glands. DHEA is the pre-

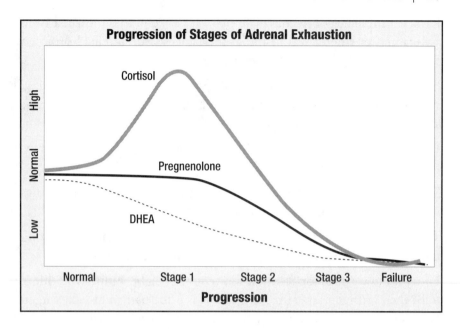

You secrete DHEA when times are good — when you are well fed, secure and free of stressors. The more DHEA in your body, the less effect stress will have on you.

If you want to turn back the effects of our stressful modern environment, you can supplement with DHEA. I use it at my Wellness Clinic regularly. DHEA therapy has successfully treated many of my patients who suffer from lack of energy, depression and chronic fatigue syndrome.

It is important for you to get your DHEA levels checked. Your doctor can perform the simple test. After your levels have been checked, you can determine optimal dosing. A common starting dose that I use is 10 mg. daily. DHEA is absorbed well and can be taken at any time but best mimics the natural daily fluctuation when taken first thing in the morning.

Step 4) Take time out for yourself. Participate in a meditative practice like yoga or tai chi to release any pent up stress and emotions.

These were the tools the ancients used to slow their brain waves and feel a sense of calm and joy.

In fact, simple yoga breathing can help. It's a technique I learned from a yoga master when I was in India. It balances your adrenal hormones and makes you relax and recuperate.

Before you begin, sit in a comfortable spot, and control your breathing. Bring it back to deep breaths, in and out. Breathe in through your nose and out through your mouth.

First: Empty your lungs until there's no more air. Exhale completely. Force out every drop.

Second: Inhale deeply for at least a slow count of four. Fill your lungs until you can't inhale any more.

Third: Hold your breath for at least a slow count of seven. Anticipating the exhalation like this creates a calming and rebalancing effect.

Fourth: Now exhale for at least a slow count of eight. Empty your lungs fully, then push out any remaining air. This is the part we usually forget, but it's the most crucial. As you exhale, you will feel yourself relax.

By adding this exercise to your daily routine you'll not only boost your immune system, you'll also effectively deal with problems like stress, anxiety and isolation that cause adrenal burnout.

---

[1] Jones TW, Boulware SD, Kraemer DT, Caprio S, Sherwin RS, Tamborlane WV. "Independent effects of youth and poor diabetes control on responses to hypogly-cemia in children." *Diabetes*. 1991 Mar;40(3):358-63

[2] Melov S, Tarnopolsky, M, Beckman K, et al. "Resistance exercise reverses aging in human skeletal muscle." *PLoS ONE*. 2007;2:e465.

Chapter 4

Attention Women: Good News from Research

Times are getting better for women. New studies are providing new opportunities for women who want better — and safer — choices to the health concerns that matter most.

I will show you some of the latest breakthrough ideas. You'll find out how to prevent breast cancer and what to do if you have fibroids. I'll also show you how to sidestep some bad advice coming from the big drug makers.

Better than a Mammogram

Doctors in Boston recently introduced a new test for breast cancer. This simple urine test may offer a safe, non-invasive way to accurately assess a woman's risk of breast cancer.

Dr. Pories of Beth Israel Deaconess Hospital in Boston shared the results of her latest study at a recent breast cancer symposium. Her team found that urinary levels of two biomarkers (M MP-9 and ADAM12) are reliable predictors of increased risk of breast cancer.

In her study, she compared levels of these markers in both women with breast cancer and women without. One hundrred percent of the urine samples that tested positive for MMP-9 and ADAM 12 belonged to women with breast cancer.

Women Are Saying No to Drugs

A new unofficial poll suggests that women don't want the toxic and potentially dangerous drug *Tamoxifen* to prevent breast cancer.

When given the option, most women choose safer, more natural ways to avoid breast cancer. Many were concerned about the drug's side effects and the reliability of studies.

Most women preferred to make changes in their diet, exercise more and try alternative therapies.

Avoid Fibroid Surgery with New Technique

Surgery used to be the only option for uterine fibroids. Now a new procedure provides women with a noninvasive treatment.

Focused ultrasound is used together with an MRI to direct the beam. The availability of 3-D scanning allows the doctor to find the target with safety and precision.

The technique provides relief for one year and beyond, *without* serious side effects.

Doctor Sings Praises of Dangerous Drug

I recently came across an article written by a doctor endorsing the use of the antidepressant *Paroxetine* in pregnant women. That's not unusual. Doctors regularly prescribe antidepressants during a woman's first trimester.

But this particular doctor supported the use of the drug in spite of the FDA issuing a strong warning that Paroxetine can cause birth defects in newborns. "The benefits of using Paroxetine outweigh the risk to the unborn baby," he claimed.

Is it any wonder that this doctor is a paid consultant of GlaxoSmithKline, the maker of Paroxetine?

Lifetime Exercise the Best Way to Beat Breast Cancer

New research shows that women who exercise throughout their lives have a 20% to 30% lower risk of breast cancer than women who don't exercise.

The benefit holds true for all women, regardless of race or ethnicity. In the study, exercise was defined as three or more hours a week over a woman's lifetime.

Dr. Bernstein speaking in the *Journal of the National Cancer Institute* said that her biggest challenge was motivating women to become physically active.

Chapter 5

How to Avoid the Dangers of Contaminated Food

When there are outbreaks of E. coli, people become quite ill and sometimes die. Bacterial contamination results in grocery stores pulling products from their shelves. In recent years, infectious contamination has hit even quality restaurants, health-food stores and organic produce farmers.

Yet as I will show you, there are easy and effective steps you can take to reduce your exposure and lower your threat from these infectious agents in our food.

What Are Infectious Diseases and How Do They Spread?

Infectious diseases are illnesses caused by bacteria, viruses and other microbes.

Infectious diseases have historically been the leading cause of death worldwide and are still the third leading cause of death in the U.S. — where the annual cost of medical care for treating them is estimated at $120 billion.[1]

You can get infectious diseases by at least four routes:

- Direct contact with an infected person or animal.

- Ingesting contaminated food or water.

- Insects like mosquitoes or ticks.

- Contaminated surroundings like animal droppings or even air.[2]

Illnesses contracted from eating contaminated food are known as 'foodborne' illnesses.

What Are the Most Common Foodborne Illnesses?

Most foodborne infections are caused by the bacteria E. coli 0157:H7, Salmonella and Campylobacter or by a group of viruses called Norwalk viruses.[3]

BUG	Major Symptoms	Source of Outbreaks
coli 0157:H7	Severe diarrhea, abdominal pain, vomiting (accompanied by little or no fever)	Undercooked beef, unpasteurized (raw) milk or eggs
Salmonella	Diarrhea, fever, abdominal cramps	Eggs, poultry, unpasteurized (raw) milk or juice, cheese, raw produce
Campylobacter	Diarrhea (often bloody), cramps, vomiting	Undercooked poultry, unpasteurized (raw) milk contaminated water
Norwalk viruses	Nausea, vomiting, abdominal cramping, diarrhea	Poorly-cooked shellfish, ready-to-eat foods such as salads and sandwiches touched by infected handlers

Since foodborne outbreaks are becoming more common, it's helpful to learn the red flags associated with each illness and the steps you can take to avoid them.

E. coili 0157:H7 is one of hundreds of strains of the bacterium *Escherichia coli.* Most strains are harmless and live in the intestines of healthy humans and animals. However, this particular strain produces a powerful toxin that can cause severe illness.[4]

The vast majority of *E. coli 0157:H7* outbreaks are associated with eating undercooked, contaminated ground beef (or swimming in sewage-contaminated water). However, past outbreaks of *E. coil 0157:H7* in organic spinach and bagged produce underscore the possible association with all kinds of foods.

Other spreaders of *E. coil* have included Taco Bell, Wendy's, Dole and a large California organic spinach farm. In 2013 E. coli infections resulted in ground beef from Wolverine Packing Co., raw clover sprouts from Idaho, and salads and wraps from Glass Onion Foods being pulled from supermarket shelves.

Salmonella (discovered by an American scientist named Salmon) is actually a group of bacteria that cause diarrhea, fever and abdominal cramps.

In recent years, a new strain of antibiotic-resistant *Salmonella*-much of it from ground beef-has emerged and become more of a problem over the last decade. If you have poor underlying health or weakened immune systems, *Salmonella* can invade the bloodstream and cause life-threatening infections.

Campylobacter is one of the most common bacterial causes of diarrhea in the United States — as well as the underlying cause of ulcers and intestinal distress.[5] It usually does not pose a threat to your life. The key is to stay well-hydrated by drinking lots of water.

Noroviruses — though hard to diagnose they are extremely common foodborne illnesses. Infected kitchen workers can contaminate a salad or sandwich as they prepare it, if they have the virus on their hands.

In addition, Noroviruses can be extremely dangerous — particularly among the elderly. Outbreaks have occurred in restaurants, nursing homes and cruise ships.

Just how common are they?

- Roughly 76 million Americans become sick;
- More than 325,000 are hospitalized;
- And 5,000 die each year from foodborne illness![6]

Fight Illness and Disease More Effectively and Naturally

Traditionalists consider antibiotics to be the treatment of foodborne infectious disease.

Antibiotics — drugs that kill or prevent the growth of bacteria or fungi — are second only to pain relievers as the most frequently prescribed class of drugs.[7] I believe in the power and usefulness of antibiotics, but sometimes they're overused.

The problem is that antibiotics indiscriminately kill all bacteria in the human body — both good and bad — which in some cases can open the door for fungus to spread and grow.

What most people don't realize is that your body is filled to the brim with trillions of bacteria. Lay them end to end and they would wrap around the earth 2.5 times.[8]

The vast majority are not only harmless — they're beneficial. Your body needs them to assist in the digestion of food, the production of enzymes, and the production of vitamins.

We call these helpful bacteria, and their products, *probiotics.*

An example is the *acidophilus* you find in milk and yogurt. If you're taking antibiotics for any reason, it's good to supplement with probiotics to keep your system balanced. (You can find them at any health food or nutrition store.)

Pumping Up Your Body's First Line of Defense

If you want to build the kind of body that is capable of fighting off disease-causing bacteria, there's no better solution than to strengthen your body's immune system.

The immune system is a complex of organs that work together to clear infection from your body. Ideally, you want a healthy balance of bacteria.

A lot of companies are beginning to add probiotics to their yogurts, drinks, and supplements — or at least they claim to.

To be certain you build a strong, healthy immune system capable of fighting off foodborne illness and disease this year and beyond, here are a couple of all-natural solutions to get you started:

- Natural anti-infectious herbs such as garlic or Goldenseal. The raw herb or essential oil can help ward off illness naturally and effectively. You can find odorless garlic supplements just about anywhere. Look for the active ingredient *allicin* - 180 to 200 mg. a day is an effective dose.

- Goldenseal is also commonly available. Try 250 to 500 mg. two or three times a day. Just remember to cycle your use of herbs. For example, take it for six to eight weeks, and then take a break for a few weeks before starting a new cycle.

- Add immune enhancers — such as Echinacea or the Beta Glucans — whenever you feel your immune system is challenged. They assist your body in the fight against viruses, harmful bacteria and fungi.

- If you're sick, Echinacea can effectively shorten the length of your illness. Take up to 900 mg. daily. Like all herbs, cycle its use as above. For Beta Glucans, a dose of 150 to 250 mg. a day is effective.

- Antibiotics are usually quite effective for acute or emergency cases. I reserve them for a last resort. If you develop fever, you may need one from your doctor. These are only available by prescription.

---

[1] Infectious Diseases Sourcebook: Health Reference :Series, 1st Edition. Omnigraphics. Copyright 2004, Page 9

[2] ibid, Page 3

[3] Norovirus (Norwalk virus). Foodsafety.gov. Your Gateway to Federal Food Safety Information.

[4] Infectious Diseases Sourcebook: Health Reference Series, 1st Edition. Page 75

[5] Two Win Nobel Prize for Discovering Bacterium Tied to Stomach Ailments," By Lawrence K. Altman, Published: October 4, 2005

[6] Proffitt C. Health Dept.: Norovirus Caused Olive Garden outbreak.

[7] Infectious Diseases Sourcebook: Health Reference Series, 1st Edition. Omnigraphics. Copyright: 2004, Page 4

[8] Nutrition Action Health Letter - "Bugs Are Breaking Out All Over." December 2006. Page 7.

Chapter 6

Low Testosterone Does More than Zap Energy — It Increases Risk of Death

You've heard me talk about testosterone — and how not having enough of it can rob you of your manhood. Here are just a few of the symptoms:

Reduced Sex Drive: No real desire to have sex or having to "fake" interest to keep your spouse or lover satisfied.

Loss of Muscle and Bone Density: We lose about three pounds of muscle mass per decade — resulting in a lack of strength that turns once-virile men into flabby couch potatoes.

PLUS: Wimpy erections, disturbed sleep, fatigue, irritability, feelings of depression, poor concentration and memory lapse, heart disease, etc.

But here's something you may not realize — there's new evidence to suggest that low levels of testosterone actually *increase* your risk of death.

If you're experiencing any of the side effects listed above — and feeling less of a man than you used to — there's a good chance your testosterone levels may be out of whack. But don't despair…

On a recent trip to India, I discovered an ancient herb that's been lifting men out of the doldrums — and supercharging their libidos — for thousands of years. By the time you get to the end of this article, you'll know exactly what it is and how to use it. Plus, you'll get four other herbal all-stars you can use right away.

Low Testosterone Levels May Boost the Risk of Death in Men over 40

A recent study published in *Archives of Internal Medicine* revealed that low testosterone levels may actually boost the risk of death in men over 40.[1]

"Older males with relatively low testosterone had an **88% increased risk of death** compared to those with normal testosterone levels," researchers reported.

Lead researcher Dr. Molly M. Shores of the Veterans Administration Puget Sound Health Care System and University of Washington, Seattle, concluded that "low testosterone in older men was associated with an increased risk for mortality."

Dr. Shores's findings were confirmed during follow-up. After four years, the men with low testosterone had a death rate two-thirds higher than those with normal levels.

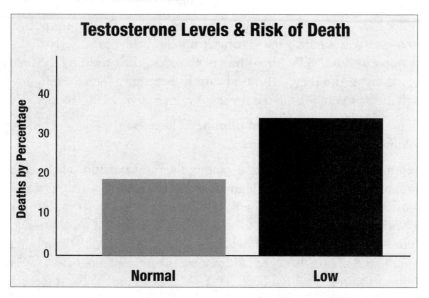

The fact that low testosterone can interfere with your ability to "perform" both in and out of the bedroom — and shorten your life — shouldn't surprise you.

For years I've been writing about the devastating effects low testosterone can have on your health and happiness. Here at my clinic, I see it firsthand in thousands of patients. The misery low testosterone levels can inflict on a man's body, mind and spirit.

In fact, men are being "feminized" by the combination of declining testosterone and rising estrogen — even young men in their 30s and sometimes in their late 20s.

These feminizing changes are due — at least in part — to the use of pesticides, chemicals and additives in the food we eat and the water we drink.

If you're worried you might have lower-than-average testosterone levels — and you'd like to learn how you can ramp up your body's production *the natural way* — here's a simple meal plan to boost testosterone and lower estrogen.

The Secret to Health, Vitality and Virility — Selecting Superior Quality Foods

Think back to the times of our ancient ancestors. Do you think cavemen ever had a hard time getting it up? Probably not. Heart disease was unheard of. And with no processed foods, their testosterone levels stayed high. And they had the advantage of eating a high protein, low-carb diet. Protein is essential for the production of sex hormones.

To get the maximum amount of protein, focus on the "big five": meat, wild fish, eggs, dairy, and nuts.

Red meat: I consider beef to be among the most nutritious foods. The protein is complete and it's a good source of creatine. Creatine makes you stronger and more energetic. Red meat is also the best source of the nutrient CoQ10, which is essential for heart health. And knowing that there's a strong connection between ED and heart disease, it makes sense that CoQ10 also plays an important role in sexual health. I recommend eating grass-fed beef. It has 20 times more of the important omega-3 fatty acids than commercial beef and none of the hormones.

Wild fish: You've probably heard that fish can be a source of mercury and other toxins. However, you can minimize these risks and enjoy the benefit of this rich source of omega-3s by choosing wild Alaskan salmon, mackerel, trout, or sardines. Chose wild over farm-raised and small over large fish. The highest levels of mercury are in swordfish, shark and king mackerel and tuna.

Eggs: Eggs are the perfect food. I eat them every day. Sure, they contain cholesterol. They don't even raise your blood cholesterol. Sure, eggs contain cholesterol. The developing embryo needs it to produced sex hormones — and so do you. But just because they contain it, this doesn't mean they'll raise your cholesterol levels. The bottom line: eggs do not cause heart disease. In fact, there was never any evidence they did.

Egg yolks have all the required fat soluble vitamins (A, D, E, and K), iron, and heart healthy omega-3 fat. The whites have all the water-soluble B vitamins and are the source of the highest quality protein on the face of the planet.

Dairy: Dairy is "liquid meat," and full of good protein. Cheese and whole milk are a great source of calcium and vitamin D. Raw, organic milk is best.

Nuts: Nuts are rich in healthy monounsaturated fat. Walnuts and almonds are among the most nutritious with omega-3 fatty acids, vitamin E, fiber, potassium, and other minerals. Other good choices are pecans, macadamias, cashews, and Brazil nuts. Enjoy them as a snack instead of chips or crackers.

Other factors like excessive drinking and smoking also have a profound effect on both your performance and stamina.

A few drinks will put you in the mood, but too many will make you useless. And smoking? Let's put it this way — the Marlboro Man doesn't see much action these days. A solid erection requires blood vessels that are flexible and able to expand. Smoking will tighten your blood vessels making them too narrow to channel the amount of blood you need for an erection.

Reignite Your Desire and Get Back in the Game

Western drugs can help you get an erection, but *loss of desire* is not something western science is equipped to deal with. Sure, your doctor may give you an antidepressant, but that will only make the problem worse. You may not realize it, but many of the active ingredients in popular antidepressants actually suppress your libido.

When I was in India, a discovered an ancient remedy they've been using since antiquity. *Ashwagandha* is a member of an elite group of herbs called *adaptogens*. These enigmatic plants have the power to normalize and balance various functions in your body. They can eliminate fatigue and help you to handle stress.

Recent studies confirm that ashwagandha helps your body make nitric oxide (NO).[2] NO relaxes smooth muscle tissue and improves blood flow. The blue little pill works on the same principle.

What's more, new research shows ashwagandha may help with anxiety and depression. In a clinical trial, doctors found that patients who took ashwagandha for five days experienced the same level of anxiety relief as those who took the prescription drugs Ativan (anti-anxiety) and Tofranil (antidepressant).

Ashwagandha is the root of the *Withania somnifera* plant.[3] Most ashwagandha products are standardized extracts of *withanolides* — the active components. The most common standard is 5%.

Ashwagandha can potentiate the effect of barbiturates.[4] If you are taking a sedative or sleeping pill, you should check with your doctor before using ashwagandha.

As a capsule, I usually start with 250 mg. a day. I use it every day for about four to six weeks, and then stop for a month. Most herbs will lose their effectiveness if you take them continuously without a break. Then, you can continue another cycle.

4 Libido-Pumping Herbal All-Stars

Ashwagandha is a great place to start. But having other strategies is important when you're using herbs. Here are a few more options for you:

Tribulus Terrestris: This reliable herb has been used in Europe for centuries to boost sex hormone levels and has been clinically proven to restore and improve libido in men. Recommendation: 250 mg. of Tribulus Terrestris daily.

Muira Puama: Recent scientific studies confirm the powerful aphrodisiac qualities of this herb. In 1990, men suffering from ED or loss of libido took Muira Puama extract. Sixty-two percent of those with loss of libido reported improvement. More than 50% of those with ED reported improvement.[5] Recommendation: 100 mg. of Muira Puama extract daily.

Yohimbe: This herb is from the inner bark of a tree, which grows in Africa. At one time, the drug made from yohimbe, *yohimbine* was the only medication approved by the FDA for the treatment of ED. Recommendation: 250 mg. of Yohimbine extract daily.

Korean Red Ginseng: This supplement is widely taken to help your body deal with stress. Ginseng also increases stamina and energy. It can even improve your testosterone levels. When you consider it also has a positive effect on blood flow, it's easy to see why ginseng would be valuable to maintain an erection. Recommendation: 250 mg. of Korean Red Ginseng daily.

A word of caution: I don't recommend taking herbal supplements continuously over a long period. Use them for four to six weeks and then take a break.

---

[1] Reinberg S. "Low Testosterone Could Increase Death Risk." *HealthDay Reporter*. August 15, 2006.

[2] Iuvone T, Esposito G, Life Sci. 2003 Feb 21;72(14):1617-25.

[3] Bhattacharya SK, Bhattacharya A, Sairam K, Ghosal S. Anxiolytic-antidepressant activity of Withania somnifera glycowithanolides: an experimental study. *Phytomedicine*. 2000 Dec;7(6):463-9.

[4] Brinker F, *Herb Contraindications and Drug Interactions.* 2001, Eclectic Medical Publications, Sandy, Oregon.

[5] Sears, Al MD, The T- Factor, pp. 38-54, 2000

PART 7

ANCIENT WISDOM FOR MODERN HEALTH AND WELLNESS

Chapter 1

Anti-Aging Reborn from Ancient India

Do you struggle with fatigue, loss of energy or no motivation? You may have become dependent on caffeine. For a better boost, I offer my patients traditional remedies from the forests of southern India. The herbs in this region are safe, reliable and proven since ancient times.

One in particular — ashwagandha — is an Ayurvedic favorite dating back thousands of years. During a trip to India, I met up with a handful of Ayurvedic doctors who gave me the inside story on this remarkable herb.

5,000-Year-Old "Formula" Reinvigorates Your Life

I began my quest to find the roots of Ayurveda in its birthplace, Kerala, in southern India. Ayurveda is the traditional medicine practiced in India. It means "the science of life." Deeply rooted in the wisdom of nature, Ayurveda sees health as the harmony of body, mind, senses and spirit — not merely the absence of symptoms.

On day two of my trip, a traditional healer introduced me to the herb ashwagandha. Used to rebuild strength and vitality, Indians from all walks of life swear by its power and effectiveness. Every village seems to claim its own unique relationship to the herb.

It was humbling to visit farmers and merchants who were preparing ashwagandha the same way their ancestors had millennia ago.

Reawaken Your Desire and Turbocharge Your Energy

Ashwagandha can help men become more potent and manly. Loss of desire is not something western science is equipped to deal with. Sure, your doctor may give you an antidepressant, but that will only make the problem worse. You may not realize it, but many of the active ingredients in popular antidepressants actually suppress your libido.

Ashwagandha is a member of an elite group of herbs called *adaptogens*. These enigmatic plants have the power to normalize and balance various functions in your body. They can eliminate fatigue and help you to handle stress.

Recent studies confirm that ashwagandha helps your body make nitric oxide (NO).[1] NO relaxes smooth muscle tissue and improves blood flow. The blue little pill that doctors prescribe works on the same principle.

What's more, new research shows ashwagandha may help with anxiety and depression. In a clinical trial, doctors found that patients who took ashwagandha for five days experienced the same level of anxiety relief as those who took the prescription drugs Ativan (anti-anxiety) and Tofranil (antidepressant).[2]

How Much Ashwagandha Should You Take?

Ashwagandha is the root of the *Withania somnifera* plant. Most ashwagandha products are standardized extracts of *withanolides* — the active components. The most common standard is 5%.

Ashwagandha can potentiate the effect of barbiturates.[3] If you are taking a sedative or sleeping pill, you should check with your doctor before using ashwagandha.

As a capsule, I usually start with 250 mg. a day. I use it every day for about four to six weeks, then stop for a month. Most herbs will lose their effectiveness if you take them continuously without a break. Then, you can continue another cycle.

---

[1] Iuvone T, Esposito G, Life Sci. 2003 Feb 21;72(14):1617-25.

[2] Bhattacharya SK, Bhattacharya A, Sairam K, Ghosal S. "Anxiolytic-antidepressant activity of Withania somnifera glycowithanolides: an experimental study." *Phytomedicine.* 2000 Dec;7(6):463-9.

[3] Brinker F, *Herb Contraindications and Drug Interactions.* 2001, Eclectic Medical Publications, Sandy, Oregon.

Chapter 2

How to Live Your Life in a "Blue Zone"

The wind made me sway a bit as I slung the little orange life jacket over my head and onto my shoulders. Without thinking I tightened the thin white nylon strap around my waist before I climbed in the boat. I don't know why. Like this tiny thing was going to save me if this boat ever flipped over. It looked like it was made for a little kid. And the life jacket wasn't very big, either.

But whatever. The waves weren't very high anywhere across the cold, dark waters that had carved out "The Lake of the Gods," as the locals called it.

The driver fired up the motor and the boat jumped forward. I thought my camera and I might get dumped in for an unexpected swim after all, just to prove me wrong, and despite the calm water. But the boat straightened out after a second, and I took a moment to look around me.

We were headed toward the tiny volcanic rock islands in the center of the lake. The sheer cliffs of the crater sliced straight down into the deep water.

The sun was bright, but I noticed there was still one stubborn cloud blocking my view of the 16,200-foot peak of Mount Cotacachi. My camera was dry, but I couldn't take a picture of it.

It didn't matter, though. Here I was, near the Equator high in the Andes Mountains and exploring a dormant (I hoped) volcano. The adrenaline was flowing, and I was doing one of my favorite things... visiting another of the world's Blue Zones.

Do you know what Blue Zones are? These are little-known but very special places tucked away around the world where the people who live there stay active and healthy well past the age of 90 and many times well over 100.

My trip to northern Ecuador was one of the best I've ever taken. I visited Cotacachi, a busy mountain village that sits between two volcanoes, Mama Cotacachi and Papa Imbabura. The main street of the town is filled with shops famous for their leather products.

They claim the people there often live past 100 because of the water. It flows down from the ice cap on top of Mount Cotacachi. They believe the water makes them stronger and able to live a long time.

When I was there, I tested it for its high mineral content. Above the town of Cotacachi the water also fills the volcanic lake called Achicocha in the local language, but called Cuicocha by the rest of the world. It feeds a river called the Ambi that townspeople use to feed their cattle and crops.

Many of the farmers I saw still work their fields by hand, and send their produce to a fantastic organic farmers' market in the village. It's part of the largest indigenous market in South America. It's full of crafts, clothing, leather, inlaid silver — almost too big of a variety to count. Over a thousand sellers gather there every Saturday.

Cotacachi is at the northern tip of a long Blue Zone called Ecuador's "Valley of Longevity," where the people often live to be over 90 and even 100 with ease. And everywhere I went, I saw it was true. These older folks weren't sitting at home, either. I got to see them because they were out and about. Many of them were still working in the leather shops, stitching and cutting and crafting some of the best leather goods I'd ever seen.

Another Blue Zone stop farther south in the Valley of Longevity is the Llanganatis region in the center of Ecuador. It's sacred to Ecuadorians, and the local legend is that the lost treasure of the Incas was buried there.

Vilcabamba, at the southern end of the valley, is also known for its long-lived people.

I haven't been to either of those places yet, but I'm hoping to go before too long. I'll tell you all about it when I go… and whether or not I find the gold!

Jamaican Secret to Long Life

Another Blue Zone I have visited is near Long Bay, on the eastern tip of Jamaica, in Portland parish. I've seen for myself the large number of people there who live to be more than 100. I was there for a funeral when the grandmother of my friend A.D. passed away, and I couldn't help but notice the grave markers. Everyone lived into their 80s and 90s.

One local named Granny Mary just passed away this year. They claim she was 128, but records in Jamaica are hard to come by. What I do know is that if you look at her children, you can see she must have been well over 100.

I don't know why they live so long, but it may be because they eat freshly caught fish for breakfast, lunch, and dinner. Omega-3-rich mackerel, tuna, snapper, cod, dolphin, shrimp, and Caribbean lobster are staples.

Omega-3 fatty acids reduce inflammation and plaque build-up in your arteries, both of which are primary causes of chronic disease. Plus, all the fish is wild caught — not farm-raised fish. Farm-raised is loaded with inflammatory arachidonic acid instead of healthy omega-3s.

On top of that, the folks in Long Bay eat a variety of fruits and vegetables with natural anti-inflammatory properties.

One is **ackee**, a fruit that is rich in omega-3s, vitamin A, zinc, and protein. Ackee is a breakfast staple commonly served with saltfish. But you need to prepare ackee properly. If it isn't cooked, it can cause vomiting and even death.

Another is **callaloo**. It looks like spinach or kale, and you'll find this green, leafy vegetable in many Jamaican dishes. It has four times the calcium, twice the iron and more than twice the vitamin A found in broccoli and spinach.

Living Healthy Past 100

I'm sure you've heard about the most famous Blue Zone, the island of Okinawa in Japan, and how long the people there live. They've done a famous study on it, called the Okinawa Centenarian Study. Okinawa has a higher percentage of 100-year-olds than almost anywhere on earth.

The people who live there aren't overweight, and they socialize constantly. For example, people come from all over the island to be a part of the world's largest tug of war every year. And it's been going on there since the 1600s!

You also may have heard that Okinawans live a long time because of *what* they eat — fish, edible marine plants and vegetables high in omega-3, minerals and vitamins that help them fight inflammation. And what they eat may be a reason for their long lives; we have no way of knowing for sure.

But what interests me most is *how* they eat.

What you probably have not heard is that Okinawans have a philosophy of eating. It's called Hara Hachi Bu, which literally means "stomach 80%." They eat until their stomachs feel 80% full, and then they stop.

In the West, we're taught to clean our plates, finish what we start and "give everything 100%."

In Okinawa, they make sure they never do this when eating.

To me, this is their longevity secret. They are practicing calorie restriction, which is a documented way to live longer.

This was discovered about 20 years ago, when researchers found a family of life-protecting genes called sirtuins (silent information protein regulators). Conditions of severe stress, such as starvation, turn the sirtuins on. And they transmit signals to every cell in your body to cancel out the effects of aging.

A Johns Hopkins University study showed that taking in fewer calories turns on the sirtuin genes, and makes organisms live longer.[1]

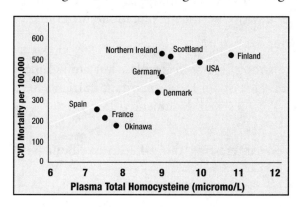

Another advantage Okinawans have is they have very low rates of heart disease. One of the reasons is that they have the lowest levels of homocysteine ever measured on Earth.

Homocysteine is a naturally occurring amino acid. But too much of it irritates the lining of your blood vessels and prevents them from dilating. This increases your risk of heart attack and stroke.

Turns out knowing your homocysteine level is even more useful than we thought. Homocysteine can predict other diseases as well. It's linked to everything from gout and psoriasis to cancer and kidney disease.

The good news is, it's easy to keep your homocysteine level low. The famous Okinawa Centenarian Study found that Okinawans keep their levels low because they eat foods high in B vitamins like folate, B6 and B12.[2]

For my patients with homocysteine levels higher than 7, I give them those same B vitamins. I also add riboflavin (B2) and trimethylglycine (TMG) which protect your blood vessels.

California Blue Zone? You're Nuts

I've read a lot of studies on places where people live a long time. Some of these studies seem to want to include Loma Linda, California. I don't know if it's just so they can claim someplace in the U.S. is a Blue Zone, or what.

I have a feeling there's another agenda there, though.

That's because they always tell you some form of, "The reason the people there live longer is because they're all vegetarians who don't drink."

Meanwhile, they only live a couple years longer than the average American, and they have to live the life of a monk to get there.

No, thank you.

Don't get me wrong. I love vegetables, but animal meat is the only good source of some of our most important nutrients like vitamin B12 and CoQ10. Plus, it's well documented that a drink a day helps you live longer.

But there is one interesting thing I learned about people in Loma

Linda. Many of them eat a serving of nuts every day. Nuts are rich in vitamins, healthy omega-3 fats, and selenium... just like the foods they eat on Okinawa. That's not a reason, but it's something to think about.

Keep the Party Going

One Blue Zone where they do not live like monks is Icaria, Greece. The people there have three-day parties, feel no stress, go to bed well after midnight and sleep late. They also drink lots of wine and socialize with everyone who visits and lives there.

And this tiny island has the highest percentage of 90-year-olds on the planet — one of every three people. Icarians also have about 20% lower rates of cancer, 50% lower rates of heart disease and almost no dementia.

A brand new study may point to why visiting friends and going to parties might keep dementia away. Cambridge University followed over 1,100 people for more than 10 years. They found that the people who were the most socially active had a 70% slower rate of cognitive decline![3]

The foods they eat on Icaria are simple, raw and whole. Milk and meat straight from the goat, raw vegetables from the garden, and olive oil with every meal.

One of the foods they eat a lot is mustard greens. High in vitamin A and vitamin K (most Americans are deficient in this nutrient), the spicy greens are good for your blood and bone strength. Icarians boil them with olive oil, garlic, and lemon.

The newest research into mustard greens tells us that they are high in *sinigrin* and *gluconasturtiin*, plant nutrients that are converted into cancer-fighting compounds in the body. In an animal study, the cancer-fighter AITC derived from sinigrin inhibited bladder cancer growth by 35%, and stopped 100% of the cancer from getting into the muscles.[4]

In a human study, AITC killed off 30% to 50% of liver cancer cells, and also stopped the cancer from spreading. Other studies show it stops colon, breast and prostate cancer cells, too.[5]

A Big Fatty Secret

Another island Blue Zone is in Sardinia off the west coast of Italy. The town of Ovodda's percentage of 100-year-olds is *six times* that of Okinawa. But where Okinawa's 100-year-olds are mostly women, men live just as long as women on Sardinia. They socialize often, and always include the elders, who are respected for their storytelling and humor.

The people there eat all fresh, local foods like pork, lamb, oily fish and shellfish prepared simply with olive oil, lemon and garlic. They drink very dark red wines with meals.

Did you know that Sardinian wine made from cannonau grapes has up to four times the flavonoids of other wines? A study in the journal *Nature* showed that Sardinian wines are high in procyanidins, the most active and beneficial of the red wine antioxidants.[6]

They also drink sheep's milk called pecorino, a raw milk rich in omega-3 fatty acids.

For dessert they eat cheese and fruit. One of the cheeses they eat is allowed to get a little rotten, because Sardinians believe the bacteria are good for your gut, which we now know is true.

For dessert, they make treats filled with pecorino cheese called Seadas. A Seada is like a fritter with cheese in the middle. And it's made with almost 100 grams of pork fat and butter, honey, lemon and eggs. Yet the people who eat them are not overweight, and live longer than anywhere on earth. Put that in your "low fat diet" and smoke it!

Sardinians also have a tradition of walking. They raise sheep there, so the shepherds walk all day, of course. But the houses and gardens are far apart, and people walk rather than ride. It's a social tradition to go for a walk with the entire family.

Sardinia also has a community festival called *Sa Sartiglia*, where masked riders gallop through the main streets of the town of Orisanto. People come from all over the island to participate.

How Do They Live So Well for So Long?

There are other places where the people claim they live to be very old: Abkhazia near Georgia, which used to be part of the Soviet Union. The

Hunza Valley in Pakistan. Bama, China, where they say the climate is ideal for human life. Even a town called Montacute in England, where they claim the secret to their longevity is their local produce grown with zero chemicals.

So what else can we learn from the longest-lived people on Earth? Can we use their secrets to live healthier for longer ourselves?

Well, here's my short list of things we can learn from Blue Zones and actually do something about.

1. Eat few if any processed foods.

2. Eat the right kinds of fat (omega-3s).

3. Take in very little sugar that is not from fruit.

4. Eat lots of real fiber (plant products).

5. Drink a moderate amount of alcohol almost every day.

6. Take in relatively few calories every day.

7. Focus on togetherness, family and community.

8. Stay very active and social, doing everything from gardening to celebrating with each other, not alone.

Celebrations, three-day parties, family fun, lots of social interaction, fresh local foods, and wine. Hmmm… seems I may have already been living in a Blue Zone.

---

[1] Mattson M. "Energy Intake, Meal Frequency and Health: A Neurobiological Perspective." *Annual Review of Nutrition*. 2005; Vol. 25: 237-260.

[2] "Okinawa Centenarian Study" Retrieved March 29, 2011.

[3] James B, Wilson R, L, Bennett D. "Late-Life Social Activity and Cognitive Decline in Old Age." *Journal of the International Neuropsychological Society*. 2011.

[4] Bhattacharya A, Li Y, Wade KL, Paonessa JD, Fahey JW, Zhang Y. "Allyl isothiocyanate-rich mustard seed powder inhibits bladder cancer growth and muscle invasion." *Carcinogenesis*. 2010 Dec;31(12):2105-10.

[5] Hwang F, Lee H. "Allyl Isothiocyanate and Its N-Acetylcysteine Conjugate Suppress Metastasis … in SK-Hep1 Human Hepatoma Cells." *Exp. Biol. Med.* 2006;231:421-430.

[6] Corder R, et al. "Oenology: Red wine procyanidins and vascular health." *Nature* 2006;444:566-7.

Chapter 3

Mysterious Magic Milk

The members of the All Russian Physician's Society were frantic. They needed the mysterious source of this magic milk called "kefir" that seemed to cure so many health problems.

But how to get it?

Desperate, they turned to the Blandov brothers. The Blandovs owned the Moscow Dairy, but also a cheese factory in the Caucasus Mountains, where kefir originated.

Please, the doctors asked, find a way to get us the source — these "kefir grains" — so we can make a steady supply of kefir for our patients.

Nikolai Blandov agreed. The Moscow Dairy would get a monopoly on producing the miracle milk. So he sent a beautiful young employee named Irina Sakharova to seduce a local prince of the Caucasus near their factory in Kislovodsk.

Her job was to wrap Prince Bek-Mirza Barchorov around her finger, and get him to give her a supply of these kefir grains.

But the prince's people believed the grains were a gift from God. He couldn't give any away without violating his religion. Irina realized her mission had failed, and she and her escorts started back for Kislovodsk.

Prince Barchorov had other ideas. He didn't want to lose Irina.

It was local custom to steal a bride, so he kidnapped Irina, to force her to marry him. The Blandovs learned of Irina's kidnapping, and hired agents who pulled off a daring rescue, capturing the beautiful Irina back from the prince.

Irina, with the help of the Blandovs, had Prince Barchorov dragged before Tsar Nicholas II. The prince offered gold and jewels to make up for his treatment of Irina… but the Tsar ordered him to pay restitution in 10 pounds of kefir grains.

This is the legend of how one of the healthiest drinks on planet earth, kefir (pronounced kuh-feer), was brought to the modern world.

The Blandovs, by the way, offered the first bottle of kefir for sale in Moscow in 1908.

No One Knows, No One's Telling

The strange thing is, despite the story of Irina and the prince, the actual origin of the kefir grains themselves is still a mystery. *No one knows where they came from.* And the mountain people aren't talking.

The people of Caucasus say the kefir grains are a gift from God, and if they reveal kefir's secret it will lose its "magic."

Some people believe kefir grains are manna, the miracle food God provided to Moses and the Jews in the Bible.

The name kefir comes from the Turkish word *keif*, which means simply "feel good." Kefir originated with the Ossetians, who became shepherds in the Caucasus Mountains between Turkey and Russia, in an area north of the country now called Georgia.

You've heard of the explorer Marco Polo? Well, he mentioned kefir in the chronicles of his travels in the East. But it was mostly forgotten after that.

Until strange stories of a magical drink made their way into Russia. There, doctors obtained it and used it to treat patients with everything from stomach aches to tuberculosis.

Whatever its origin, we know that people in Caucasus have been drinking kefir for over a thousand years. And they are known for routinely living to well over 100 years old.

Miniature Magic

Kefir grains are nothing like the foods we call grains today. Each one looks like a small version of a cauliflower. The granules are made up of colonies of healthy bacteria that grow together, symbiotically, in a culture of the milk protein casein. And it's all held together by a sugary matrix named kefiran.

The bacteria are the same types of "flora" that are an integral part of your digestive system, and may even help you make B vitamins.

Kefir is a cousin to other cultured products like yogurt, sour cream and buttermilk, except much more powerful. It's made in the old tradition of fermentation.

Today, many of the foods we eat are preserved through processing or pasteurization. This uses heat from outside sources to kill off live cultures. It also strips the food of many helpful bacteria and nutrients. For yogurt, the live flora are then added back in.

But kefir is fermented. That means preserving with the help of heat generated by the food itself, and the beneficial flora. Before refrigerators, this is how you would have made food last for a few days without spoiling.

The kefir grains contain a complex flora of lactic acid bacteria (lactobacilli, lactococci, leuconostocs), acetic acid bacteria, and yeast mixture.

When you drink kefir, the flora goes right to work for you. These mini soldiers help re-colonize the good flora in your gut. They also get rid of harmful organisms, like too much H. Pylori, the bacteria that cause ulcers.

Kefir grains also seem to have the unique ability to unlock peptides from milk.[1] In regular milk, these peptides stay hidden, or *encrypted*. But when you ferment the milk with kefir grains, it unlocks these peptides to give you benefits including:

- Lower blood pressure.
- Increased immune strength.
- Normalize cholesterol function.
- Improved protein digestion.

And despite the fact that kefir is made from milk, most people who are lactose intolerant can drink kefir easily.[2]

Kefir is also a very nutrient-dense food, so it fills you up and keeps you from getting that "empty stomach" feeling, like you get after eating processed, starchy snacks.

It can have as much as 35% protein, lots of vitamins A, B and K, and also phosphorus. Phosphorus helps you digest fats and carbohydrates to use as energy. The flora in kefir also add to your digestive enzymes, helping you break down foods and use the nutrients more efficiently.

There's no way to know for sure, but these two benefits might be why people who drink kefir say they have so much energy.

And do you want to know what my favorite thing about kefir is?

Modern science can't duplicate it. Even though they know exactly what's in kefir, they can't make the real thing.

Scientists have all the ability and technology in the world to alter molecules and make synthetic drugs. But they can't create kefir grains no matter how hard they try.

I love that.

In fact real kefir grains can only be obtained from growing and dividing already existing kefir grains.

Kefir is one of my favorite examples of how nature has science beat.

Here are four other things to love about kefir, each of which separates it from all other cultured milk products to make it unique.

- Nearly all other fermented products have only one, or at most three, kinds of flora. Kefir has four main groups, and 40 to 60 different strains of healthy bacteria and yeast.

- You never need to obtain more real kefir grains once you have some. They grow, and you divide them to make more.

- With proper care, real kefir grains last forever.

- Kefir has yeast, which means that kefir is a slightly alcoholic drink.

Depending on the fermentation process, temperature, time and the type of culture used (what you ferment the kefir in), the alcohol content will vary from 0.06% to 3% alcohol.

Shaking the container while the kefir is fermenting will give you higher alcohol content. In the Caucasus Mountains, you would have made kefir in an animal skin bag, and then hung the bag on your front door to make sure it was jostled around.

It was even a custom that everyone who came in or went out of a home with a kefir bag on the door had a responsibility to give the bag a poke or a shake to help mix it.

To make kefir today, you don't need an animal skin bag. You simply add the kefir grains to fresh milk from any source — coconut, rice, goat, cow or sheep milk — and let it ferment at room temperature for 18 to 24 hours. The next day, you have your kefir! And, if you let it ferment another 24 hours, the B vitamin content increases.

The end product is a creamy drink with a tangy, slightly sour but refreshing taste. And the great thing is, if you want you can add flavor to it by mixing in whatever kind of fruit you like.

My favorite is strawberry.

I get my kefir from Amber, my friend and farmer who also gets me my organic eggs. She makes me and my staff yogurt, too. She delivers the yogurt and kefir in these giant glass jars filled to the top... almost too good to be true.

If you don't have a local organic grower or farm that makes kefir or has kefir grains, there are now quite a few places you can get them from.

Some health food stores are starting to sell packaged brands. These are another reason why I don't trust too many foods that come in a box. That's because store-bought kefir isn't the real thing.

To package it, they have to stop the yeast process or the sealed containers would explode on the store shelves. That means it's not made from real kefir grains. They're imitations that only have a few strains of flora and no yeast activity, which gives you some of the biggest health benefits.

To obtain real kefir grains, there are two things you can do. The first is to buy them. There are many websites you can order your kefir grains from. Here are the three I think are the most reliable:

- Yemoos Nourishing Cultures http://www.yemoos.com/
- Real Kefir Grains http://www.kefirlady.com/
- Cultures for Health http://www.culturesforhealth.com/

Also, you can have your kefir grains given to you. In that case, there are two other websites you should know about. One is a directory of free and for sale kefir grains all over the U.S. (and the world):

- http://www.rejoiceinlife.com/kefir/kefirlistUSA.php

The other is a website for people who share real live kefir grains:

- http://www.torontoadvisors.com/Kefir/kefir-list.php

---

[1] Miller. N.P., Scholz-Ahrens, K.E., Roos. N. and Schrezenmcir, J., "Bioactive peptides and proteins from foods: Indication for health effects," *Eur. J. Nutra*, 2008;47:171-182

[2] Guzel-Seydim, et al., "Review: Functional Properties of Kefir," *Critical Reviews in Food Science and Nutrition* 2011;51: 261-268

Chapter 4

Inca Gold, Longevity Fruit, and the All-American Sugar

Ever feel a little bit naughty and reach for the sugar to add it to your morning yogurt, bowl of fruit, cup of coffee or afternoon snack for a decadent little sugar rush? You're not alone.

Eating is an emotional experience for most people. And modern diet advice takes all the fun out of eating. Take the advice of a nutritionist or diet guru and you'll feel like you've been locked away in a dungeon somewhere and you're only allowed to eat gruel.

My basic philosophy of eating is to eat foods that you enjoy in their natural, unadulterated forms. That means for the most part, natural sugars are good, and man-made sugars are bad.

And I hate to ruin all the fun, but refined sugar is not natural. Take a look at the following chart and you'll see all the steps it takes to make the white stuff. Not exactly straight from the field to your table.

And eating a lot of it can be dangerous. For the short rush you may get from eating it, you're exposing yourself to dozens of health threats.

- Sugary foods could make you go blind.

In a study published in *Investigative Ophthalmology & Visual Science* last year, researchers in Australia found that a high-glycemic diet increases cataract risk. They looked at the eating habits of more than 1,600 people and found that the ones who ate the most carbohydrates more than *tripled* their risk for cataracts.[1]

- Sugar will leech essential minerals right out of your system.

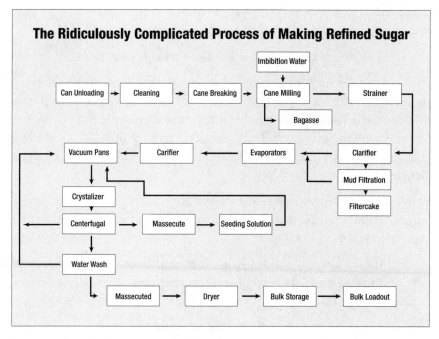

A can of soda has around nine teaspoons of processed sugar. But as little as two teaspoons of sugar throws off the natural balance of minerals in your blood, starting with depleting chromium, the mineral that helps your insulin process all that sugar in the first place.

- Sugary foods make your calcium go up, and your phosphorus go down, which can lead to calcium toxicity. You can get kidney stones, gall stones, arthritis and hardening of the arteries.

- Sugar reduces zinc absorption. Your body needs zinc for your immune system to work right.

I remember reading a study that found eating only three ounces of sugar during a meal or snack almost stops white blood cells from being able to destroy bacteria and viruses.[2] And that's ALL sugars — fructose, glucose or sucrose. This immune suppression starts about 30 minutes after you eat the sugar and can last for up to *five hours*.

What may be even worse is that when you don't have enough zinc, you can start to lose your sense of taste. That makes you want foods with more sugar and flavorings to make up for it, diminishing your taste sensation even more. It becomes a vicious cycle.

- Too much sugar in your food can shrink your bones.

In an animal study, they took bone building cells (osteoblasts) and dosed them with sugar (glucose). The more sugar they gave the cells that are supposed to build your bones, the more damage it did. There was less cell growth, more cell death, reduced activity of ALP (an enzyme that helps build bone), less calcium absorption and more free-radical damage.[3]

Another study found that refined sugar stimulates your adrenal glands to unnaturally release a cascade of hormones that can adversely affect your behavior.[4]

And all those "low fat" foods flying off store shelves just make it worse. The advertising and labels seem to promise that they're better for you because they're "fat free."

Do you know what they replaced the fat with?

Sugar. Lots of it.

Many reduced fat and fat-free foods are basically the original food with the fat removed but with refined sugar added. Eat the reduced fat food and you're taking in more sugar without even knowing it.

And "health" drinks are the worst. These things have heaping servings of refined sugar in them. The name "Vitamin Water" sure sounds healthy, until you see that a bottle has 32 grams of sugar. That's like eight sugar packets.

SoBe Green Tea seems like it should be healthy. It's green tea, right?

Sixty one grams of sugar per bottle. That's like eating four slices of cherry pie!

But what are you going to do, make all your food and drinks bland and tasteless? Then you will be eating like you're trapped in a dungeon.

Fortunately, not everything that's sweet is the enemy.

I've traveled all over the world looking for natural products I can bring back to my clinic to help my patients. And along the way I've found some delicious and healthy alternatives to refined cane sugar that don't spike your blood sugar and cause health disasters.

One thing to remember is that no matter what their makers say, Rapadura, Panela, Sucanat, Muscavado, Turbinado, Jaggery, palm sugar and "organic raw" sugar act the same in your body as plain old cane sugar. They're less refined, so they may still have some minerals in them, but does anyone eat sugar for its health benefits?

Here are some you've probably never heard of, but that I recommend to sweeten your foods and drinks:

Save Your Stomach with Peru's Favorite Sugar — When I was traveling in the mountains of Peru I learned about Yacon, a fruit-like vegetable called the "jewel of the Andes." Ancient Incas used to eat the roots for endurance and to keep from getting thirsty.

Yacon is good for diabetics because it has fructooligosaccharides, a kind of sugar you can't digest, so it doesn't affect blood sugar. But what I like about it is that yacon has inulin, a prebiotic. It helps you digest other foods and enhances immunity because it promotes beneficial bacteria in your intestines.[5] It has an apple/caramel/honey flavor that you can try as a dressing, or add it to your morning coffee or tea.

Discover Incan "Gold" — Lucuma is a fruit grown in the high valleys along the coast of Peru and its sugar tastes sort of like maple syrup. But where maple syrup has to be heated and processed to get maple sugar, lucuma is just dried and ground. So it keeps all its nutrients and antioxidants.

Lucuma was called "Gold of the Incas." In South America they use it to make ice cream, and to sweeten milk. But you can also add it to water to make juice, or even use it as a sugar replacement when you bake. They grow some in Hawaii and California now, but you can find authentic lucuma in a Peruvian restaurant or a Latin market near you.

Protect Yourself With Sugar? — Erythritol has a chemical-sounding name, but it's really just a type of sugar alcohol, or *polyol* which occurs naturally in fruits and vegetables. It's easy to digest, yet it's not metabolized by your body. That means it's teeth-friendly, and blood sugar friendly.

Erythritol also has another benefit — it's an antioxidant. Studies show it has a protective effect against oxidative stress on the lining of your blood vessels.[6]

I don't think erythritol's polyol cousin xylitol is too bad. But some studies have shown problems at high doses. Also, a lot of what you can buy at the store is overly processed, and made cheaply from Chinese corn instead of from its real source — the xylan fiber of the birch tree. Stick with erythritol.

Use China's Ancient Sugar — Momordica (Luo Han Guo) is a low-glycemic sugar substitute that's almost unknown in America, but it's 250–300 times sweeter than sugar and loaded with vitamin C. The Chinese have been using the dark brown juice from the fruit they call the "longevity fruit" for thousands of years.

Like honey, studies show that powder from momordica helps heal cuts and wounds.[7] It can also help keep your teeth healthy. It's a zero on the glycemic index, and has a little bit of a caramel flavor, so it tastes great in tea.

Try the All-American Sweetener — Folks in the southern United States have been making syrup from sweet sorghum stalks for almost 300 years.[8] They use sorghum syrup as a substitute for sugar and to brew gluten-free beer.

Sorghum syrup is full of vitamin B6, iron, calcium, magnesium, potassium and selenium. But maybe the best thing about sorghum syrup is that you don't have to put it in the refrigerator, and it won't mold. And if it crystallizes like honey, just heat it a tiny bit to return it to a liquid.

Sweeten Summer Drinks with My Grandmother's Secret: Here are two ideas you can use to make water a little more fun and tasty in the summer, so you don't have to settle for those sugar-water drinks from the store.

If you have kids, you can take whatever fruits they like the best — watermelon, pineapple or even strawberries — and add them to a large pitcher of water the night before. The next day, you'll have a perfectly naturally-sweetened fruit-flavored drink.

Or you can try my grandmother's wonderful natural solution. She called it "summer lemonade." She made it from fresh squeezed lemons, water and a splash of apple juice. She served it over ice with a slice of orange and a slice of lime.

---

[1] Chung-Jung Chiu. "Dietary Carbohydrate in Relation to Cortical and Nuclear Lens Opacities in the Melbourne Visual Impairment Project." *Investigative Ophthalmology & Visual Science*, June 2010, Vol. 51, No. 6.

[2] Ringsdorf, WM Jr., Cheraskin, E. Ramsay RR Jr. "Sucrose, Neutrophilic Phagocytosis and Resistance to Disease." *Dent Surv.* 1976 Dec; 52(12):46-8.

[3] Zhen D, Chen Y, Tang X. "Metformin reverses the deleterious effects of high glucose on osteoblast function." *J Diabetes Complications.* 2010 Sep-Oct;24(5):334-44. Epub 2009 Jul 22.

[4] Jones TW, Boulware SD, Kraemer DT, Caprio S, Sherwin RS, Tamborlane WV. "Independent effects of youth and poor diabetes control on responses to hypoglycemia in children." *Diabetes.* 1991 Mar;40(3):358-63.

[5] Stoyanova S, Geuns J, Hideg E, Van Den Ende W. "The food additives inulin and stevioside counteract oxidative stress." *Int J Food Sci Nutr.* 2011 May;62(3):207-14.

[6] Den Hartog G.J.M. et al. "Erythritol is a sweet antioxidant." *Nutrition*, 2009; 1-10.

[7] Prasad V, Jain V, Girish D, Dorle AK. "Wound-healing property of Momordica charantia L. fruit powder." *J Herb Pharmacother.* 2006;6(3-4):105-15.

[8] D.J. Undersander, W. E. Lueschen, L.H. Smith, A.R. Kaminski, J.D. Doll, K.A. Kelling, and E.S. Oplinger. "Sorghum—for Syrup." *U of Wisc. Alt. Field Crops Manual.* Nov. 1990.

Chapter 5

The Pleasure Prescription —
When to Say "No" to Drugs and Surgery

"That's a cake?"

My assistant S.D. just chuckled. Everyone was asking her that same question.

"It looks like a sculpture. Are you sure we can eat it?" My researcher K.D. took out his phone and snapped a photo.

S.D. told him, "It even comes with instructions on how to cut it after we sing Happy Birthday to Dr. Sears."

That was a fun cake. It looked so real. It had a couple of old-time doctors' briefcases, a globe marked with all of the places I've traveled to, a couple of stethoscopes that looked like you could use them, and even a copy of my PACE™ book!

You know I don't usually recommend eating sweets like that. But cake is an important symbol of celebration and coming together in America. Plus it's a little bit of decadent pleasure, which is also important from time to time.

Besides cake, we also had hula dancers, tropical cocktails and a big Polynesian island buffet.

I like Polynesian food because they've mixed in foods from other cultures but kept their native foods as the main focus of their meals.

I also liked the idea of having a Polynesian party because togetherness and pleasure are very important in their culture.

And that's what I want to talk to you about today. It's called The "Pleasure Prescription."

"Aloha!"

The Polynesians have a whole different set of values for social interactions.

They don't value things like independence. Your strength of character is not judged by how you soldier on and get through things without complaint, but by your cooperative behavior. To be amiable is very highly regarded. So they don't have some of the issues that we have in that they are first and foremost polite.

Dr. Paul Pearsall explains it this way in his book, *The Pleasure Prescription*. He writes that Polynesians live by their understanding of *aloha*. It's the drive to do what's healthful and pleasurable. *Alo* means share, and *ha* means breath. So *aloha* means to share the breath of life.

A Better Life in the Modern World

They strive for the relaxation, happiness and long life that come from sharing. Dr. Pearsall counsels people about how to do better with their relationships and how to have a more healthy and pleasurable life in today's world by learning from the Polynesians. And it's exceptionally good advice.

Pearsall describes the five principles that make up *aloha*.

They are five terms that we don't even have in English that describe their simple, harmonious and gentle take on life:

Ahonui: This means to be patient, but to persevere in that patience.

Lokahi: This is unity, but in the sense of harmoniousness.

Olu'olu: To be pleasantly agreeable.

Ha'aha'a: This means humility, with a sense of careful modesty.

Akahai: A gentle kindness that includes tenderness and consideration toward everyone.

When I think about those, I realize that virtually every person I've ever had a problem with didn't have those things. They didn't have patience, they weren't agreeable, they didn't have humility, and they weren't kind. And you know, you run into that a lot.

Most of us will live longer than our great-grandparents, but how are we getting there? Did you know that how you feel about yourself and how well you expect to live may be more important than any assessment made by a doctor?[1]

It's true. In one study, people who thought of their health status as "poor" died early at almost *three times* the rate as those who said they felt their health was "excellent."[2]

And in a review, researchers looked at 30 studies on self-reported health and how well people lived. They found that self-reported well-being can actually control how other risks affect you.

It seems the ancient Polynesians knew this.

They have developed their own "health care" system for living together, solving problems, and finding pleasure in living that you and I can emulate.

Here is Dr. Pearsall's prescription for how to have a better, longer and more pleasurable life the Polynesian way:

1) A penny for your patience. To Polynesians, the secret to a joyful life is to realize that you don't develop patience because you have time to spare. Rather, you realize you have more than enough time because you have patience.

Here's an easy way to learn to be persistent in your patience. Put three pennies in your pocket. Every time you become irritated or impatient with someone else or even yourself, put your hand in your pocket; gently turn one of the pennies while you count to ten. Then take out that penny and leave it for someone to find.

At the end of each day, see how many pennies you have left. If you have any, add them to the three you put in your pocket the next day. If your pocket jingles by the end of the week, congratulations! You're developing a good sense of *ahonui*.

2) Listen to the message. The Polynesians believe that all things on earth think, feel, and communicate in ways we haven't discovered yet and maybe can't even imagine. There is no separation, only unity.

To have a greater sense of harmony with others; try to spend five minutes each day sitting quietly with someone. Don't *try* to make a connection, just let it happen. Then talk about it, and you'll see how powerful nonverbal communication can be. You'll be on your way to building *lokahi*.

3) Confess instead of express. In the West we hear often how good it is to "express your feelings." But Polynesians believe that how much pleasure you get out of life is in direct proportion to how little anger you show.

To help your body and mind deal with times when you're angry or feel anger coming on, write it down. Write down what your mind thinks is the source of your anger, then stop. Go back a few days later and read it when your mind is calmer. This is confessing your anger, instead of expressing it.

Ancient Polynesians knew that anger has a long fuse, and you have to let all the hormones that build up inside you diffuse before you can look at what happened. No one is ever happy after they've been angry. The pleasurable life is one with *olu'olu*, which you'll have room for when there's no more anger.

4) Share some humble pie. A strong self-image isn't necessarily the best way to health and happiness in today's world. The Polynesians feel you need a core of stable features instead. They include accepting your appearance and respecting your family and origins. That way, you can fill several roles in your community, and grow through those in which you might not be as good while still succeeding in others you excel in.

To gain humility, Polynesians have an exercise where they go the entire day without saying the words "I," "me," or "mine." You can substitute something else, or say nothing at all. You'll notice it's tough in modern society.

But at the end of the day, you might discover it was one of the most stress-free days you've ever had. You might also find that as you use those pronouns less, so will others. You may start to feel a greater sense of *ha'aha'a*, but also more connected to others (*lokahi*) and more kind and considerate, which is the fifth principle of *aloha*, called *akahai*.

5) Try a little tenderness. This part of *aloha* is about giving and helping, sharing the breath of life, and being considerate and altruistic.

There are four ways to do this:

1. Help strangers — Commit to helping one person you don't know each day.

2. Make personal contact — Help people one on one. Don't mail in your donation.

3. Build your core, give your energy — Take care of yourself so that you have energy to help others.

4. Be a partner — Help for help's sake. Helping is giving.

You don't have to fix, or be the rescuer. Caring enough to be there is what makes people feel better. That's *akahai.*

---

[1] Mossey JM, Shapiro E. "Self-rated health: a predictor of mortality among the elderly." *Am J Public Health.* 1982 Aug;72(8):800-8.

[2] ibid.

PART 8

WHERE TO AVOID
TRADITIONAL MEDICINE

Chapter 1

Too Much Stress! How to Beat It — Even When Nothing Else Works

You know what constant stress feels like: Anxiety, worry, irritation and nagging fatigue that just won't go away. If you suffer under the weight of these symptoms, it's easy to despair. But don't! You may have a very treatable condition.

Most doctors don't even realize that these symptoms — taken together — add up to a real condition. Many will simply write a prescription for antidepressants or anxiety drugs. It is one of the most commonly overlooked and misdiagnosed problems in the U.S. today.[1]

It is due to the overtaxing of your adrenal glands by the modern world of constant sensory bombardment and chronic stressors. Too much stress for too long and you get stuck in "fight or flight."

But you don't need drugs to overcome the debilitating effects of low energy and constant fatigue. I'll give you some insight into the problem and tell you how to proceed.

The Modern World Can Put Your Body into a State of Constant Distress

Tens of thousands of years ago, when our ancient ancestors walked the Earth, life was very different. Loud noises were rare. The world was a lot "calmer." Sure, there was the stress of finding food. And escaping from predators could have been horrendously stressful — but almost always quite brief. In general, we spent most of our time in an atmosphere that was relaxed.

That was the environment that shaped our evolution. And our bodies are not much different today, even though our culture and technologies have changed drastically.

In our modern world, you are constantly bombarded by sirens, stereos, televisions, street noise, telephones, and crowds of busy people, sometimes yelling and screaming — not to mention the challenge of making money, raising children, managing your career and enduring the violence-filled evening news.

In physiological terms, these stresses cause changes in your body. The adrenal glands, which make adrenaline and cortisol, get to the point where they are constantly excited and distressed. Your bloodstream becomes flooded with not only adrenaline from short-term stress, but cortisol from long-term stress as well.

Cortisol is your body's chronic stress hormone. It gives your body the chance to pool all of its resources to deal with a crisis. And adrenaline gives you short bursts of energy to help get yourself out of trouble. The two of these hormones together create your "fight or flight" response.

Under these conditions, your body is not focused on long-term health and maintenance. It's only concerned with the crisis in front of you. But when your body gets stuck in fight or flight mode, it drains your energy and eliminates your natural balance and ability to adapt to change.

Hormones are extremely powerful. A little goes a long way. And when your adrenal glands get stuck in the "on" position, it can literally wipe you out. Your body simply isn't equipped to be stressed all the time. It prevents your body from performing other vital functions like building your immune system or laying down new bone or muscle.

At any given moment, your body is performing thousands of tasks and carrying out all sorts of remarkable feats. This is all part of its daily maintenance. But when the alarm bells sound, all energies are diverted into dealing with the crisis at hand.

In our caveman days, these stresses were short-lived. If you were chasing down an animal during the hunt, your adrenaline was pumping — but usually for a matter of seconds and rarely longer than 15 or 20 minutes at a time. But these days, our bodies can get trapped in a cycle of never-ending stress. And that means that we don't give our bodies a chance to attend to all the other long-term maintenance issues it's responsible for.

Imagine you're running a business. You have hundreds of things you're responsible for on a daily basis. But what if one of your employees is so disruptive, he constantly creates fires that you have to spend all your time and energy to put out? You won't be in business for very long.

With your body, if all its resources are constantly diverted to an immediate problem, it can't sustain optimal health and fitness for very long. Sickness, depression and disease are right around the corner.

Take the Quiz: Do you have Adrenal Fatigue?

Q: I catch colds or other infections (cold sores, yeast or bladder infections, eye infections, boils, sinus infections) easily.

❏ True ❏ False

Q: I'm gaining weight around my middle.

❏ True ❏ False

Q: I have strong cravings for sweet or salty foods.

❏ True ❏ False

Q: I feel overwhelmed or stressed by work, family, and other responsibilities.

❏ True ❏ False

Q: I'm often irritable, impatient, or pessimistic.

❏ True ❏ False

Q: I often have trouble waking in the morning, even though I went to bed at a reasonable hour.

❏ True ❏ False

Q: I often feel tired after exercise, rather than energized.

❏ True ❏ False

Q: I have developed allergies, asthma, hay fever, skin rashes (hives, eczema, psoriasis, rosacea, acne), arthritis, autoimmune disease, or other inflammatory conditions and/or I've taken anti-inflammatories or steroid drugs.

❏ True ❏ False

The more true answers you selected, the more likely you are to have adrenal fatigue.

Get Your Energy Back by Following These Simple Steps

You can take action right away. First, you can go to your local health food store and pick up a bottle of low-dose DHEA. I call DHEA the "anti-stress hormone."

DHEA stands for *dehydroepiandrosterone*. But don't let that tongue-twisting name bother you; everyone refers to it as DHEA. It is the most abundant product of the adrenal glands when your health is stable.

DHEA is the precursor used by your body in producing sex hormones like testosterone, estrogen and progesterone. It is produced in large quantities when you're young, but dwindles with age. <u>DHEA is the natural counter to cortisol</u>.

Some of the other benefits of DHEA include:

- Less stress.
- Enhanced energy.
- A boost in immune system function.
- Reduced body fat.
- Increased libido.
- Sharper memory.
- Prevention of wrinkles and the signs of physical aging.[2]

You secrete DHEA when times are good — when you're well fed, secure and free of stress. But when you are under stress, you suppress DHEA and secrete adrenaline and cortisol from the adrenals instead. This combined action puts off all long-term repair and maintenance.

Every problem or injury goes unhealed and unaddressed.

One of the problems with over-the-counter DHEA is finding doses that are low enough. Most people make the mistake of taking too much. And this can be a problem. As I said earlier, hormones are very powerful. Having too much can be as problematic as not having enough.

Start with just 5 mg. a day. See how you feel. If you need to, you can bump it up to 10 mg. a day. And if you feel like you could benefit from more, have a blood test to check your levels. Do NOT take more than 10-mg. a day without consulting a doctor and having your levels checked first.

Additionally, you can raise your levels of DHEA with your actions. They can also be helpful in lowering your levels of cortisol. Here are a few of my favorite forms of stress-reduction that will help:

- Martial Arts;
- Meditation;
- Acupuncture;
- Yoga;
- Massage;
- My PACE™ exercise program.

---

[1] Wilson, James and Wright, Jonathan. Adrenal Fatigue: The 21st-Century Stress Syndrome. Santa Rosa: Smart Publications, 2002

[2] Adapted from Regelson W and Colman C, The Super-Hormone Promise, Pocket Books: New York 1996

Chapter 2

Warning! Mad Scientists at Work — on Your Blood Pressure

A Swiss biotechnology company wants to launch a "vaccine" against high blood pressure.[1] The idea is to "trick" your body into attacking itself. There's obviously something seriously wrong with this picture but it does give me something to talk about to help you get — and keep — a healthy blood pressure in a much safer way.

Here's how this treatment works.

There's a hormone your body makes closely linked to blood pressure called "angiotensin II." It binds to receptors in the lining of your blood vessels, causing them to tighten up.

That may sound like a bad thing at first, but you need angiotensin II in critical situations when your blood pressure suddenly drops. A serious injury, major dehydration, or anything that causes you to go into shock can make your blood pressure so low you could die. Angiotensin II comes to the rescue by naturally restoring blood pressure to safe levels.

Scientists have figured out a way to make a synthetic version of angiotensin II with a slightly different molecular make-up. The synthetic version is designed to "look" like a virus. Then they inject it into your bloodstream and "fool" your body into thinking it's getting attacked by a foreign invader.

Your immune system naturally kicks into gear. As it fights off the fake hormone, it attacks the real one at the same time. Your natural antibodies lock onto angiotensin II, so the real thing won't work. This is what causes your blood pressure to drop.

Just hope you don't have this stuff in your bloodstream if you get into a car accident or sustain a dangerous fall. Your body won't have any way to keep your blood pressure up — and save your life.

This treatment may actually worsen the problem and wind up causing heart disease because one of the main causes of arterial damage and heart disease is inflammation.

When the delicate tissue lining in your arteries becomes inflamed, it's vulnerable to all kinds of damage. Scar tissue forms and then bad stuff passing through your bloodstream gets caught on it, like a net in a stream. Cellular waste, calcium, and even healthy compounds like cholesterol and fat build up and become plaque.

When your body unleashes white blood cells to deal with an invader, they send for reinforcements using a class of hormones called "cytokines." One of the side effects of high levels of cytokines and an immune system working overtime is inflammation of tissue across your entire body.

This is a great example of the law of unintended consequences at work in so much of modern medical treatments. If you mobilize your immune system to attack your body, chances are you're going to worsen inflammation.

Practical, Natural, Effective and Safe

High blood pressure is not some isolated event that calls for targeted treatment. This isn't to say it's not a serious condition. Leave it untreated and you put yourself at risk for:

- Clogged arteries;
- Organ damage (kidneys, eyes, brain);
- Heart attack;
- Stroke.

It's also not a limited problem, either. About one in ten Americans has high blood pressure. And your risk goes up as you age. Yet you can lower your blood pressure safely with a few simple changes. Here are 10 surefire tips:

- **Throw out the cigarettes.** Nicotine makes your heart beat faster and your blood vessels constrict. In fact, if you smoke, you're five times more likely to have a heart attack and sixteen times more likely to suffer a stroke.

- **Shed the pounds.** If you're within a normal weight range, you don't have to worry about this step. But if you aren't, chances are you've got high blood pressure. About half of all people with high blood pressure are overweight.

- **Avoid these over-the-counter medicines.** Antihistamines, decongestants, cold remedies, and appetite suppressants may contain compounds that raise your blood pressure.

- **Watch your caffeine intake.** These get your heart racing, as you know, and can also lead to chronic hypertension.

- **Exercise.** But do it the right way. "Cardio" or endurance training will wind up stressing your body out. It responds by releasing cortisol, a hormone that increases blood pressure and weakens immunity. Short bursts of intense activity followed by rest is the best method for heart health, greater lean muscle mass... and low blood pressure. My PACE™ fitness program's a great way to do this.

- **Eat Cayenne.** Cayenne peppers contain a compound called "capsaicin." This is a natural, mild blood thinner that reduces clotting factors in your bloodstream that may lead to high blood pressure. The hotter the pepper, the better. Cayenne's also rich in vitamins E and C. Taken together, these three compounds will help you improve circulation, fight inflammation, clear congestion and boost immunity.

- **Snack on Celery.** Celery (including the oil and seeds) helps to lower blood pressure by relaxing the smooth muscles that line your blood vessels. As few as four stalks a day are all it takes to get the benefit.

- **Go Heavy on the Garlic.** Garlic's a great way to lower blood pressure. It's what's known as a "vasodilator," which means it opens your blood vessels up. A 12-week German study found that even powdered garlic significantly lowered blood pressure and improved cholesterol and triglyceride profiles.[2]

- **Keep your potassium levels high.** Diets low in potassium often lead to high blood pressure. The best way to get enough is to eat the right foods. Your muscles need a lot of it for efficient power generation. In fact, one of the signs of low potassium is muscle cramping. Here are a few potassium-rich foods:

Food	Potassium levels (mg.)
Figs (10 pieces, dried)	1,352
Avocado (whole or one cup)	1,319
Sun Dried Tomatoes (1/2 cup)	1,272
Pistachios (1 cup)	1,241
Apricots (1 cup)	1,222
Winter Squash (1 cup, mashed)	1,070
Almonds (1 cup, unsalted)	1,039
Pumpkin seeds (1/2 cup)	945
Bananas (1 large)	467

Get your calcium and magnesium. Low levels of both can lead to high blood pressure. Luckily, it's easy to get both through diet alone. Here are some foods rich in calcium and magnesium:

Calcium-Rich Foods	Magnesium-Rich Foods
Milk (1 cup)	Almonds (1 cup)
Yogurt (1 cup)	Tofu (1/2 cup)
Salmon (3 ounces)	Cashews (1 cup)
Cheese (1 ounce)	

---

[1] Sternberg S. "Blood pressure vaccine maybe on way." Health & Behavior. *USA Today.* 2/3/08.

[2] Auer, et al. "Hypertension and hyperlipidaemia: Garlic helps in mild cases." *British Journal of Clinical Practical Supplements.* 1990. 69:3-6

Chapter 3

But…Will She Get Better without Surgery?

"She needs to have it removed."

"But she's not dehydrated. She doesn't have any tenderness or Murphy's sign. She doesn't have an acute abdomen…"

In fact, A.D. didn't have any of the emergency symptoms they taught us in medical school.

"She must have colicystitis. She should have her gallbladder taken out."

"Well, what's the likelihood that if she doesn't have it removed, that her gallbladder will recover?"

"I wouldn't know."

At first I thought he was joking. I suppressed my chuckling when I saw he wasn't kidding. "You're a GI specialist…"

"You don't understand… I wouldn't know if she'd recover because I've never seen anybody with these symptoms who I've sent to have their gallbladder removed who hasn't had the surgery."

"What?"

This was the third GI doctor we'd been to, and the only thing any of them recommended was surgery. "How can you recommend surgery without considering the question of whether or not it's going to get better without surgery?"

"She has zero ejection fraction in her gallbladder. Normal is 35%. If someone has 34% I send them for surgery. If you don't want to do that… well, good luck."

No effort to save A.D.'s gallbladder. No care, no discussion, no attempt to find the cause of the problem.

I would have to do the research myself.

After a few days of some pretty intense reading, I discovered a little-known study.

A doctor put 69 people who were having gallbladder attacks on an elimination diet to determine their food allergies.

Here's the most embarrassing part to us doctors: Six of them had **already had their gallbladders removed** and were still having the exact same symptoms!

All 69 people — 100% of them — were totally symptom-free after they stopped eating foods they were allergic to.[1]

And all 69 had their symptoms come back when they started eating those foods again.

It made sense. When you have food allergies, your body treats those foods like a toxin. The lining of your gastrointestinal tract becomes inflamed in much the same way your sinuses become inflamed when you have respiratory allergies.

That inflammation causes the gallbladder's ejection fraction to go down — in other words, it doesn't empty out very well. It can look like you have colicystitis or gallbladder disease.

After I read the study, I had her blood drawn at my clinic to see if she had any food allergies. We found that she had a high percentage of a two different kinds of white blood cells — *granulocytes* and *eosinophils.*

That's exactly what you would have with an allergic reaction. So we did tests for a lot of food allergies, and discovered that A.D. is allergic to pork.

So I asked her if she had eaten any pork lately. Here's what she said:

"Oh wow. I ate the most ham I've ever eaten in my life! I bought this big ham, and made a stew from it and it was so delicious. I cut up the skin with all the fat still on it and put that in there because that's the part I like the most.

"My friends loved it! So I threw a party the next night and made the same thing for them. I ate another huge helping…"

The doctors didn't know that because they never bothered to ask her about her diet. Every GI specialist recommended gallbladder surgery without a word about what she might have eaten.

My clinical nurse M.T. drew A.D.'s blood, and when I told her what we were looking for M.T. said, "The same thing happened to me."

"I was pregnant and had the same symptoms. I had this craving for tuna salad and it had to have a lot of mayonnaise in it. I'd sit there and eat the stuff by the spoonful. After doing that for like two weeks I started to get pain. I went to my doctor.

"He sent me to a GI specialist, and he said 'Remove your gallbladder.'

"My doctor didn't want to do it during the pregnancy and wanted to put it off. The GI doctor said, 'No problem. It's not urgent. She has no emergent signs, but obviously she's going to need her gallbladder taken out. So just have it taken out after her pregnancy.'

"But when my craving went away and I stopped eating the mayonnaise, my symptoms went away. Never had them since."

Her gallbladder would be gone right now. And she'd be on medication the rest of her life. Without asking her anything about what she might have eaten. And there was zero effort or consideration by the doctors about whether or not — or how — someone can get better without surgery. It doesn't even come up in their minds.

And this is happening everywhere.

How could you care about your patient, and not ever in your professional career consider the question of whether this patient would get better without surgery before you refer them to surgery?

If you're going to refer them to surgery because of some algorithm — we did our job, we did the test, we did the ultrasound, it produced this result, that means they go to surgery — do you really care about the people who are coming in for help?

You cannot care and think that way.

They don't have any faith in nature or your body. They learn to do a differential diagnosis, and what you do about it always has to end in a drug therapy or an operation. Anything else is not worthy of consideration. To talk about what caused the problem is not part of the algorithm.

I think you have to say that these doctors are doing their job, but they don't think their job is really to empathize and take that suffering on themselves. Like when a friend comes to you for advice and you feel obligated.

They're not feeling that. It's so disconnected and removed from the patient. They just do this pattern of diagnosis that they learned in a class.

So think about what that means when a doctor says that he wouldn't know. When I think about all the people he sent to surgery, to me, it seemed like he really didn't care about the outcome of his patients.

Because if a doctor sends you to surgery, aren't you going to make the assumption that he's pretty certain you won't get better without the surgery? Otherwise, most people would think he wouldn't be recommending the operation in the first place.

But what most people don't know is that your gallbladder is not some useless organ. It helps you absorb the fat soluble vitamins A, D, E and K as well as the essential fatty acids omega-3 and omega-6.

And your stomach is a living system. You could almost think of your gut as a second brain. It's an integral part of your immune system and your body's intelligence. Most doctors completely ignore this.

But I tend to trust nature, and your body's ability to heal itself, until I'm proven wrong.

So if you've eaten and you have:

- A metallic taste, itching or swelling in your mouth;
- Difficulty swallowing or breathing;
- Nausea, vomiting, cramps diarrhea, or abdominal pain;
- Dizziness or lightheadedness...

You may be having an allergic reaction. These kinds of reactions can be very serious, and you should go to your doctor or the hospital if you're in pain. But mention to the medical professional what you may have eaten.

In the gallbladder study, the foods that caused the most allergic reactions were:

Food	Pct. of people with allergy
Eggs	92.8 %
Pork	63.8 %
Onions	52.2 %
Chicken/Turkey	34.8 %
Milk	24.6 %
Coffee	21.7 %
Oranges	18.8 %

Corn, beans, nuts, apples, tomatoes, peas, cabbage, spices, peanuts, fish, and rye also caused gallbladder attacks.

If you think you may have a food allergy, stop eating each of these foods one at a time and see if the reaction disappears. If you're still not sure, add each food back in to what you eat to see if the allergic reaction develops again.

To help protect your stomach and gallbladder, and keep your immune system and digestive system in top shape, I recommend these three things every day:

1. A Little Relaxation — Magnesium can stimulate gallbladder contraction and relaxes the muscles. One study looked at 42,075 men and followed them for 13 years. It found that those who took in the most magnesium (454 mg. a day) were 28% less likely to develop gallbladder problems compared to men with the lowest intake (262 mg.).[2]

In most cases, an effective dose is 400–500 mg. daily. If you have kidney problems or high-degree heart block, don't take any magnesium supplements until you talk to your doctor.

2. Calm Your Insides — Ginger keeps your digestion moving along smoothly. When researchers tested it with a group of healthy volunteers, their stomach contractions increased and food moved through more quickly.[3]

You can take dried ginger powder, but you'd need about 6,000 milligrams a day. An easier way to take ginger is a liquid extract. A half teaspoon a day should do the trick.

3. Fuel Your Flora — Glutamine is an amino acid that your immune and digestive systems rely heavily on. But did you know that the friendly little defenders in your gut called "microflora" can use it for fuel? Your microflora help protect your intestines from bad stuff that might be in your food. What's more, they help turn glutamine into glutathione, one of your body's most powerful antioxidants.[4] Take one gram (1,000 mg.) of L-glutamine three times a day.

---

[1] Breneman JC. "Allergy elimination diet as the most effective gallbladder diet." *Ann Allergy.* 1968 Feb;26(2):83-7.

[2] Tsai CJ, Leitzmann MF, Willett WC, et al. "Long-Term Effect of Magnesium Consumption on the Risk of Symptomatic Gallstone Disease Among Men." *Am J Gastro.* February 2008;103(2): 375-382.

[3] Wu KL, et al. "Effects of ginger on gastric emptying and motility in healthy humans." *Eur J Gastroenterol Hepatol.* 2008 May;20(5):436-40.

[4] Bergen W, Wu G. "Intestinal Nitrogen Recycling and Utilization in Health and Disease." *J. Nutr.* May 2009 vol. 139 no. 5 821-825.

PART 9

THROW AWAY YOUR JOGGING SHOES

Chapter 1

Beyond Aerobics — Your Native Fat Burner

Back in the late 1960s, Dr. Kenneth Cooper published *Aerobics* as the "perfect" way to "train" your heart. He thought that *medium intensity* aerobic exercise practiced three or four times a week was all you needed for heart health.

Today, we know the reality is different. A recent study by Harvard researchers shows that those who do short-duration, high-intensity workouts, reduce their risk of heart disease by ***100% more*** than those who practice aerobic exercise.[1]

A study published in the *Archives of Internal Medicine* showed that men and women who exercised at a higher intensity had lower blood pressure, lower triglycerides (blood fat), higher HDL (good cholesterol) and less body fat.[2]

What's more, *medium intensity* does not train your "high-energy output system" — your ability to get extra power fast. And that's exactly what we're missing in our modern world.

Forget Aerobics — Discover Your *REAL* Fat-Burning Zone

A few years ago, a patient of mine — B.P. — came to me saying that his cardiologist told him to never exceed his "aerobic threshold" when he exercised. But that's exactly what you need to do. By exceeding your aerobic capacity, you generate *real* heart and lung strength.

To better understand what your aerobic threshold is, we need to take a closer look at metabolism…

Aerobic means "with oxygen." So your aerobic metabolism combines oxygen with carbs, fats and proteins to make energy. Because walking is not a strenuous activity, you have plenty of oxygen available to make more and more energy. Using this model, you could walk for hours and not get too tired.

Jogging is a typical aerobic exercise because it can be sustained with oxygen metabolism (aerobic metabolism). But what happens when your body can't get enough oxygen from aerobic metabolism alone?

To answer that, let's say you start sprinting. You can't sustain that high output with oxygen alone. *That's the point at which the anaerobic system starts.* This is also known as crossing your **aerobic threshold**.

Anaerobic means "without oxygen." This system converts carbs — and some fats — into energy without using any oxygen at all. This will sustain you as you sprint. But obviously, you can't run at your peak output for very long.

When you pant after the exercise you've created an **oxygen debt**. This occurs when you ask your lungs for more oxygen than they can supply at that moment — like when you're sprinting.

Understanding when the anaerobic system kicks in is critical. When you're using your anaerobic system, you are training your *high-energy output system.*

When this happens, you are successfully building up reserve capacity in your heart, expanding your lung volume, triggering the production of growth hormone, and melting away fat.

And all these years, doctors, trainers and fitness "gurus" have been telling you to never cross that aerobic threshold!

But let's take this a step further — and this is the big misunderstanding that I want to set straight: *Aerobic and anaerobic can only be used to describe metabolism.* Aerobic and anaerobic shouldn't be applied to exercise. This is where modern exercise science has steered us in the wrong direction. It's possible for your cells to make energy without oxygen — but it's impossible for you to *exercise* without oxygen.

In essence, there's no such thing as anaerobic exercise. When you're sprinting, your body will start its anaerobic metabolism, but you are still breathing — still using oxygen. In fact, when your anaerobic system kicks in, your aerobic system is still functioning. *One does not replace the other.*

You either go at a rate you can sustain with oxygen or you exceed that rate, in which case you use both energy systems.

It's more appropriate to say that you've crossed over into your **supra-aerobic zone**.

By pushing yourself into your **supra-aerobic zone**, you're going to increase your ability to get high energy fast. This strengthens your heart, lungs and muscles.

Melt Away Extra Fat in Just 12 Minutes a Day

Remember — aerobic exercise is low to medium output held for an extended period. Supra-aerobic exercise is high output, but short in duration. Why is this important? For one thing, *it restores an element of your native environment.*

Our ancestors lived in a world where their food fought back. Predators attacked without notice. They had to run or fight — fast and hard. These short bursts of high-output activity fine-tuned our ancient ancestors and kept them fit. We still have the same physiology yet have lost that kind of challenge.

To move your workout into the anaerobic range, the key feature is this — you want to create an "oxygen debt" as I described earlier. Simply exercise at a pace you can't sustain for more than a short period. Ask your lungs for more oxygen than they can provide.

The difference between the oxygen you need and the oxygen you get is your oxygen debt. This will cause you to pant and continue to breathe hard even after you've stopped the exertion until you replace the oxygen you're lacking.

Here's another example. Let's say you pedal as fast as you can on a bike for 15 seconds. When you stop, you continue to pant. This is the kind of high-output challenge you can't sustain for very long. You have reached a **supra-aerobic zone**. This is very different from doing an aerobic workout for 45 minutes.

This is the basis of my PACE™ program. I began using most of this program 25 years ago. More recently, I added *progressivity* to increase the benefits.

By making small changes in the same direction, your workouts can produce remarkable results. And you only need 12 minutes to achieve the desired effect.

In a matter of weeks, you can:

- Lose pounds of belly fat.
- Build functional new muscle.
- Reverse heart disease.
- Build energy reserves available on demand.
- Strengthen your immune system.
- Reverse many of the changes of aging.

---

[1] Lee I., et al. *Circulation* 2003 Mar 4; 1087 (8): 2220-6.

[2] Williams P. Relationships of heart disease risk factors to exercise quantity and intensity. *Arch Intern Med.* 1998;158:237-245.

Chapter 2

The Key to Fitness — Advancing to the Next Level

Last month, I told you about pushing past your aerobic threshold and entering your *real* fat-burning zone. Now that you have a good foundation, you can start to add the elements that make PACE™ uniquely effective.

In a nutshell, you'll use this system to practice and train your ability to use energy at a *higher rate* — this is your **high-energy output system** we talked about last month. And you'll practice and train getting to that higher output *faster*.

Why bother?

Because if you never challenge your current aerobic capacity, breathing rate, cardiac output or the maximal metabolic rate that you can achieve, these systems will inevitably decline — in the same way that muscles you don't challenge will weaken and atrophy.

If you've ever broken a bone and worn a cast, you know how fast and far muscles you're not using shrink. Your physiology and "metabolic fitness" adapt and respond in the same way.

The training of your high-energy output system is critical to your health improvement, disease resistance, fat-fighting, energizing and anti-aging capacities. It's incredible that no popular exercise program has ever specifically addressed this issue.

On the surface, it would be dangerous — even foolhardy — to go on an intense exercise rampage to challenge your heart, lung, vascular and metabolic capacities. What you need is a plan to build these capacities safely and effectively.

PACE™ is the first and only program conceived, designed, tested and proven to achieve this most important of all fitness goals. It does this for you by measuring where you are, then making progressive, small, incremental changes over time.

It is a flexible plan that works equally well for athletic power lifters, marathoners, extremely deconditioned couch potatoes, overly aerobicized fitness buffs, elders and even heart patients in rehabilitation. It is effective and safe *because* of its flexibility.

It's flexible because it's not focused on what you do as much as the direction of your change over time.

The key is to start with a brief exertion that is comfortable for you at your current capacity. It's not so important how hard you exert yourself today. It's that little bit that you do next week that you didn't do this week. This is the element of ***progressivity***.

That tiny incremental change compounds — like interest on capital — to have an amazing and powerful effect over time. By changing your program through time, you work with your metabolism and your inborn adaptive response to coach your body to change.

The Four-Week Progression: Your Easy 12-Minute PACE™ Program

Here's a simple program to use progressivity in the right direction. In the 12-minute program below, you're going to focus on gradually increasing the challenge as you progress.

To aid in this effort, and to make your body accept the proper signal to gear up your metabolism, this program also simultaneously decreases the duration of the exercise period. This has synergistic power that will surprise you.

Weeks	Warm-up	Set 1		Set 2		Set 3	
		Exertion	Recovery	Exertion	Recovery	Exertion	Recovery
1	3 min	6 min	3 min				
2	2 min	3 min	2 min	3 min	2 min		
3	2 min	2 min	2 min	2 min	2 min	2 min	2 min
4	3 min	1 min	2 min	1 min	2 min	1 min	2 min

Notice the *progressive* feature of this workout. Over time, the **duration** of each exertion period *decreases*. This *progressivity in the right direction* toward maximal capacity is the heart of PACE™.

During Week 1, you're going to take it easy and just do one warm up for three minutes and then one exercise set at a <u>low to moderate</u> intensity. Just do what feels comfortable. If you are not in very good shape, just start with walking.

Go slow for the warm-up, pick up the pace of your walk a little during the exertion period and drop to a slow pace again during the recovery. During each recovery period focus on returning your breathing rate to near your resting rate — about 12 to 16 breaths per minute is ideal.

Try and do this 20-minute interval at least three times during the first week. <u>But each time you do it, slightly</u> *increase* <u>the intensity level</u>. By the end of the first week, you should feel like you've given yourself a slight challenge you were able to accomplish.

NOTE: How you adjust the intensity will depend on what instrument you're using. If you're on a stationary bike, increase the level on the control panel so it becomes harder to pedal. If you're on an elliptical, boost the incline so it's harder to run.

How hard you push yourself should depend on your current level of conditioning. At this beginning stage, don't push yourself too hard. This is just a warm-up.

During Week 2, you'll add another exercise set. But the duration of your exertion periods will decrease. After a two-minute warm up, you'll do a three-minute exertion period. As you start, notice how fast you're going and how long it takes for your heart and lungs to meet the challenge.

When three minutes is up, begin your recovery. If you need to stop, that's okay. Otherwise, your recovery period should be a slow, easy pace. If you're on an elliptical machine for example, you should slow down so you feel like you're walking.

As always during your recovery period, focus on your heart rate slowing down. If you start to pant, let it happen. Feel your lungs quickly fill up and release. Allow your body to come back to a state of rest.

During Week 3, you'll start with a two-minute warm up and then a two-minute exertion period. <u>But this time, increase the intensity to give yourself more of a challenge</u>.

When two minutes is up, begin your recovery. Repeat this process for exercise Sets 2 and 3. During Week 3, try and repeat this workout three or four times.

When you hit Week 4, you're going to do three exercise sets as in Week 3. Except this time, you're going to reduce the exertion periods to just one minute each, followed by two-minute recovery periods.

Apply the same principles. Take your warm-up at a low to moderate intensity. Then turn up the intensity when you start your first exertion period.

Remember, don't stress yourself. It's not necessary to work that intensely. <u>By decreasing the duration, it will actually feel easier as the four weeks progress</u>. Part of the PACE™ program is realizing that real progress can be made in just minutes a day.

Chapter 3

Stop "Aerobicising" — Meet a Girl's New Best Friend

Most women spend hours every week watching their weight and taking care of their health. If you do, I applaud your effort. But if you are like my patients, you don't realize that for maximum weight loss, minimal aging and the best-looking body, much of your effort is taking you in the wrong direction.

I'll show you why aerobics is working against you to accelerate your aging, and how to reverse it and get that killer body you've always wanted.

Your Fat-Free Body Takes Just Minutes a Day

Let me start by telling you about a simple study I did on a couple of young women. They are identical twins. One twin followed my PACE™ program. It's based on alternating periods of **exertion** and **recovery** for about 10 minutes a day. The other followed a traditional aerobic exercise program. I tracked their progress over 16 weeks.

At the end of the study, the twin doing interval training lost 18 pounds of fat and increased her muscle mass by eight pounds. The twin doing long bouts of aerobic exercise lost only seven pounds of fat and actually lost two pounds of muscle mass. By the end of the study, the twin using my PACE™ program had much better muscle tone, and an overall healthier look. The amount of time she spent working out was about one fifth that as the other twin.

Aerobics Won't Help You Lose Weight — and Studies Prove It

My study isn't the only one that shows aerobic exercise is a dismal failure when it comes to weight loss. Researchers at George Washington University looked closely at how well diet, aerobic exercise, and dieting combined with aerobics work to help you lose weight.

These researchers analyzed 25 years' worth of study results to see what is most effective for weight loss. I bet you'll be surprised at what they found.

People using diet alone to lose weight lost an average of 10.7 pounds. People using both together lost an average of 11 pounds.[1] That's right — adding aerobic exercise to a weight loss diet makes hardly any difference at all. It's no wonder aerobics leave you feeling disappointed and frustrated. It's just a poor weight loss tool.

Now contrast this to the results of my PACE™ program from my twin study.

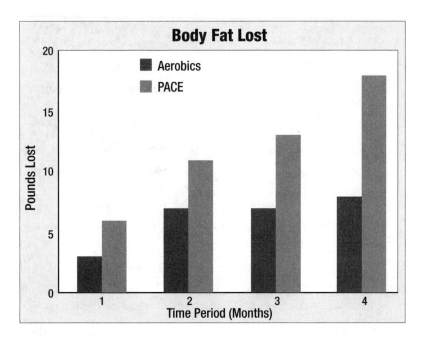

Over four months, the "PACE™" twin lost over 18 pounds of fat. The "aerobics" twin lost just seven pounds. And the "aerobics" twin also lost two pounds of critical muscle mass. What's more, the PACE™ twin's workouts lasted less than 15 minutes. Her "aerobic" sister sweated for hours.

A Better Way to Lose Weight — *Fast!*

What works when it comes to weight loss is a different kind of activity.

Researchers from Laval University in Quebec compared long duration cardio exercise with short duration high intensity workouts. For 20 weeks, half the participants did five 45-minute workouts a week at moderate intensity. The other half did 19 high intensity interval workouts (like my PACE™ program) over the course of 15 weeks.

Although the second group spent less time exercising, and only did half the work as the first group, they increased their aerobic capacity by 30%. What's more, the second group lost nine times as much body fat as the first group.[2] That's right — they lost **nine times more fat.**

So what is PACE™? Well first of all, it's simple, fun, and it's easy to stick with. PACE™ stands for **P**rogressively **A**ccelerating **C**ardiopulmonary **E**xertion. It's a way to work out that uses short duration bursts that slowly get stronger as you get more fit.

Start Today—You'll See Dramatic Results within Weeks

Warm Up	Set 1		Set 2		Set 3		Set4	
	Exertion	Recovery	Exertion	Recovery	Exertion	Recovery	Exertion	Recovery
2 min	1 min	1 min	1 min	1 min	1 min	1 min	1 min	1 min

Exertion periods are always followed by *recovery periods*. Together, they make an *exercise set*. So let's use this 10-minute program to get a better idea of how it works.

Look at the program chart above. After an easy warm-up, your first minute is an exertion period. For the next 60 seconds, you're going to exercise at a pace that gives your heart and lungs a challenge.

If you're new to exercise, or feel out-of-shape, take it easy for the first two weeks. The speed and intensity of your exertion period should be fast enough for you to break a sweat, but not so intense that you can't finish the 10-minute program.

Let's say you're in the gym and you decide to try the stationary bike. First, make sure you're comfortable. Adjust the seat and choose a level of resistance that will give you a slight challenge. On a stationary bike, the resistance will make it harder to pedal.

Begin to pedal and make note of the time. Your first exertion period is just 60 seconds so time yourself accordingly.

After your first exertion period, begin your first recovery period. During your recovery period, slow down to an easy pace — as if you're walking. If you need to stop, you can. Otherwise, simply slow down and go at a slow, easy speed. This gives your body a chance to rest and recover.

Your recovery periods are crucial. They're more than just empty spaces between the repetition intervals. Recovery is the flip side of exertion. Training your body to recover is one of the keys to your success.

During your recovery periods, focus on your breath and feel your heart rate starting to slow down. Feel your heart and breath returning to a resting level before you move on.

Now that you have a feel for it, repeat the process. Start your next exertion period and follow it with a recovery period. You'll soon get into the groove of exercising in short bursts followed by periods of rest.

Getting your feet wet with the basics will help you get started right away. What's more, it will prepare you for a deeper level of your PACE™ program, which adds other dimensions like acceleration, intensity and duration.

---

[1] Miller WC, Koceja DM, Hamilton EJ. "A meta-analysis of the past 25 years of weight loss research using diet, exercise or diet plus exercise intervention." Int J Obes Relat Metab Disord. 1997 Oct;21(10):941-7.

[2] Tremblay A, Simoneau JA, Bouchard C. "Impact of exercise intensity on body fatness and skeletal muscle metabolism." Metabolism. 1994 Jul;43(7):814-8.

PART 10

CALCIUM DOING MORE HARM THAN GOOD?

Chapter 1

Calcium Increases Risk of Bone Fracture

The Harvard Nurses Study followed 77,761 nurses for 12 years, examining the link between dietary calcium and bone fractures. You might be surprised, but nurses who had the highest calcium intake actually had an increased risk of bone fracture.[1]

One thing is certain: when it comes to making your bones stronger, taking calcium is not the answer. Fortunately, there are alternatives to calcium that do work. I'll tell you my experience and how you can use what I've learned to keep bones as strong as steel until the day they put you in the earth.

Why Don't Calcium Supplements Work?

As you age, there's a slowing down in the ability of your bones to grow new tissue. What's more, your bones can lose their natural calcium through the action of cells that take calcium away from your bone fluid and transfer it to your blood.

And when your bones become more brittle and your muscle strength decreases, you're more at risk for falls and broken bones.

Taking calcium supplements isn't the best way to guard against these dangers because **hormones control the amount of calcium that sticks to your bones**. Falling estrogen and testosterone levels cause calcium to drop away from your bones. Hormones counteract the short-term rise in bone density you get from taking calcium. Your bones will actually become more brittle than before.

For years I've been pointing out to my patients that while the U.S. has the highest intake of calcium, our rates of osteoporosis are the highest in the world. Countries with lower intakes of calcium have lower rates of hip fracture and osteoporosis.[2]

And calcium supplements also interfere with the absorption of other minerals, which can then create deficiencies in these other minerals that you wouldn't otherwise have.

If that isn't enough, there is evidence that men who take high amounts of calcium increase their chance of developing prostate cancer.[3]

Here's the good news: there's an effective way to combat brittle bones. It's an element found in the earth's crust.

Boost Your Bone Strength with This Natural Element

It's called strontium. If it rings any bells for you, it may from news reports early in the Cold War that mentioned the radioactive properties of a different form of the element, strontium-90.

The form we're interested in is strontium ranelate. The National Cancer Institute lists it as an element that lowers the risk of bone fractures.[4] How? By helping to protect against bone loss and helping new bone tissue to grow.

All of us are eager to prevent debilitating injuries that restrict our mobility and reduce our independence, such as spine and hip fractures.

Researchers have found that strontium is effective in preventing both.

In one study, with a daily oral dose of 2g of strontium ranelate (providing 680 mg. of strontium), elderly women with osteoporosis reduced the risk of vertebral fractures by 40–50%. In another, their risk of hip fracture went down 36% with strontium supplement.[5]

And strontium ranelate was the only treatment proven to be effective in preventing vertebral and hip fractures in women 80 and above.[6]

Because of its chemical similarity, strontium can act as a substitute for calcium, helping to strengthen bones and teeth. Evidence also suggests that strontium can help guide calcium into bones.[7]

Researchers are looking into exactly how strontium improves our bone strength. Bone is made of an inner spongy core similar to a honeycomb and a tougher outer layer. One recent study showed that strontium may improve your bone's mechanical strength by thickening the outer layer and improving the structure of the inner layer.[8]

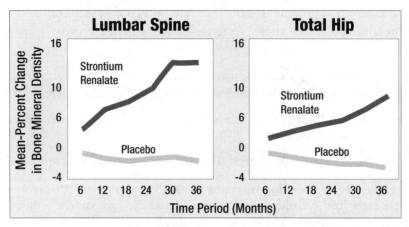

Adapted from Neuiner et al. 350 (5): 459, Figure 3, "Effects of Stronium Ranelate on Bone Mineral Density in all Patients Receiving 2g a day or oral strontium ranelate," *New England Journal of Medicine*, Jan 29, 2004

Strontium also showed promise in combating metastatic bone cancer, cancer that has spread to the bones.

People with this condition can have bones so weak they collapse just by bearing the weight of the body. X-rays of patients who had taken strontium for over three months showed new mineral deposits in the parts of the bone that had been eaten away by the cancer.[9]

Preserve Your Independence

We all want to continue living independent lives even as we age. To do this, we need strong bones that can keep us upright and mobile. Strontium can help us preserve our independence by preventing fractures and keeping our bones sturdy.

Strontium is naturally present in soils, so people used to obtain it in the foods and water they consumed. But due to the commercialization of agriculture, the minerals in our soil have become severely depleted. It is now very difficult to get sufficient amounts of minerals from just diet alone. There is no RDA for strontium. However, **a safe and effective dosage that I recommend is 680 mg. per day**, the amount used in the above-mentioned study.

It's important to remember that bone power is not gained through strontium alone. Here are a few simple things you can add to boost your bone strength:

- Exercise. This is a sure way to make your bones denser and stronger. The best way to increase bone density and reduce fractures is body-weight exercises (like calisthenics) and short bursts of high intensity exercise (like sprints). Try it two or three times a week.

- Take vitamin D. Most people don't realize it, but vitamin D is also a hormone. It directs your calcium metabolism. It helps your body absorb it into the bone. Your skin makes vitamin D in response to ultraviolet light from sunlight. Few foods contain vitamin D except dairy and eggs. I recommend taking 400 IU per day of a vitamin D supplement.

- Eat your greens. They contain vitamin K, which regulates calcium while stabilizing bones. And it regulates blood clotting. The best sources are spinach, kale, collard greens, mustard greens and broccoli.

- Eat foods rich in B-complex vitamins. Your body uses B vitamins in bone building. The best sources are liver, eggs, lean meats, raw nuts, asparagus, broccoli and bananas.

---

[1] Feskanich D, Willett WC, et al. "Milk, dietary calcium, and bone fractures in women: a 12-year prospective study." *Am J Public Health.* 1997 Jun;87(6):992-7

[2] Millstine D, Bergstrom L, et al. "Calcium: Too Much of a Good Thing?" *Journal of Women's Health.* November 22, 2013.

[3] Chan JM, Stampfer MJ, et al. "Dairy products, calcium, and prostate cancer risk in the Physicians' Health Study." *American Journal of Clinical Nutrition.* October 2001.

[4] "Handout on Health: Osteoporosis." National Institute of Arthritis and Musculo-skeletal and Skin Diseases. August 2014.

[5] "Strontium Ranelate" International Osteoporosis Foundation.

[6] Blake G.M., and Fogelman, I. "Strontium ranelate: a novel treatment for post-menopausal osteoporosis: a review of safety and efficacy." *Clin Interv Aging.* 2006 Dec; 1(4): 367-375.

[7] Dean W, MD. "Strontium: Breakthrough Against Osteoporosis." World Health Network. May 5, 2004.

[8] Zacchetti G, Dayer R, et al. "Systemic Treatment with Strontium Ranelate Accelerates the Filling of a Bone Defect and Improves the Material Level Properties of the Healing Bone." *BioMed Research International.* Published 28 August 2014.

[9] Dean W, MD. "Strontium: Breakthrough Against Osteoporosis." World Health Network. May 5, 2004.

Chapter 2

Use Nature's "Glue" for Stronger Bones

In spite of what you hear on TV, calcium supplements have little to do with the strength of your bones.

Taking calcium supplements will give you a short-term boost in bone density, but that's it. Over time, your hormones will work against the extra calcium and actually leave your bones more brittle than before.

Consider this: the U.S. has the highest intake of calcium, yet our rates of osteoporosis are the highest in the world. Countries with lower intakes of calcium have lower rates of hip fracture and osteoporosis.[1]

A lack of calcium isn't why your bones become weak.

Osteoporosis is caused by a number of factors. I've written to you about vitamin D3 and PACE™-style exercise. Both are critical for strong bones and a steel-like frame.

But here's something I bet your doctor never told you: there's a commonly overlooked vitamin that acts as a "glue" to build strong, healthy, impact-resistant bones.

One Japanese study found this "glue" to be just as effective as drugs used to prevent bone fractures.

In the study, women taking a 45 mg. dose of this "glue" only had a fracture rate of 8%. Those taking the drug Didronel had a fracture rate of 8.7%. And get this…

The fracture rate in the placebo group was almost three times as high (a whopping 21%).[2]

Did Your Doctor Tell You about This?

Most doctors and the media still insist you pop calcium pills and drink plenty of milk.

But here's what they usually miss:

It doesn't matter how much calcium you consume. If your body isn't metabolizing that calcium properly, it's not doing your bones any good.

A major key in preventing osteoporosis — and even reversing it — is to simply make sure your body regulates calcium properly.

Fortunately, the solution is simple.

I'm talking about vitamin K2.

Vitamin K naturally comes in two forms.

The first is vitamin K1. This is the type normally found in green, leafy vegetables and helps mainly with blood clotting.

Vitamin K2, on the other hand, is responsible for regulating calcium.

It's in charge of telling your body when to fuse the calcium into your bones to make them stronger and denser.

Chances Are You're Not Getting Enough

Your bone is a complex structure. It's composed of mineral crystals and cells that are bound together by matrix proteins.

The most important of these is the calcium-regulating protein osteocalcin. It's under vitamin K2's control.

It tells the osteocalcin proteins to go through a process called carboxylation. Once carboxylated, they can create new bone tissue.

The trouble starts when you don't get enough K2.

When levels of this critical vitamin are low, osteocalcin can't undergo carboxylation.

The end result?

It can't glue itself to the bone and create new bone tissue. Over time, the bone becomes porous and weak, making it prone to fracture.

The scary part is that it's all too easy to be K2-deficient. That's because it occurs in very small quantities in the diet compared to K1.

Because of this, most people get 10 times more K1 in their diets than K2. The good news is, there are a few K2-rich sources of food that are accessible and cheap. I'll share those with you in just a moment.

But first, you should know that frail bones aren't the only reason you want to make sure you're getting adequate amounts of K2…

Osteoporosis Means Bad News for Your Heart

The connection isn't obvious, but your bone health and heart health are linked.

A team of scientists from California studied plaque tissue from arteries. Inside they found several key components that are critical to bone formation.[3]

Why is this important?

Osteoporosis doesn't just mean weak bones. It's a risk factor for heart disease.

See, K2 also controls another important bone-building protein known as matrix GLA-protein.

Without K2, matrix GLA-protein can't undergo the same carboxylation process that osteocalcin undergoes. New research is showing this plays a role in calcification of the arteries.

For example, researchers bred mice to lack the matrix GLA-protein. The mice died within a few weeks after birth due to the unrestrained calcium deposits in their arteries.[4]

In humans, the effects of a lack of vitamin K2 are similar.

One study followed a group of people taking the popular blood-thinning drug Coumadin (warfarin), which blocks vitamin K1 and K2. They were compared against a group not taking the drug.

The findings were astonishing.

Not only did those taking Coumadin suffer more bone fractures, they had two times as many calcium deposits in their heart valves and arteries.[5]

This Overlooked Nutrient Could Save Your Life

The evidence is overwhelming. Vitamin K2 not only protects your bones, but it's also a potent heart-defender.

This became clear in the Rotterdam Heart Study. Dutch researchers followed 4,800 participants over the course of seven years.

Those with the highest levels of vitamin K2 had a 57% reduced death rate from heart disease than those who had the lowest levels. This relationship did not hold true with vitamin K1.[6]

What's more, this same study found that getting enough K2 in your diet can reduce severe aortic calcification by 52% and overall mortality by 26%.

With findings like these, it's surprising vitamin K2 hasn't gotten much press.

Six Easy Ways to Get More of Nature's "Glue"

You don't need much vitamin K2 to reap the benefits. Here are a few ways to make sure you're getting enough to keep your bones strong and your heart healthy:

1. Egg Yolks — I've been telling my patients for years to eat them. Eggs are not the enemy. So eat them without fear. Not only will you get a good dose of K2, but you'll also get plenty of vitamins and nutrients. Whenever possible, choose cage-free, vegetarian-fed eggs.

2. Organ Meats — If you've got a taste for it, liver is an excellent choice. Personally, I love liver and onions. Make sure you get your organ meats from grass-fed, free-range cattle.

3. Natto — This ancient Japanese dish contains, by far, the highest concentrations of K2. Natto is made of soybeans that have been fermented with the bacterium *Bacillus subtilis*. In Japan, it's a popular breakfast food. Some grocery stores usually carry it. But you can also check local Asian markets in your area. I must warn you though, natto is an acquired taste.

4. Traditionally Fermented Cheese — Two cheeses in particular have moderately high amounts of K2. Swiss Emmental and Norwegian Jarlsberg.

5. Menaquinone (MK-7) — Supplementing is always a good option. Make sure it's the MK-7 form of vitamin K2. This is usually made out of a natto extract. Be sure to choose a supplement that's been extracted from non-genetically modified (non-GMO) soybeans. You can find MK-7 at your local health-food store. I recommend 45 to 90 mcg. per day.

---

[1] Millstine D, Bergstrom L, et al. "Calcium: Too Much of a Good Thing?" *Journal of Women's Health*. November 22, 2013.

[2] Frisoli A Jr, Chaves PH, Pinheiro, MM, et al. "The effect of nandrolone decanoate on bone mineral density, muscle mass, and hemoglobin levels in elderly women with osteoporosis: a double-blind, randomized, placebo-controlled clinical trial." *J Gerontol A Biol Sci Med Sci*. May;60(5):648-53.

[3] Bostrom K, Watson KE, Horn S, et al. Bone morphogenetic protein expression in human atherosclerotic lesions. J Clin Invest. 1993 Apr;91(4):1800-9.

[4] Luo G, Ducy P, McKee MD, et al. Spontaneous calcification of arteries and cartilage in mice lacking matrix GLA protein. Nature. 1997 Mar 6;386(6620):78-81.

[5] Barclay L, MD. "Vitamin K & Warfarin." *Life Extension Magazine*. June 2007.

[6] Geleijnse JM, Vermeer C, Grobbee DE, et al. Dietary intake of menaquinone is associated with a reduced risk of coronary heart disease: the Rotterdam Study. J Nutr. 2004 Nov;134(11):3100-5.

Chapter 3

How to Build Strong Bones
That Last a Lifetime

I have some news for you that goes against almost everything you hear on CBS News, or read on WebMD — *osteoporosis isn't caused by a lack of calcium.*

Mainstream medicine still has its head in the sand on this. I read a study from the *Journal of the American Dietetic Association* claiming — again — that you aren't getting enough calcium, and that calcium is what prevents osteoporosis.

Don't get me wrong — calcium is critical for making bone. But you're getting enough calcium. It's in almost everything you can think of — bread, milk, orange juice, pasta, yogurt, toothpaste, chewing gum, snack crackers, and granola bars. It's even in your water, depending on where you live. That's a lot of calcium.

In fact, two studies back up what I've known for years. Higher calcium intake doesn't prevent fractures due to bone loss,[1] and can damage your heart.

A brand new study looked at over 195,000 women and found that drinking milk fortified with calcium had zero effect on the risk for hip fractures.[2]

Another new study in the journal *Osteoporosis International* found that taking calcium supplements meant a 27-31% increase in risk of heart attack and up to a 20% increased risk of stroke. The authors even suggest you use "other osteoporosis treatments that are available without calcium."[3]

A third study that just came out a few days ago looked at 61,443 women, who were followed for almost 20 years. It found that increasing your daily calcium has no effect on fractures later in life. The women who took in the most calcium *did not reduce the risk of fractures of any type, or of osteoporosis.*[4]

If things keep going the way they're going today, you have a one in four chance of an osteoporosis-related bone break after you turn 50.

It's worse if you're a woman. You have a one in two chance of fracture. You're at greater risk because women lose bone mass a little faster than men until they're 65. After that, everyone loses bone at about the same rate.

And a broken bone has a huge effect on your life. You could be in constant pain, lose mobility, have a long-term disability, or completely lose your independence.

Instead of taking in more calcium, let me show you how you can build bones that will last a lifetime.

But first I want to tell you a little bit about how your body makes bone.

Your bones have cells called *osteoclasts.* Their job is to remove old bone tissue. This makes room for your bones to grow strong because other cells called *osteoblasts* then rebuild them.

With osteoporosis and other bone diseases, there is an imbalance — either your osteoblasts aren't making new cells fast enough, or osteoclasts are removing too much bone tissue.

Some very common medications can also make your bones weaker and more likely to break. For example:

- The newest drugs meant to improve bone density actually cause bone breaks. Bisphosphonates like Fosamax, Boniva, Reclast and Actonel are supposed to help stop you from getting bone fractures as you get older.

Researchers studied women taking these medications who experienced some sort of fracture. *Over 65%* had the same rare fracture in the same area of their thigh bones. And these were the women who had been on the drugs for the longest time.[5]

- If you use cortisone for your asthma or arthritis for longer than only three months, it increases risk of fracture regardless of bone density.[6]

- Acid reflux medications like Nexium and Prevacid increase risk of hip fracture. A review so new it hasn't even been published yet looked at over 230,000 fracture cases. These medications, called proton pump inhibitors, upped the odds of suffering a hip fracture by 25%. The odds of getting a spinal fracture increased by 50%![7]

- Antidepressants like Paxil and Prozac (called SSRIs) contribute to bone loss and a higher risk for fractures. That's because antidepressants increase serotonin levels, and too much serotonin restrains osteoblasts from making new bone.

The journal *Bone* published a study on almost 80,000 people and found SSRI users had almost twice the risk of osteoporosis-related fractures as those who didn't use those medications. Even people who used non-SSRI antidepressants had around a 40% higher risk for a break.[8]

- Long-term therapy with antiepileptic drugs (phenobarbital) can cause the metabolic bone disease osteomalacia. This causes "soft bones" and increases fractures. In one study, antiepileptic drugs reduced both neck and hip bone density, and caused significant bone loss.[9]

- Another study from *Bone* done just last month found that the odds of getting a fracture were 56% higher for people who use acetaminophen (Tylenol, Excedrin) compared with people who don't. Adjusting for age, bone mineral density, weight, smoking, calcium and other factors didn't change the results.[10]

It's another example of how modern medicine doesn't learn from its mistakes. They refuse to take a whole-body approach to healing. Instead they opt to treat individual symptoms with drugs designed only for those symptoms, regardless of how they affect the rest of your body.

This is why in my practice, I seldom use these drugs. I've helped thousands of patients — both men and women — increase their bone mass and strength naturally. Here's what I tell them:

Step 1) Use This Hormonal Secret to Build Bones of Steel: Hormones control the amount of calcium that sticks to your bones. You can take all the calcium you want, but if your estrogen and testosterone levels fall, calcium will drop away from your bones.

In women, estrogens are the main regulators of bone breakdown. And the hormone progesterone controls the rate of new bone deposits. The higher the progesterone level the more bone formation. But the most powerful bone builder in both men and women is testosterone. Testosterone is central for achieving maximal bone mass and strength.

Maintaining healthy levels of hormones in your body will keep your bones strong.

There is an easy and inexpensive hormone precursor that has been shown to improve the levels of other sex hormones. It's called DHEA (Dehydroepiandrosterone). It is involved in the manufacturing of most major sex hormones in the body, like estrogen and testosterone. DHEA treatments are becoming more common.

You can purchase it over the counter, but I don't advise that anyone take DHEA without having their blood levels checked. You will have to ask your doctor to measure it. You just can't count on maintaining good bone health without good hormonal health.

In addition to healthy hormone levels, here are some other ways to help you keep your bone strength, and your independence:

Step 2) Drive Down Cortisol to Form More Bone: There is a membrane that lines the outer surface of your bones called the *periosteum*. Its cells turn into osteoblast cells that make new bone. The "stress" hormone cortisol reduces bone density by stopping those cells from becoming osteoblasts. That's why the higher your cortisol levels, the lower your bone density and the faster you lose bone. Cortisol also reduces calcium absorption.

Both mental and physical stress increase cortisol, and those stressors are constant in the modern world. Also, most hormones decline with age, but cortisol increases.

To lower cortisol naturally so you can keep your bones strong, the easiest thing to do is counter cortisol with physical exertion.

My program is designed specifically to return your body and metabolism to their natural states. With PACE™, you incrementally challenge your body and restore your native metabolism and hormone levels.

The other benefit you get from PACE™ is that weight-bearing exercise is one of the most effective ways to increase your bone strength and help prevent fractures. These include walking, bicycling, sprints, swimming or weight training. Focus on increasing intensity, not duration, in all of these exercises.

Another way to turn back the effects of our stressful modern environment is to supplement with DHEA. I use it at my Wellness Clinic regularly. I call it the "anti-stress hormone." You secrete DHEA when times are good — when you are well-fed, secure and free of stressors.

The more DHEA in your body, the less effect stress will have on you. That's because DHEA is the antidote to cortisol.

It's important for you to get your DHEA levels checked. Your doctor can perform the simple test.

A common dose that I use is 5–10 mg. daily, but no more than that. You can take it any time but it best mimics your natural daily levels when you take it first thing in the morning.

Step 3) Soak up the Sun and Build Better Bones: Vitamin D is a vitamin and a hormone. It directs how much calcium you store in your bones so you can use it when you need it. Too little vitamin D can lead to thin, brittle bones and osteoporosis.

By preventing bone loss, vitamin D:

- Reduces risk of breaking a bone in any part of the body by 33%.

- Reduces risk of a breaking a hip by 69%.

- Reduces risk of having constant bone pain — a condition called osteomalacia.

Your best source of vitamin D is sunshine. You don't need more than 20 minutes out in the sun to get all your vitamin D for the day. But since we spend most of our time inside in the modern world, you might have to get your vitamin D from other sources. Food sources of vitamin D include salmon, mackerel, tuna fish, sardines, eggs, beef, and cheese.

Of course, you can also get vitamin D from supplements. Cod liver oil is by far the best source. Take up to one tablespoon a day.

Step 4) Make "Superior" Bones with Vitamin K: I've helped hundreds of patients regulate their calcium and stabilize their bones using vitamin K. A new study completed last month found that high vitamin K intake means higher bone mineral density, and less bone loss with aging.[11] The authors wrote that vitamin K gave people "superior bone properties."

Foods with vitamin K include dark leafy vegetables like kale, spinach and collard greens. Parsley and green olives also have vitamin K, as do the spices basil and thyme. I recommend at least 90 mcg. a day.

Step 5) Protect Your Bones with Selenium: Just 55 micrograms a day can help reduce your risk of osteoporosis by up to 15%.

A study gave two groups of animals a drug that causes osteoporosis. They treated one group with selenium. When researchers looked at the leg bones, those from the selenium group were protected, and looked almost like normal bone.[12]

The best source of selenium is Brazil nuts, which contain a whopping 544 micrograms in just one ounce. You can also get selenium from red meat, tuna, eggs, and walnuts.

Step 6) Harden Your Bones with Boron: It's crucial to bone strength, with increasing benefits as people age. Boron keeps bones from losing calcium and magnesium. The best way to get it from food is by eating nuts, plums, prunes, red grapes, raisins, apples, pears, and avocados. One thing I sometimes tell patients is to make all-natural trail mix from their snack food of choice. All those raisins and nuts are a great source of boron. Get between three and six mg. per day.

Step 7) Ramp Up Energy to Make New Bone: It takes a lot of energy for your body to produce bone. Osteoblasts use a hormone called osteocalcin to tell your body to make that energy so the osteoblasts can do their job.

There's only one problem — leptin. This hormone, that increases when you gain weight, interferes with osteocalcin and inhibits new bone formation.

Fortunately, there's a solution for leptin. The herb *irvingia gabonensis*, from the forests of West Africa, helps leptin work normally.

One study measured the effect of irvingia on fat cells. They injected the cells with irvingia and found that the herb significantly reduced leptin production, and leptin levels. Those given the most irvingia cut their leptin levels by over 60% in just 12 to 24 hours.[13]

Another irvingia study found that people taking the seed extract were able to drop their leptin levels by 49%.[14]

I recommend 150 mg. of irvingia seed extract twice a day before meals.

[1] Freskanich, D., et al., "Milk, dietary calcium, and bone fractures in women: a 12-year prospective study," *American Journal of Public Health* June 1997; 87(6): 992-997

[2] Bischoff-Ferrari, HA, et al., "Milk intake and risk of hip fracture in men and women: A meta-analysis of prospective cohort studies," *J. Bone Miner Res.* Apr. 2011;26(4):833-9

[3] Reid, I.R., Bolland, M.J., Avenell, A., Grey, A., "Cardiovascular effects of calcium supplementation," *Osteoporos Int.* March 16, 2011

[4] Warensjo, E., Byberg, L., Melhus, H., et al., "Dietary calcium intake and risk of fracture and osteoporosis: prospective longitudinal cohort study," *BMJ* May 2011; 342

[5] Lenart, B., Lorich, D., Lane, J., et al., "Atypical Fractures of the Femoral Diaphysis in Postmenopausal Women Taking Alendronate," *New England Journal of Medicine* 2008

[6] Aubry-Rozier, B., Lamy, O., Dudler, J., "Prevention of cortisone-induced osteoporosis: who, when and what?" *Rev. Med. Suisse* Feb. 10, 2010;6(235):307-13

[7] Ngamruengphong, S., Leontiadis, G.I., Radhi, S., et al., "Proton Pump Inhibitors and Risk of Fracture: A Systematic Review and Meta-Analysis of Observational Studies," *Am. J. Gastroenterol.* April 12, 2011

[8] Verdel, B.M., Souverein, P.C., Egberts, T.C., et al., "Use of antidepressant drugs and risk of osteoporotic and non-osteoporotic fractures," *Bone* Sept. 2010;47(3):604-9

[9] Andress, D.L., Ozuna, J., Tirschwell, D., et al., "Antiepileptic drug-induced bone loss in young male patients who have seizures," *Arch. Neurol.* May 2002;59(5):781-6

[10] Williams, L.J., Pasco, J.A., Henry, M.J., et al., "Paracetamol (acetaminophen) use, fracture and bone mineral density," *Bone* March 17, 2011

[11] Bulló, M., Estruch, R., Salas-Salvadó, J., "Dietary vitamin K intake is associated with bone quantitative ultrasound measurements but not with bone peripheral biochemical markers in elderly men and women," *Bone* April 5, 2011

[12] Turan, B., Can, B., Delilbasi, E., "Selenium combined with vitamin E and vitamin C restores structural alterations of bones in heparin-induced osteoporosis," *Clin. Rheumatol.* Dec. 2003;22(6):432-6

[13] Oben, Julius E., Ngondi, Judith L., Blum, Kenneth, "Inhibition of Irvingia gabonensis seed extract (OB131) on adipogenesis as mediated via down regulation of the PPARgamma and Leptin genes and up-regulation of the adiponectin gene," *Lipids Health Dis.* 2008;7:44

[14] Ngondi, et al., "IGOB131, a novel seed extract of the West African plant Irvingia gabonensis, significantly reduces body weight..." *Lipids in Health and in Disease,* March 2, 2009